Spine Imaging

Spine Imaging

A Case-Based Guide to Imaging and Management

Edited by

Shivani Gupta, MD
Clinical Instructor in Radiology
University of British Columbia
Diagnostic Neuroradiologist
Abbotsford Regional Hospital and
Cancer Center
Fraser Health Authority
Abbotsford, BC, Canada

Daniel M. Sciubba, MD
Associate Professor of Neurosurgery,
Oncology, and Orthopedic Surgery
Director, Spine Tumor and Spinal
Deformity Research
Department of Neurosurgery
Johns Hopkins University
Baltimore, Maryland

Mark M. Mikhael, MD
Reconstructive Spine Surgeon
Illinois Bone and Joint Institute
Division of Spine Surgery
NorthShore University Health System
Clinician Educator
Department of Orthopedic Surgery
Pritzker School of Medicine
University of Chicago
Chicago, Illinois

Savvas Nicolaou, MD
Associate Professor of Radiology
Director of Emergency/Trauma Imaging
Vancouver General Hospital
University of British Columbia
Vancouver, BC, Canada

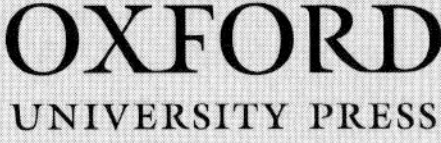

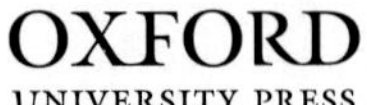

Oxford University Press is a department of the University of Oxford. It furthers
the University's objective of excellence in research, scholarship, and education
by publishing worldwide.Oxford is a registered trade mark of Oxford University
Press in the UK and certain other countries.

Published in the United States of America by Oxford University Press
198 Madison Avenue, New York, NY 10016, United States of America.

Library of Congress Cataloging-in-Publication Data
Names: Gupta, Shivani, 1981–, editor. | Sciubba, Daniel M., editor. |
Mikhael, Mark M., editor. | Nicolaou, Savvas, editor.
Title: Spine imaging : a case-based guide to imaging and management / edited
by Shivani Gupta, Daniel M. Sciubba, Mark M. Mikhael, Savvas Nicolaou.
Description: Oxford; New York: Oxford University Press, [2016] | Includes
bibliographical references and index.
Identifiers: LCCN 2015017610 | ISBN 9780199393947 (alk. paper)
Subjects: | MESH: Spinal Diseases—diagnosis—Atlases. | Spinal
Diseases—diagnosis—Case Reports. | Diagnostic Imaging—Atlases. |
Diagnostic Imaging—Case Reports. | Spinal Cord
Diseases—diagnosis—Atlases. | Spinal Cord Diseases—diagnosis—Case
Reports. | Spinal Diseases—therapy—Atlases. | Spinal
Diseases—therapy—Case Reports.
Classification: LCC RD768 | NLM WE 17 | DDC 616.7/30754—dc23 LC record available at http://lccn.loc.
gov/2015017610

9 8 7 6 5 4 3 2 1
Printed by Sheridan, USA

This book is dedicated to my family, whose support and love are a large never-ending well.
—Shivani Gupta

To my supportive wife, Karrie, and my three wonderful children, Hayley, Camryn, and Duncan, who have all sacrificed so much in allowing me to pursue my clinical and academic endeavors.
—Daniel M. Sciubba

To my wife, Noha, and kids, Elizabeth and Magdalena. Thank you for your kindness and patience.
—Mark M. Mikhael

I dedicate my work to my lovely wife Sonya, my mother Androulla, my deceased father Charalambous, my brothers Nick and George and a special thank you and gratitude to the assistance I received from Ismail Tawakol and Shamir Rai in creating this work.
—Savvas Nicolaou

Preface

This text represents a collaborative effort across specialties. We have put together a collective work from Neuroradiology, Orthopedic Surgery, and Neurosurgery in order to provide the most complete overview of multiple spinal entities. We hope that this text will serve as a valuable resource to medical students, mid-level providers, residents, surgeons, and radiologists in order to highlight and illustrate examples of various spinal conditions with a quick reference to etiology and management principles.

The purpose of this book was not to create an extensive text but to provide the reader with relevant, concise information that can be practically used on a daily basis. The collaboration among radiologists, orthopedic surgeons, and neurosurgeons has proven to be valuable, as we have learned from one another to create a case-based format that highlights important points when dealing with spine pathology.

This book seeks to become a go-to resource for all providers involved in spine care. It reviews the imaging characteristics of all spinal pathologies, yet also does not encumber the reader with an overwhelming encyclopedic approach. With clearly illustrated patient vignettes combined with short, but relevant didactic information, the book provides an efficient and thorough explanation of all spinal pathologies likely to present to a clinic, emergency department, or imaging center. Moreover, this book serves as an ideal review book during examination preparation for radiologists, neurosurgeons, orthopedic surgeons, pain management physicians, rehabilitation physicians, physician assistants, and physical therapists.

We hope readers will gain an adequate understanding of various spine pathologies, and learn about both the imaging and management behind each entity. We also hope it will serve as in important review text for those studying for board examinations.

Contents

Contributors

Vikas Agarwal, MD
Assistant Professor of Radiology
Director, Spine Intervention
University of Pittsburgh Medical Center
Pittsburgh, Pennsylvania

Remi M. Ajiboye, MD
Resident Physician
Department of Orthopedic Surgery
UCLA Medical Center
Los Angeles, California

Ismail Tawakol Ali
Clinical Fellow
Emergency and Trauma Radiology
University of British Columbia
Vancouver General Hospital
Vancouver, BC, Canada

Bita Ameri
Diagnostic Radiology Department
Newark Beth Israel Medical Center
Newark, New Jersey

Martin Arrigan
Fellow in Diagnostic Neuroradiology
Vancouver General Hospital
Vancouver, BC, Canada

Jaspreet Bajwa
Medical Student
Graduate Entry Medical School
University of Limerick
Limerick, Ireland

Manpreet Bajwa
Medical Student
Royal College of Surgeons of Ireland
Dublin, Ireland

Bavrina Bigjahan, MS
Department of Radiology
Division of Neuroradiology
Keck School of Medicine
University of Southern California
Los Angeles, California

Joseph Boonsiri, MD
Department of Radiology
University of Pittsburgh Medical Center
Pittsburgh, Pennsylvania

Camilo G. Borrero
Department of Radiology
University of Pittsburgh Medical Center
Pittsburgh, Pennsylvania

Cynthia A. Britton, MD
Professor of Clinical Radiology
Department of Radiology
University of Pittsburgh Medical Center
Pittsburgh, Pennsylvania

Jaysson T. Brooks, MD
Resident Physician
Department of Orthopaedic Surgery
The Johns Hopkins University School of
Medicine
Baltimore, Maryland

Mauricio Castillo, MD, FACR
Professor and Chief of Neuroradiology
University of North Carolina, Chapel Hill
Chapel Hill, North Carolina

Keith A. Cauley, MD PhD
Associate Professor of Radiology
Columbia-Presbyterian Medical Center
New York, New York

Paul Celestre, MD
Department of Orthopedic Surgery
Ocshner Clinic
New Orleans, Louisiana

Safia Cheeney, MD
Resident
Department of Radiology
University of Washington School of Medicine
Seattle, Washington

Francisco Chiang, MD
Department of Radiology
Division of Neuroradiology
University of North Carolina
Chapel Hill, North Carolina

Brad Currier, MD
Professor of Orthopedics
Director, Spine Surgery Fellowship Program
Mayo Clinic College of Medicine
Rochester, Minnesota

Francesco D'Amore, MD
Division of Neuroradiology
Department of Radiology
Keck School of Medicine
University of Southern California
Los Angeles, California

Sylvie Destian, MD
Professor of Clinical Radiology
SUNY Upstate Medical University
Syracuse, New York

Philip Dougherty, MD
Resident
Department of Radiology
University of Washington School of Medicine
Seattle, Washington

Christopher G. Filippi, MD
Professor of Radiology
Hofstra North Shore-LIJ School of Medicine
Manhasset, New York

Kathleen R. Fink, MD
Assistant Professor of Neuroradiology
Department of Radiology
University of Washington
Seattle, Washington

Eric Friedberg, MD
Assistant Professor of Radiology and Imaging
Sciences
Emory University School of Medicine
Atlanta, Georgia

Ernst Garcon, MD
Neuroradiologist
Department of Radiology
Columbia University Medical Center
New York, New York

Shivani Gupta, MD
Clinical Instructor in Radiology
University of British Columbia
Diagnostic Neuroradiologist
Abbotsford Regional Hospital and Cancer Center
Fraser Health Authority
Abbotsford, BC, Canada

Yazeed Gussous, MD
Physician
Orthopedic Surgery
Mayo Clinic
Rochester, Minnesota

Paul Harkey, MD
Assistant Professor of Radiology and Imaging
Sciences
Emory University School of Medicine
Atlanta, Georgia

Daniel Helmy
Division of Neuroradiology
Department of Radiology
Keck School of Medicine
University of Southern California
Los Angeles, California

Manraj Kanwal Singh Heran, MD, FRCPC
Associate Professor of Diagnostic and Therapeutic
Neuroradiology
University of British Columbia
Vancouver General Hospital
Pediatric Interventional Radiology
British Columbia Children's Hospital
Vancouver, BC, Canada

Justin Morris Honce, MD
Department of Radiology
University of Colorado School of Medicine
Aurora, Colorado

Nima Jadidi
Radiology Residency Program
Upstate University Hospital
SUNY Upstate Medical University
Syracuse, New York

A. Jay Khanna, MD, MBA
Professor of Orthopedic Surgery and Biomedical
Engineering
Vice Chair of Professional Development
Department of Orthopedic Surgery
Johns Hopkins University
Baltimore, Maryland

Sara E. Kingston
Fourth Year Medical Student
Keck School of Medicine
University of Southern California
Los Angeles, California

Anant Krishnan, MD
Department of Diagnostic Radiology and Molecular
Imaging
Beaumont Health–Royal Oak
Associate Professor of Radiology
Oakland University William Beaumont School of
Medicine
Royal Oak, Michigan

H. Kate Lee, MD
Hofstra North Shore
LIJ School of Medicine
Manhasset, New York

Bruce Lehnert, MD
Assistant Professor of Radiology
Department of Radiology
University of Washington
Harborview Medical Center
Seattle, Washington

Alexander Lerner, MD
Assistant Professor of Clinical Radiology
Department of Radiology
Keck School of Medicine
University of Southern California
USC Norris Comprehensive Cancer Center and
Hospital
Los Angeles, California

Malisa S. Lester, MD
Assistant Professor of Radiology
Neuroradiology Section
Northwestern University Feinberg School of
Medicine
Chicago, Illinois

Chia-Shang J. Liu, MD
Department of Radiology
Division of Neuroradiology
Keck School of Medicine
University of Southern California
Los Angeles, California

Pedro Lourenco
Department of Radiology
University of British Columbia
Vancouver, BC, Canada

Rakesh Mannava, MD
Department of Radiology
University of Pittsburgh Medical Center
Pittsburgh, Pennsylvania

Joseph M. Mettenburg, MD, PhD
Assistant Professor of Radiology
University of Pittsburgh Medical Center
Pittsburgh, Pennsylvania

Mark M. Mikhael, MD
Reconstructive Spine Surgeon
Illinois Bone and Joint Institute
Division of Spine Surgery
NorthShore University Health System
Clinician Educator
Department of Orthopedic Surgery
Pritzker School of Medicine
University of Chicago
Chicago, Illinois

Michelle Naidich, MD
Assistant Professor of Radiology
Neuroradiology Section
Department of Radiology
Northwestern University Feinberg School of
Medicine
Chicago, Illinois

Ahmad Nassr, MD
Associate Professor of Orthopedic Surgery
Mayo Clinic
Rochester, Minnesota

Megha Nayyar
Keck School of Medicine
Los Angeles, California

Brian Neuman, MD
Assistant Professor of Orthopaedic Surgery
Orthopedic Spine Surgery
Johns Hopkins University
Baltimore, Maryland

Emily Nguyen, MD
Orthopedic Surgeon
Mayo Clinic Health System
Austin, Minnesota

Quynh Nguyen
Department of Radiology
Department of Orthopedics and Sports Medicine
University of Washington
Harborview Medical Center
Seattle, Washington

Savvas Nicolaou, MD
Associate Professor of Radiology
Director of Emergency/Trauma Imaging
Vancouver General Hospital
University of British Columbia
Vancouver, BC, Canada

Tao Ouyang, MD
Neuroradiologist
Department of Radiology
Penn State Hershey Radiology
Hershey, Pennsylvania

Daniel Park, MD
Assistant Professor of Orthopedic Surgery
Oakland Univerisity-Beaumont Hospital
Southfield, Michigan

Brandon C. Perry, MD
Resident
University of Washington School of Medicine
Seattle, Washington

Shamir Rai
Resident
Department of Radiology
University of British Columbia
Vancouver, BC, Canada

Anandh Rajamohan, MD
Department of Radiology
Division of Neuroradiology
Keck Hospital of USC
Los Angeles, California

David Rodriguez, MD
Resident, Department of Radiology
University of Pittsburgh Medical Center
Pittsburgh, Pennsylvania

Daniel M. Sciubba, MD
Associate Professor of Neurosurgery, Oncology, and
Orthopedic Surgery
Director, Spine Tumor and Spinal Deformity
Research
Department of Neurosurgery
Johns Hopkins University
Baltimore, Maryland

Arjun Sebastian
Department of Orthopedic Surgery
Mayo Clinic
Rochester, Minnesota

Arya N. Shamie, MD
Professor and Chief of Orthopedic Spine Surgery
David Geffen School of Medicine at UCLA
Los Angeles, California
Professor (Hon.)
Zhejiang University
Hangzhou, China

Gary Shapiro, MD
Clinical Assistant Professor of Orthopedic Surgery
The University of Chicago Medical Center
Illinois Bone and Joint Institute
Glenview, Illinois

Mark S. Shiroishi, MD
Assistant Professor of Radiology
Division of Neuroradiology
Keck School of Medicine
University of Southern California
Los Angeles, California

Richard Silbergleit, MD
Vice Chief of Diagnostic Radiology and Molecular
Imaging
Beaumont Health–Royal Oak
Professor of Radiology
Oakland University William Beaumont School of
Medicine
Royal Oak, Michigan

Lakshmanan Sivasundaram, BS
Department of Radiology
Division of Neuroradiology
Keck School of Medicine
University of Southern California
Los Angeles, California

Freddie R. Swain
Muscoloskeletal/Emergency Radiology Radiologist
Kettering Network Radiologists, Inc.
Kettering, Ohio

Gustavo A. Tedesqui, MD
Department of Neuroradiology
University of North Carolina
Chapel Hill, North Carolina

Daniel S. Treister
University of Southern California Keck School of
Medicine
Los Angeles, California

Tina Raman, MD
Department of Orthopaedic Surgery
The Johns Hopkins University
Baltimore, Maryland

Daniel Varon, MD
Neuroradiologist
Colombia

Nupur Verma, MD
Fellow
Trauma and Emergency Radiology
University of Washington
Harborview Medical Center
Seattle, Washington

Cornelia Wenokor, MD
Assistant Professor
Department of Radiology
New Jersey Medical School
Rutgers, The State University of New Jersey
Newark, New Jersey

Section 1   **Trauma**

Safia Cheeney and Kathleen R. Fink

History

▶ A 13-year-old male presents to the emergency department with upper and lower extremity weakness after a snowboarding accident (Figures 1.1 and 1.2).

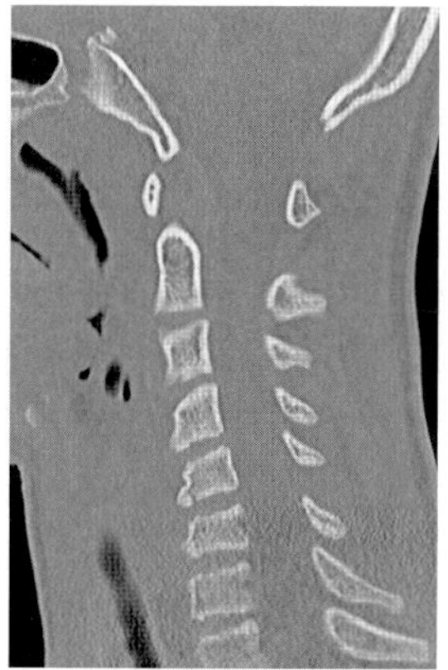

Figure 1.1

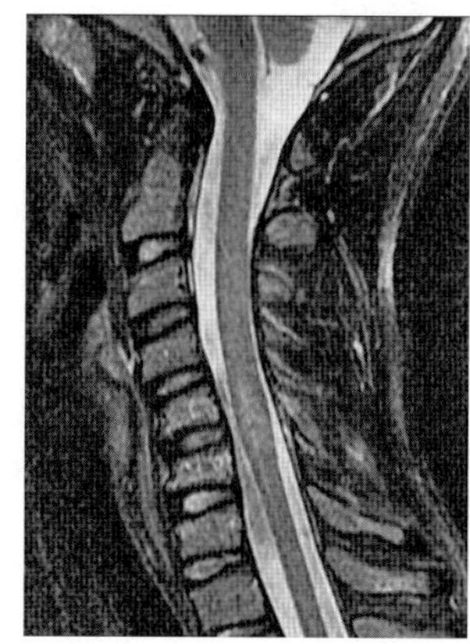

Figure 1.2

Chapter 1 **Spinal Cord Injury**

Findings

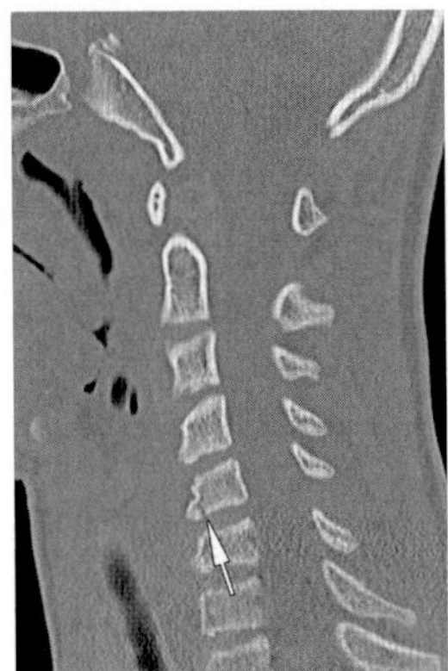

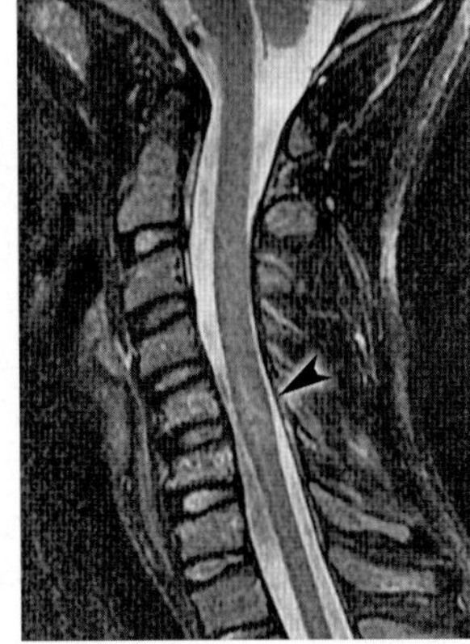

Figure 1.3

Figure 1.4

Sagittal computed tomography (CT) of the cervical spine (Figure 1.3) demonstrates a C5 anterior inferior corner fracture (arrow). Sagittal fat-suppressed T2-weighted magnetic resonance imaging (MRI) (Figure 1.4) shows focal cord expansion with increased cord signal consistent with cord contusion (arrowhead).

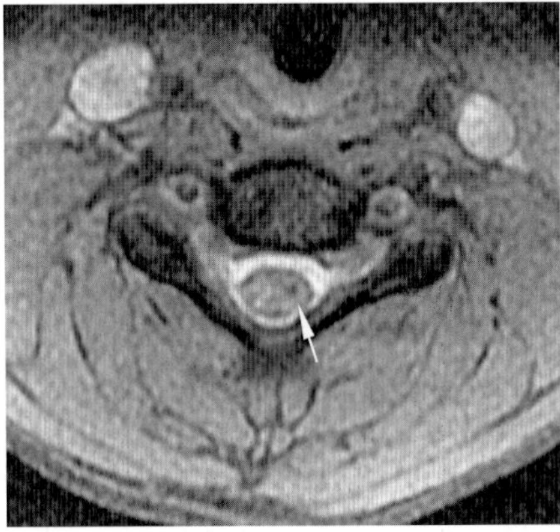

Figure 1.5

An axial gradient recalled echo (GRE)-weighted sequence (Figure 1.5) demonstrates a focal area of susceptibility artifact in the spinal cord (arrow), indicating petechial cord hemorrhage.

Differential Diagnosis

In the setting of trauma, a focal cord abnormality may reflect:
- ► Cord contusion
- ► Cord hemorrhage
- ► Cord transection

Discussion

In this case, a hyperflexion injury at C5–C6 resulted in a C5 anterior teardrop fracture, with associated cord contusion and hemorrhage. Although a wide range of pathologies can result in focal cord expansion and edema, including demyelination, transverse myelitis, infarction, and neoplasm, among others, in the setting of significant trauma, the differential diagnosis becomes limited to acute cord injuries.

Radiological Evaluation

CT and radiographs are the first-line imaging modalities used to evaluate the spine in the setting of trauma. Radiographic findings that suggest serious ligamentous injury or instability include vertebral body or facet subluxation, increased interlaminar space, an abnormally wide bony spinal canal, and fracture disrupting the posterior vertebral body line. CT provides a more detailed evaluation of the vertebral column in multiple planes and allows for better visualization of fractures and soft tissue injury.

MRI is indicated in acute spine trauma if there are neurological deficits or a clinically suspected injury to ligaments, or for treatment planning. It allows classification of spinal cord injury, allows identification of epidural hematoma, and is helpful in evaluating ligamentous or disk injury. Specifically, the sagittal T2-weighted sequence is very sensitive in evaluating cord edema and hemorrhage.

Four patterns of posttraumatic cord signal in T2-weighted MRI have been shown to correlate with neurological outcome: (1) normal cord signal, (2) single-level edema, (3) multilevel edema, and (4) mixed hemorrhage and edema. In severe cases, the cord can be transected.

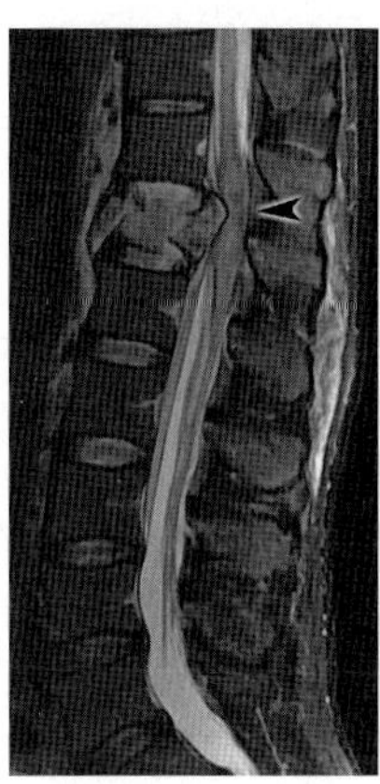 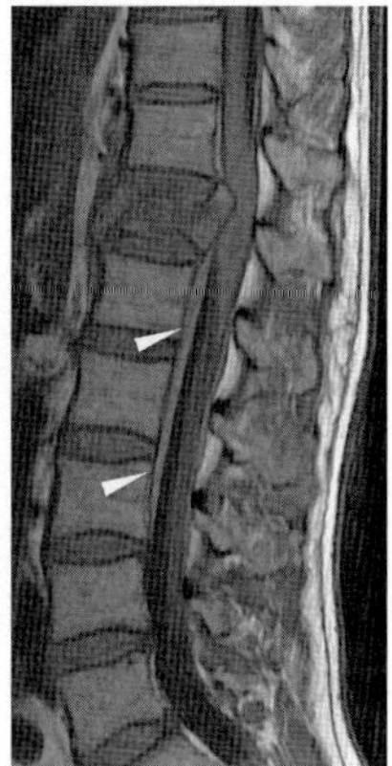

Figure 1.6   Figure 1.7

Burst fracture of T12 with retropulsed fragments causing spinal canal narrowing and cord compression. T2 fat-suppressed MRI (Figure 1.6) shows an expanded cord with single-level heterogeneous T2 signal hyperintensity consistent with edema (arrowhead). There was no blooming on the GRE sequence to indicate spinal cord hemorrhage (not shown). Sagittal T1-weighted MRI (Figure 1.7) shows anterior epidural hematoma (arrowheads).

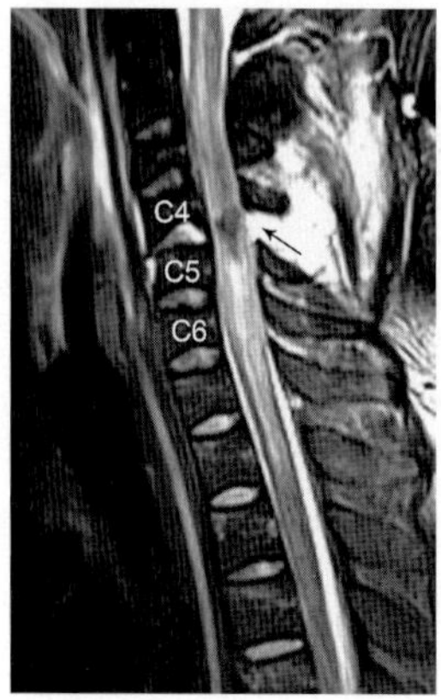
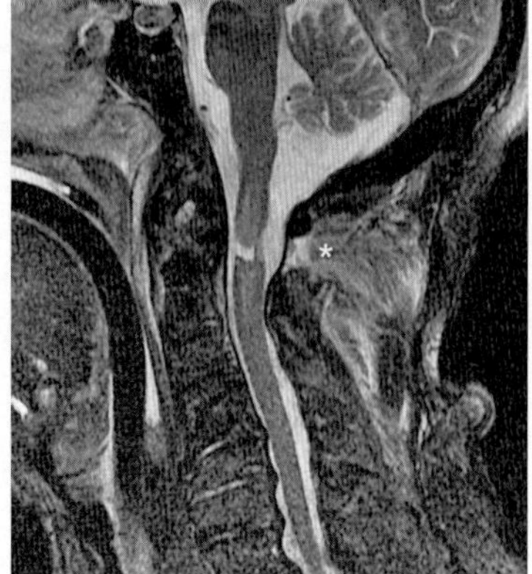

Figure 1.8   Figure 1.9

Cord contusion. Sagittal short TI inversion recovery (STIR) MRI (Figure 1.8) shows multilevel cord edema extending from C3 through T1. Focal hemorrhage at the level of C4/C5 manifests as signal dropout. Note the disruption of the ligamentum flavum (arrow).

Sagittal T2-weighted MRI (Figure 1.9) shows cord edema with transection at the C1–C2 level. Note the abnormal signal in the interspinous tissues (*).

Management

Early identification of a spinal cord injury is necessary to ensure early stabilization of the spine and prompt surgical consult.

Teaching Points

- ▶ Radiographs and CT are the best initial examinations for the evaluation of bony structures.
- ▶ If a spinal cord injury is suspected, MRI is the most sensitive examination to evaluate the extent of injury and to look for associated findings such as epidural hematoma and the status of the ligamentous structures and disks.
- ▶ Sagittal T2-weighted imaging of the spinal cord is an important sequence to evaluate for cord edema and hemorrhage.

Further Reading

1. Daffner RH, Deeb ZL, Goldberg AL, et al. The radiologic assessment of post-traumatic vertebral stability. Skeletal Radiol 1990;19(2):103–108.
2. Scarabino T, Salvolni U, and Jinkins R. *Emergency Neuroradiology*. Berlin, Germany: Springer, 2006.
3. Bozzo A, Marcoux J, Radhakrishna M, et al. The role of magnetic resonance imaging in the management of acute spinal cord injury. J Neurotrauma 2011;28:1401–1411.

Francisco Chiang, Mark M. Mikhael, and Mauricio Castillo

History

▶ A 48-year-old male presents with acute onset of back pain (**Figures 2.1 and 2.2**).

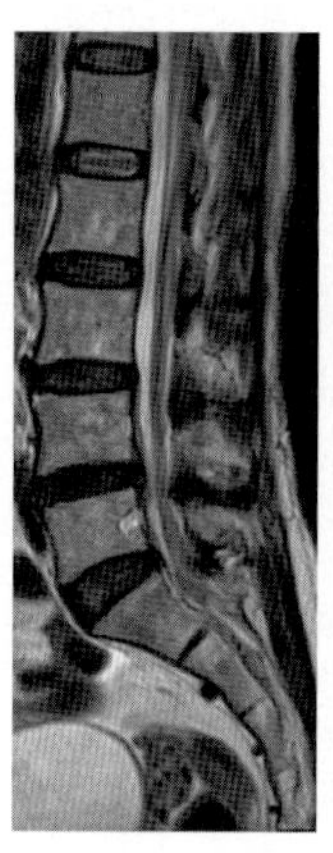

Figure 2.1

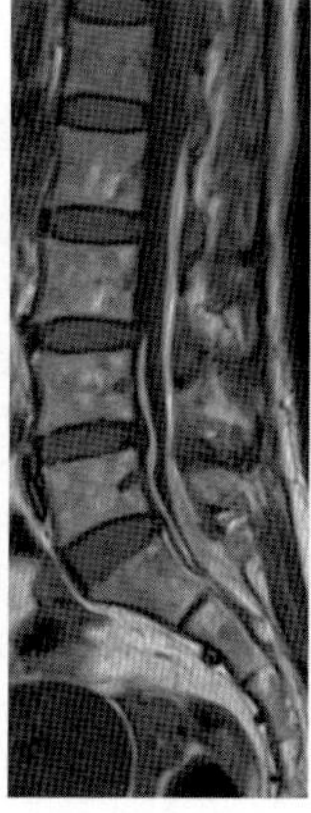

Figure 2.2

Chapter 2 Spontaneous Epidural Hematoma

Findings

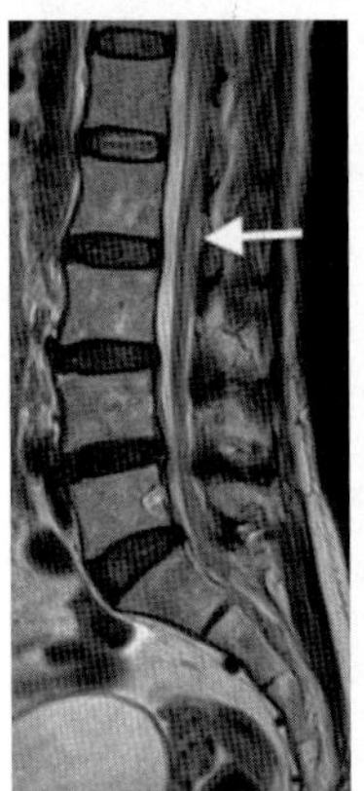
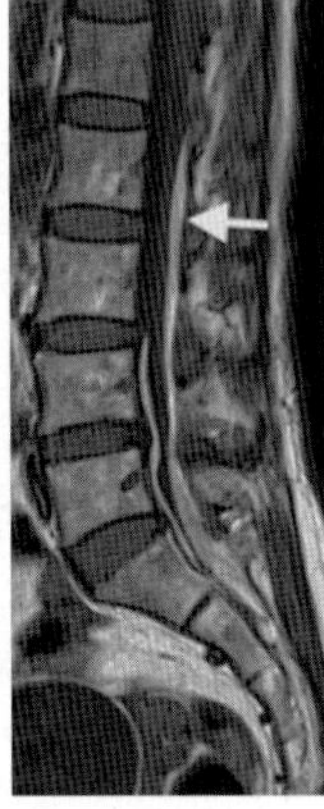

Figure 2.3   Figure 2.4

Epidural hematoma. A midsagittal T2-weighted sagittal MR image (**Figure 2.3**) shows a long segment
hypointense lesion (arrow) in the posterior epidural space without anterior displacement of the thecal sac.
A midsagittal T1-weighted sagittal MR image (**Figure 2.4**) shows that the lesion (arrow) is hyperintense
and extends to the lower anterior epidural space filling the lower spinal canal. The signal characteristics are
compatible with early subacute (intracellular methemoglobin) hemorrhage in the epidural space.

Differential Diagnosis

► Epidural metastasis
► Epidural abscess
► Epidural lipomatosis
► Lymphoma

Discussion

Spontaneous epidural hematoma is defined as an accumulation of blood in the epidural space, without a
history of trauma or recent surgical intervention. It is thought to result from venous hemorrhage. The majority
of epidural hematomas are spontaneous, unlike subdural hematomas of the spine that tend to be traumatic.
Spontaneous epidural hematomas are more common in the thoracic and lumbar spine than in the cervical
spine and are usually long, involving multiple levels. Patients are usually children or adults (50–60 years).

Radiological Evaluation

An epidural spinal hematoma usually appears as a broad-based lentiform or biconvex lesion that involves
multiple levels and has variable degrees of cord compression on axial images. On CT, it usually appears as
a hyperdense epidural mass with attenuation similar to that of the intervertebral discs, usually between 60
and 70 HU. On MRI, the signal varies depending on the age of the hematoma. In hyperacute hematomas,
the signal is isointense on T1WI and mildly hyperintense on T2WI. After that, from 6 to 72 hours, the signal
changes and hypointensity on T2WI appears. In the subacute stage, formation of methemoglobin produces
a high signal on T1WI relative to the spinal cord, while the T2 signal continues to be low such as seen in our
patient (**Figures 2.5 and 2.6**). T1 fat suppressed images can be used to differentiate blood from epidural fat as
the signal intensity spof the latter decreases. Finally, chronic hematomas are typically of low signal intensity on
all MRI sequences.

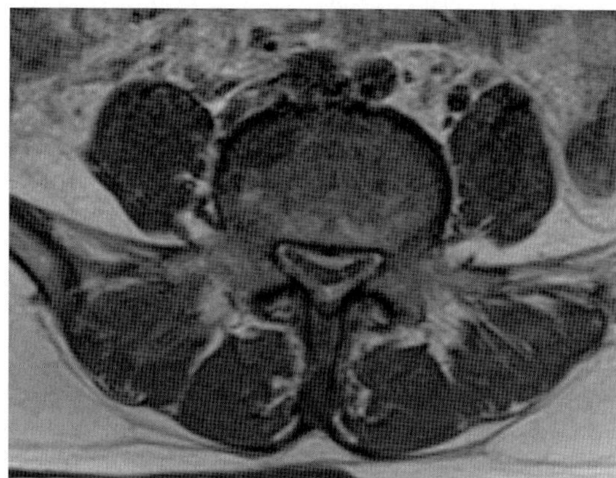

Figure 2.5

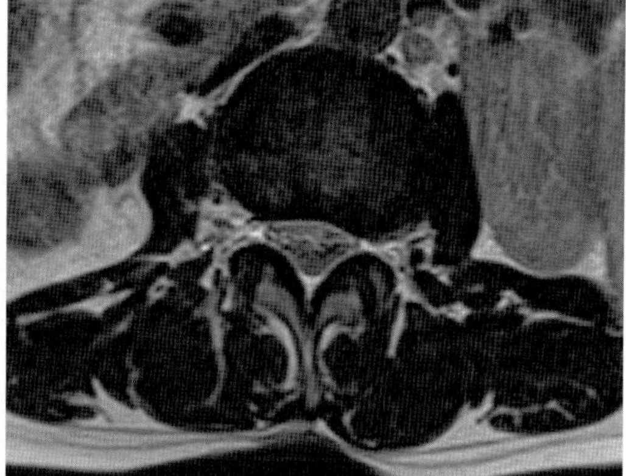

Figure 2.6

Subacute epidural hematoma. Axial T1WI (**Figure 2.5**) shows a hyperintense hematoma in the ventral epidural space that produces mild compression of the thecal sac. An axial T2WI (**Figure 2.6**) at a different level in the same patient shows a mildly hypointense anterior epidural hematoma that displaces the thecal sac.

Management

Epidural hematomas may resolve spontaneously with favorable outcome. In patients with cord compression or severe thecal sac compression around the cauda equina causing neurological injury, decompressive laminectomies and hematoma evacuation may be performed. Cord edema and inflammation can be reduced using intravenous dexamethasone or hypothermia. If an underlying coagulopathy is suspected, correction with vitamin K, protamine sulfate, and platelet transfusions may be used.

Teaching Points

▶ Spontaneous epidural hematomas are more common than traumatic or iatrogenic epidural hematomas.
▶ Epidural hematomas appear as lentiform or biconvex long epidural lesions with a variable signal on MRI.

Further Reading

1. Sklar EM, Post JM, and Falcone S. MRI of acute spinal epidural hematomas. J Comput Assist Tomogr 1999;23:238–243.
2. Patel H, et al. Spontaneous spinal epidural hematoma in children. Pediatr Neurol 1998;19(4):302–307.
3. Cuenca PJ, Tulley EB, Devita D, and Stone A. Delayed traumatic spinal epidural hematoma with spontaneous resolution of symptoms. J Emerg Med 2004;27:37–41.
4. Dorsay TA, et al. MR imaging of epidural hematoma in the lumbar spine. Skeletal Radiol 2002;31(12):677–685.
5. Fukui MB, Swarnkar AS, and Williams RL. Acute spontaneous spinal epidural hematomas. AJNR Am J Neuroradiol 1999;20:1365–1372.
6. Holtas S, Heiling M, and Lonntoft M. Spontaneous spinal epidural hematoma: Findings at MR imaging and clinical correlation. Radiology 1996;199:409–413.
7. Groen RJ and Ponssen H. The spontaneous spinal epidural hematoma: A study of the etiology. J Neurol Sci 1990;98:121–138.

Chapter 3

Cornelia Wenokor, Gary Shapiro, and Daniel Park

History

▶ A 35-year-old construction worker fell off a scaffolding. He complained of back pain, but had no neurological deficits on examination and was ambulatory (**Figures 3.1 and 3.2**).

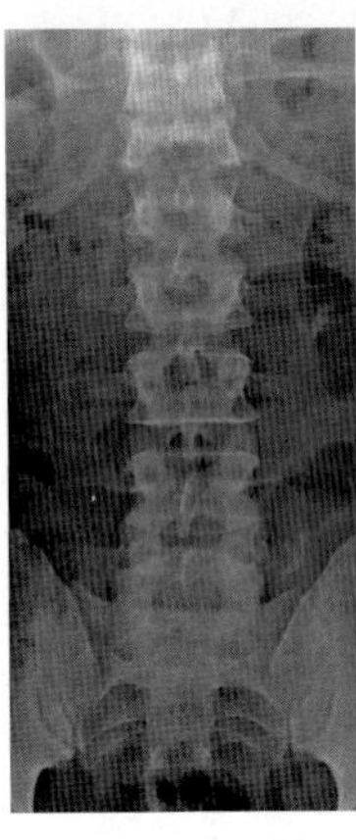 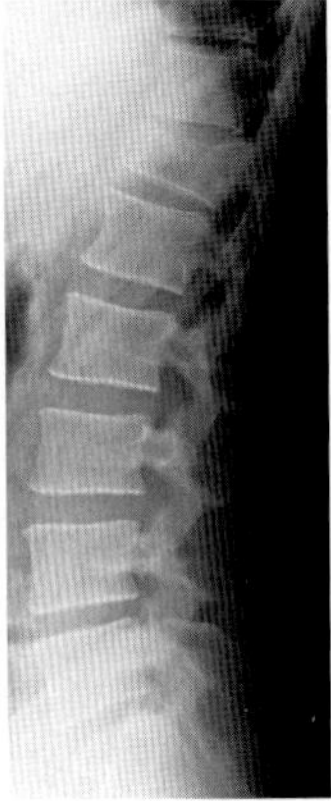

Figure 3.1　　　　Figure 3.2

Findings

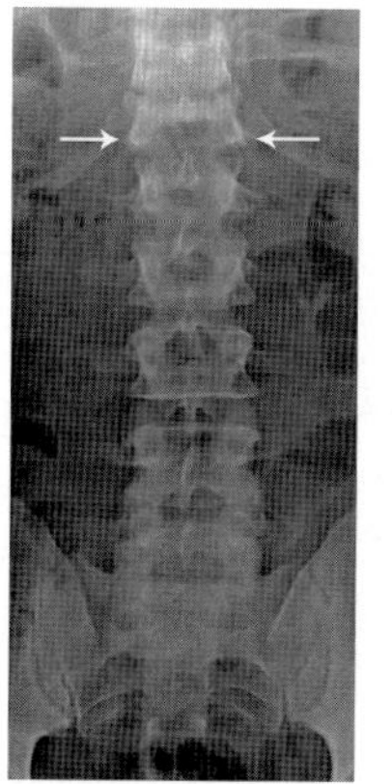 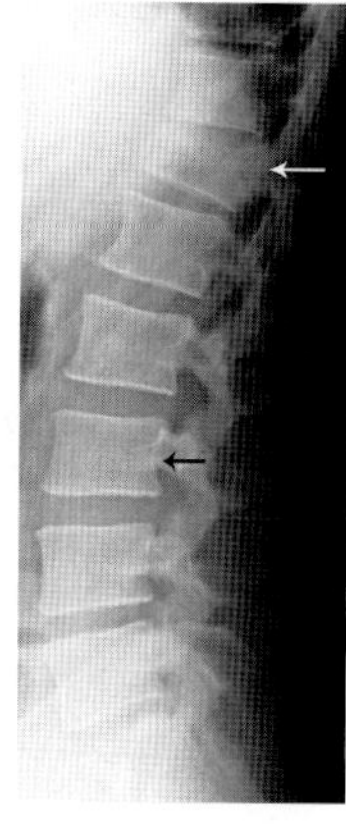

Figure 3.3   Figure 3.4

Burst fracture. On the radiographs (**Figures 3.3 and 3.4**), there is an anterior wedge deformity of T12, with decreased height on both the anteroposterior (AP) and lateral view. The AP view shows a subtle increase in the interpedicular distance and overall width of T12 (arrows). Additionally, on the lateral view there is loss of the normal posterior vertebral body concavity of L1, secondary to posterior displacement of a fracture fragment. Compare this to the remainder of the spine (black arrow at L3), where there is posterior body concavity.

Axial and sagittal CT images (**Figures 3.5 and 3.6**) demonstrate a posterior superior fracture fragment displaced into the spinal canal, resulting in significant spinal canal narrowing. There is anterior wedging of T12 and comminution. The axial view (**Figure 3.5**) shows subtle splaying of the pedicles.

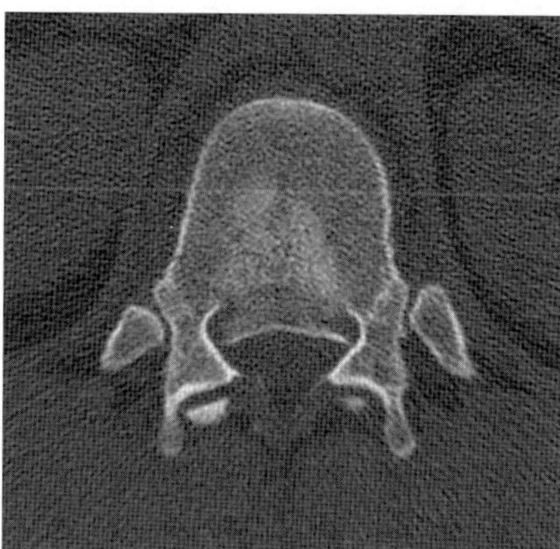 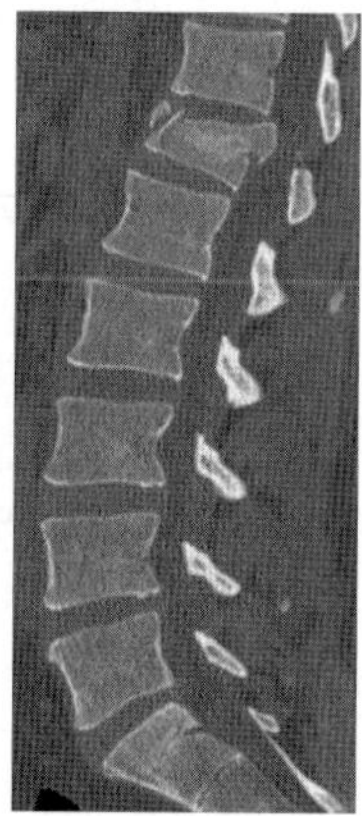

Figure 3.5   Figure 3.6

Sagittal and axial T2-weighted MR (**Figures 3.7 and 3.8**) demonstrate a retropulsed fracture fragment into the spinal canal, causing spinal stenosis. There is bone marrow edema and soft tissue edema. Figure 3.8 also shows disruption of the posterior ligamentous complex (arrow).

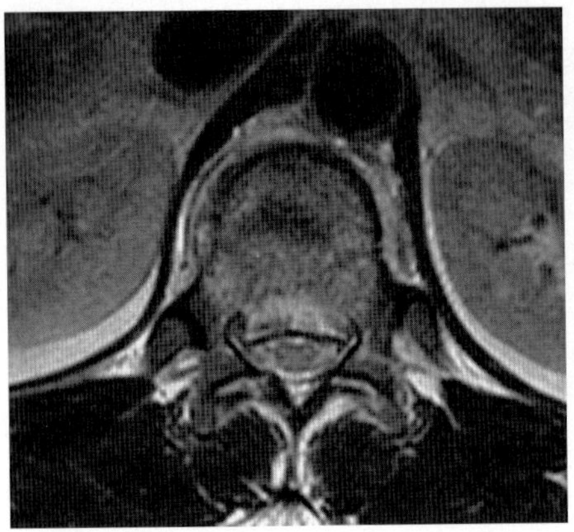

Figure 3.7

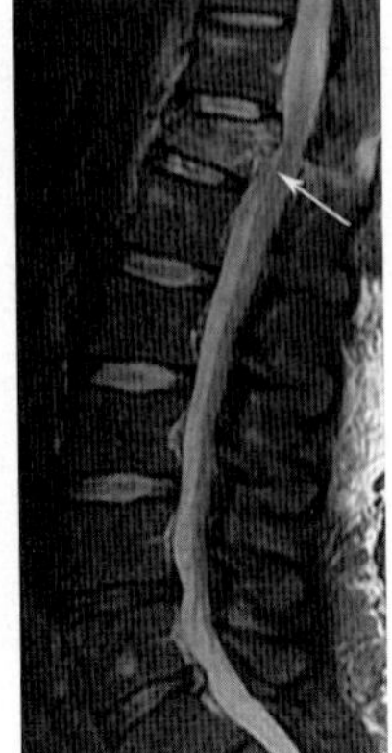

Figure 3.8

Differential Diagnosis

▶ Compression fracture
▶ Chance fracture

Discussion

A burst fracture is a specific type of compression fracture with retropulsion of a posterosuperior fracture fragment into the spinal canal. It occurs after axial loading, for example, after a patient falls from a significant height and lands on the feet or with a high energy compression injury. Both the anterior and middle column of the spine are disrupted. The energy gets transferred to the intervertebral disc, increasing pressure in the nucleus pulposus, and causes hoop stress upon the annulus fibrosus, dissipating from the center to the periphery. Burst fractures can be stable or unstable and may have associated injury to the spinal cord, conus medullaris, or cauda equina.

Radiological Evaluation

Radiographic findings include a compression fracture with retropulsion of bone into the spinal canal, widening of the interpedicular distance, and loss of posterior vertebral body height. CT imaging is important to determine the degree of retropulsion of bone into the spinal canal and to detect the presence of additional osseous trauma. Magnetic resonance imaging (MRI) is optimal to determine soft tissue abnormalities, including injury to the cord.

Management

The majority of thoracolumbar burst fractures can be treated nonoperatively with a brace when the patient is neurologically intact. A thoracolumbosacral brace (TLSO) is usually the treatment of choice for thoracolumbar burst fractures if nonoperative treatment is pursued. If the fracture is in the lower lumbar spine, a thigh extension may be needed.

Absolute indications for surgical treatment are biomechanical instability, neurological impairment with nerve compression, and progressive neurological decline. Relative indications include an inability to brace due to body habitus, progressive deformity despite bracing, and multifractures. Controversy arises when deciding a burst fracture is considered "unstable." Classically, greater than 50% vertebral body height, angulation >20 degrees, and canal compromise >30% were taught; however, recently, the importance of the posterior ligamentous complex (PLC) has been the focus. Advanced imaging is critical in determining the competency of the PLC. If the PLC is disrupted, surgeons favor surgical stabilization in many instances. The Thoracolumbar Injury Classification and Severity Score (TLICS) has recently been utilized by surgeons to determine if surgery is needed. This score is based on morphology of the injury, integrity of the PLC, and neurological status.

If surgery is indicated, treatment options can be anterior only, posterior only, or anterior posterior (**Figures 3.9 and 3.10**). Typically if the PLC is out, a posterior or combined approach is indicated. An anterior approach is indicated if there is incomplete spinal cord injury with significant canal compromise; however, many surgeons are now able to perform anterior decompression through a posterior approach.

Postoperative appearance after a burst fracture (**Figures 3.9 and 3.10**). Coronal and sagittal reformatted CT images of the lumbar spine are shown in a different patient after stabilization of an L1 burst fracture, demonstrating corpectomy of L1, placement of a stackable carbon fiber cage with bone grafting, and screw rod fixation from T12 to L3. Also note a superior endplate compression fracture of L3 (white arrows) and a chronic compression fracture of L4 (black arrow).

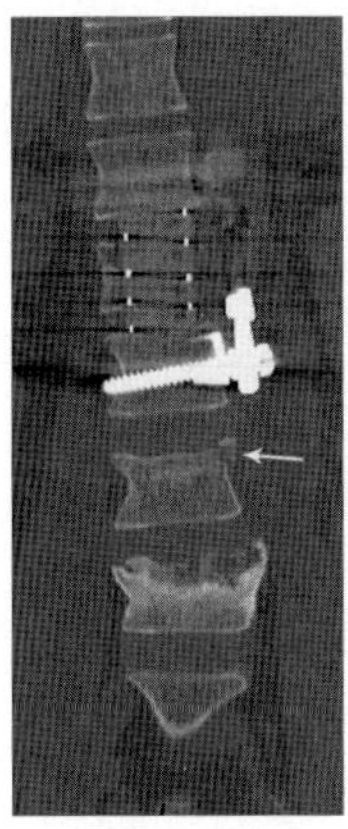 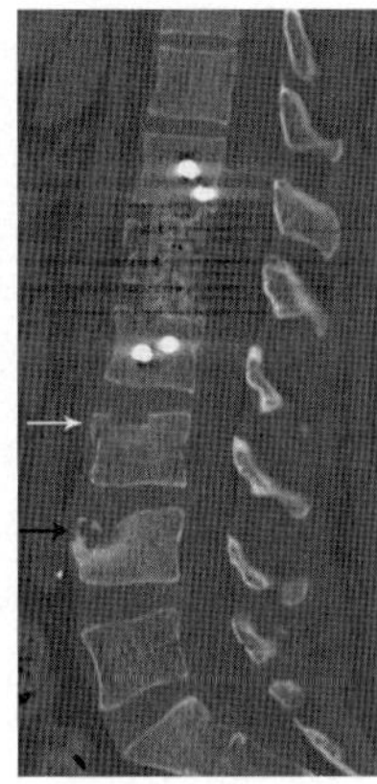

Figure 3.9   Figure 3.10

Teaching Points

- ► Unstable burst fractures have an increased incidence of developing posttraumatic kyphosis and progression of neurological symptoms.
- ► Most commonly the thoracolumbar spine is involved (T12–L2), as the rib cage provides additional stability and the vertebrae in the lower lumbar spine are larger, the ligaments are stronger and the psoas muscle is more substantial, helping in force distribution. Additionally, the facets joints are more sagittally oriented, allowing for more flexion, extension, and sliding motion.
- ► Signs of instability include disruption of the posterior ligamentous complex and a neurological deficit.

Further Reading

1. Shuman WP, Rogers JV, Sickler ME, et al. Thoracolumbar burst fractures: CT dimensions of the spinal canal relative to postsurgical improvement. AJR Am J Roentgenol 1985;145(2):337–341.
2. Atlas SW, Regenbogen V, Rogers LF, et al. The radiographic characterization of burst fractures of the spine. AJR Am J Roentgenol 1986;147(3):575–582.
3. Vaccaro AR, et al. A New classification of thoracolumbar injuries. Spine 2005;30(20):2325–2333.

Chapter 4

Pedro Lourenco and Manraj Kanwal Singh Heran

History

► A 73-year-old male presents with back pain 2 weeks after minor trauma (**Figures 4.1, 4.2, 4.3, 4.4, and 4.5**).

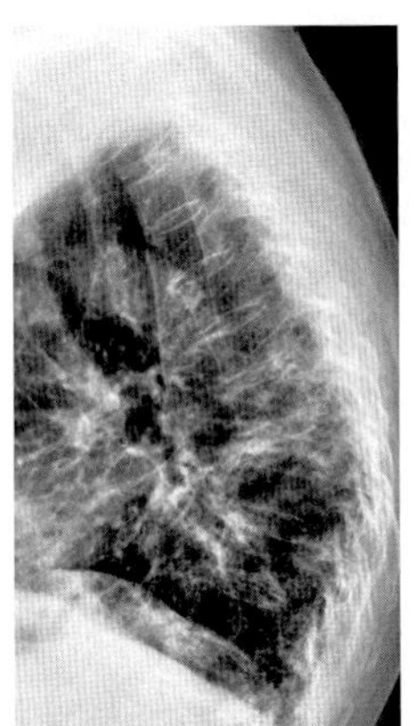

Figure 4.1

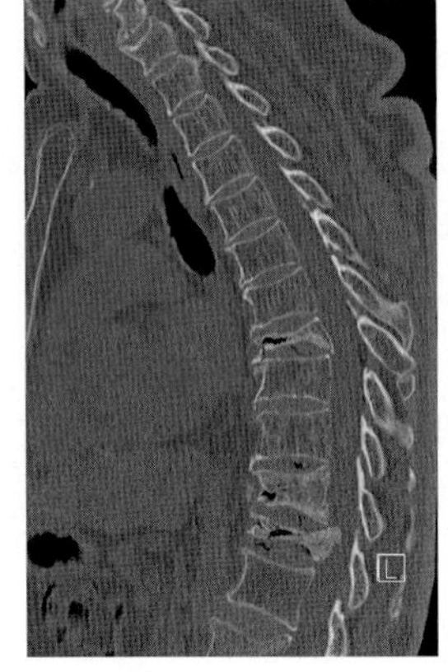

Figure 4.2

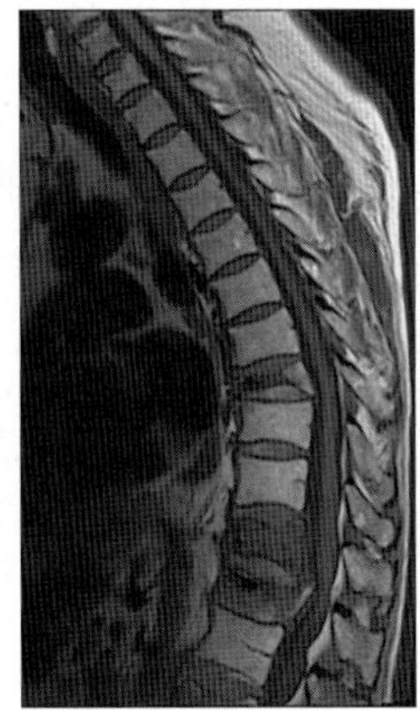

Figure 4.3

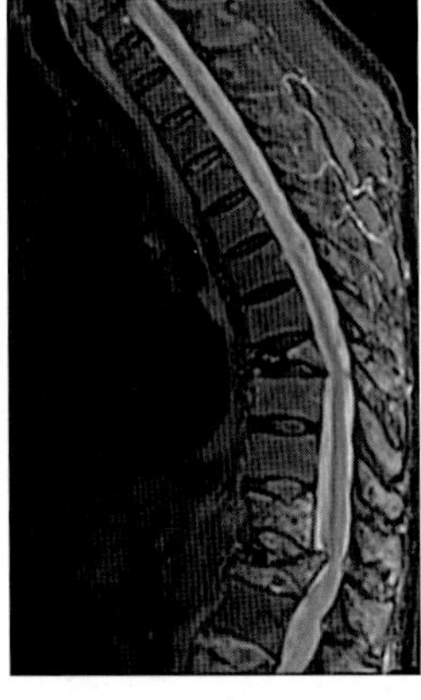

Figure 4.4

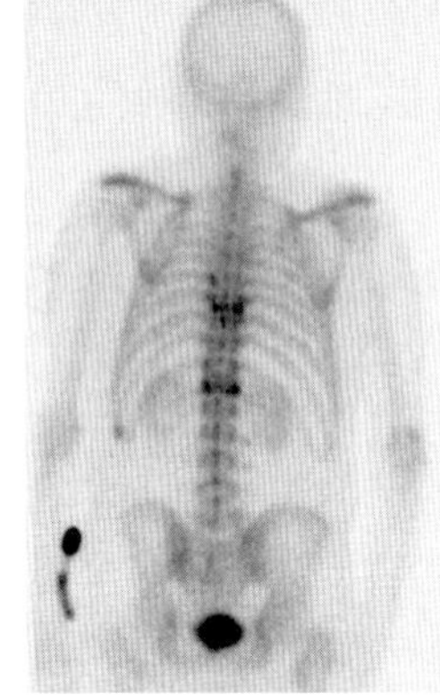

Figure 4.5

Chapter 4 Vertebral Compression Fractures and Vertebra Plana

Findings

Compression fractures. Lateral chest X-ray demonstrates a wedge compression fracture of T8 (**Figure 4.1**). A sagittal CT reformation (**Figure 4.2**) demonstrates wedge compression fractures at T8, T11, and T12, all containing intravertebral gas. T1WI and T2WI MR images (**Figures 4.3 and 4.4**) demonstrate decreased T1 and increased T2 signal at the affected levels, characteristic of bone marrow edema. A nuclear bone scan (**Figure 4.5**) demonstrates increased uptake at the T8 and T12 levels.

Differential Diagnosis

The differential diagnosis for the etiology of vertebral compression fractures can be divided into osteoporotic versus nonosteoporotic. Nonosteoporotic etiologies include trauma, metastasis, myeloma, lymphoma, leukemia, osteomyelitis, Paget disease (Chapter 50), Scheuermann disease (Chapter 78), and Langerhans cell histiocytosis (Chapter 45).

Discussion

Vertebral compression fractures (VCFs) are a common cause of back pain. The diagnosis of a traumatic VCF is facilitated by the existence of a traumatic event. However, many pathological conditions also contribute to the development of a VCF, and can be separated into osteoporotic and nonosteoporotic etiologies.

Osteoporotic VCFs are frequent, reported in up to 1.2 per 1000 adults aged >85 years in the United States. Osteoporosis is associated with advanced age, postmenopausal state, and prolonged corticosteroid therapy. Pathological VCFs due to malignancy are also common.

Kummel disease is delayed avascular necrosis of a vertebral body after minor trauma, representing vertebral nonunion and a subsequent VCF. Refer to Case 76 for further imaging findings and management of Kummel disease.

Approximately two-thirds of VCFs are asymptomatic. Symptomatic patients often present with acute back pain after low-impact movements, such as coughing or lifting. The quality of pain is variable, and often radiates abdominally in the distribution of the involved nerve roots. Insidious height loss can also be observed. In rare cases, VCFs can result in spinal canal or foraminal narrowing, resulting in radiculopathy, spinal compression, or cauda equina syndrome.

Radiological Evaluation

Loss of anterior vertebral body height is typical, with posterior cortex preservation, resulting in a wedge-shaped appearance and increased kyphosis. Complete vertebral body height ("vertebra plana") loss can also occur. The mid thoracic to upper lumbar spine and multilevel involvement are common. In an acute VCF, the paravertebral stripe may be lost due to adjacent hematoma. Perivertebral soft-tissue stranding can also be seen in an acute VCF on CT. CT is also helpful in evaluating for bone fragments projecting into the spinal canal, differentiating a compression fracture from a burst fracture (**Figures 4.6, 4.7, and 4.8**).

MR can demonstrate bone marrow edema, characterized as a low T1WI and high T2WI signal, which normalize over time. This is often a helpful finding when trying to determine whether a compression fracture is acute or chronic (**Figures 4.9, 4.10, 4.11, and 4.12**).

A nuclear medicine bone scan is nonspecific, but helpful in determining an actively healing VCF, by demonstrating positive flow, blood pool, and increased activity, which may persist for months to years.

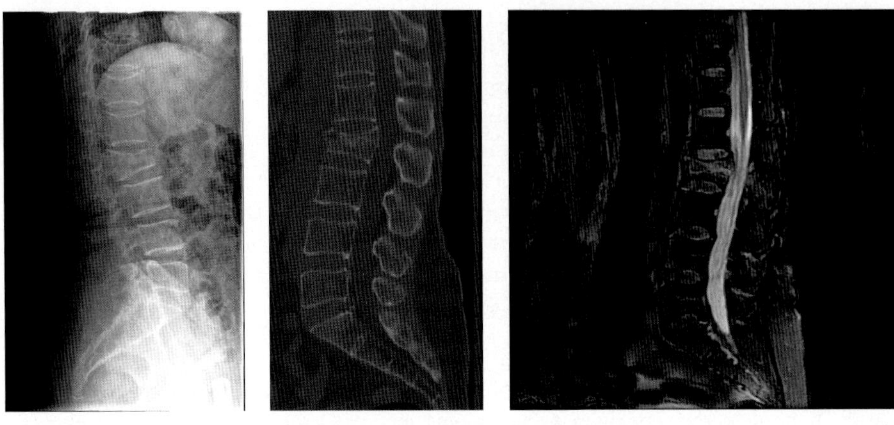

Figure 4.6	Figure 4.7	Figure 4.8

L2 burst fracture in a 67-year-old patient (Figures 4.6, 4.7, and 4.8). A lateral view of the lumbar spine (Figure 4.6) demonstrates a compression deformity of L2. However, a sagittal CT (Figure 4.7) and a fat-sagittal T2-weighted MR image (Figure 4.8) better delineate the retropulsion of bone into the spinal canal, thereby indicating a burst fracture as opposed to a compression fracture. Refer to Case 3 for further discussion of burst fractures.

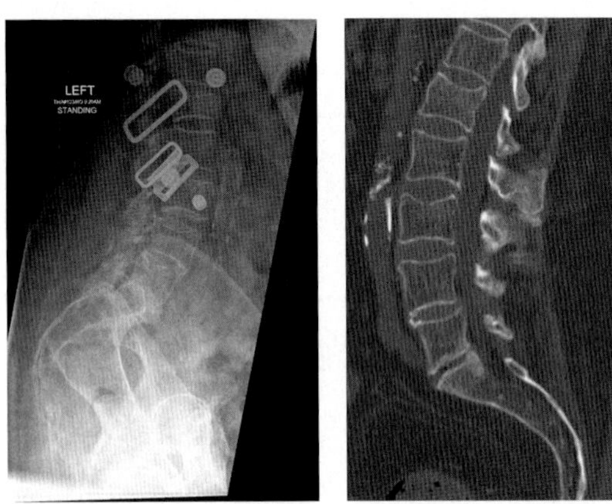

Figure 4.9	Figure 4.10

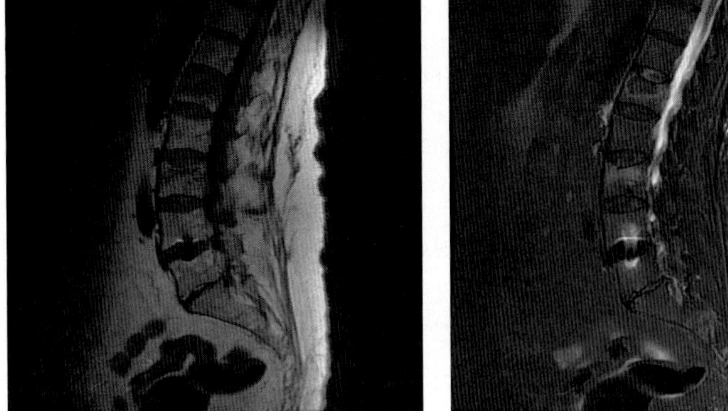

Figure 4.11	Figure 4.12

L1 and L3 compression deformities in an 89-year-old patient (Figures 4.9, 4.10, 4.11, and 4.12). A lateral radiograph of the lumbar spine (Figure 4.9) demonstrates a compression deformity at L1 of indeterminate age. L3 is poorly seen. A subsequent CT sagittal reformat (Figure 4.10) demonstrates subtle deformities at both

L1 and L3, both of which could easily be overlooked. In this case, MRI is helpful in determining the acuity of both VCFs. Sagittal T1 (Figure 4.11) and STIR (Figure 4.12) weighted images depict an abnormal bone marrow signal at both L1 and L3 (hypointense on T1WI and hyperintense on STIR), suggesting acute fractures. Abnormal signal overlying the L4/L5 disc space was an artifact.

Management

Treatment depends on the severity of the disease and should also be aimed at the underlying disease. Initial management includes analgesia and physical therapy.

Symptomatic relief can also be achieved by percutaneous cement augmentation procedures such as vertebroplasty or kyphoplasty. Selective nerve-root blocks or epidural steroid injections may also be of benefit.

Teaching Points

▶ The etiology of a VCF can broadly be defined as osteoporotic versus nonosteoporotic.
▶ Osteoporosis is the most common cause of a VCF.
▶ Treatment typically is conservative, but should also address the underlying disease process. Other image-guided therapies may also be of benefit in selected cases.

Further Reading

1. Lenchik L, et al. Diagnosis of osteoporotic vertebral fractures: Importance of recognition and description by radiologists. AJR Am J Roentgenol 2004;183(4):949–958.
2. Vogt TM, et al. Vertebral fracture prevalence among women screened for the Fracture Intervention Trial and a simple clinical tool to screen for undiagnosed vertebral fractures. Fracture Intervention Trial Research Group. Mayo Clin Proc 2000;75(9):888–896.

Chapter 5

H. Kate Lee

History

▶ A 65-year-old male presents with neck pain status post-motor vehicle accident (MVA) (**Figures 5.1, 5.2, 5.3, and 5.4**).

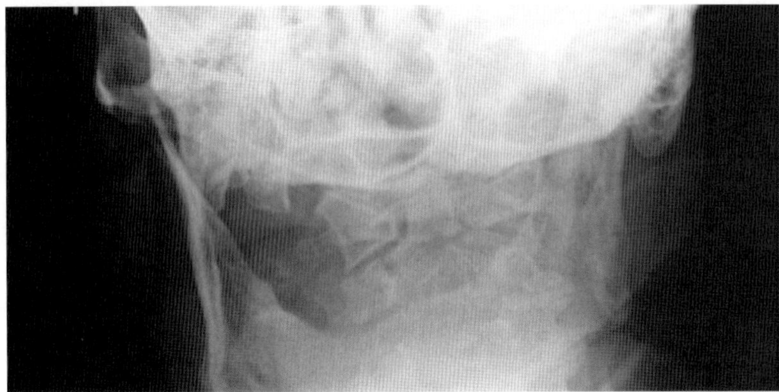

Figure 5.1

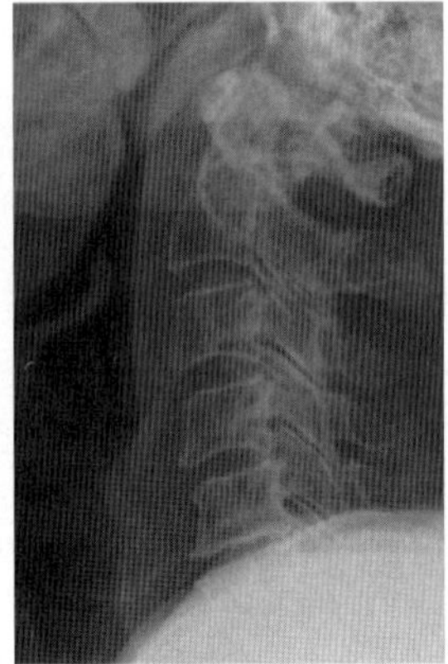

Figure 5.2

Findings

C2 Fracture. An open mouth view (Figure 5.1) of the cervical spine radiographs demonstrates a lucency in the C2 body and incompletely aligned C1 and C2 lateral masses, especially on the right. A lateral cervical spine radiograph (Figure 5.2) demonstrates a lucency through the C2 body with cortical irregularity along the anterior cortex. These findings indicate a C2 fracture.

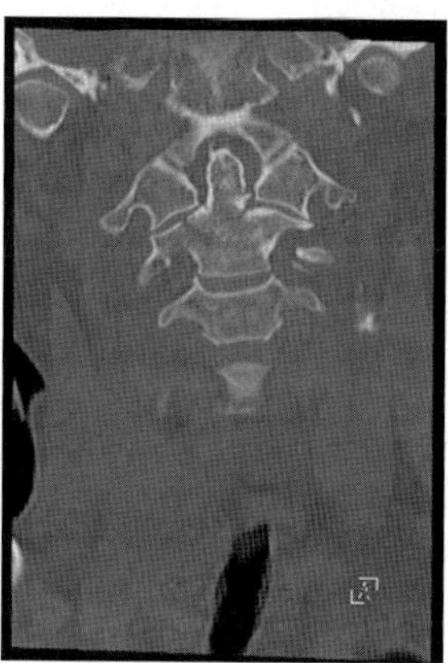

Figure 5.3

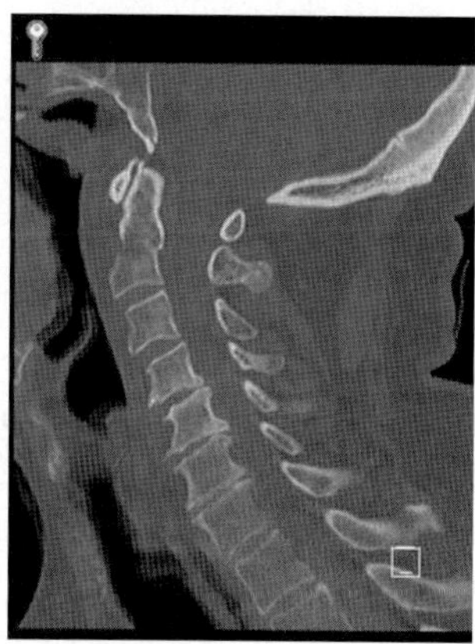

Figure 5.4

Coronal and sagittal CT reconstructions (Figures 5.3 and 5.4) confirm a Type III dens fracture. The inferior C2 body is mildly anteriorly displaced with respect to the odontoid process.

Differential Diagnosis

► Mach line: artifactual lucency from a superimposed occiput base traversing the base of the dens.

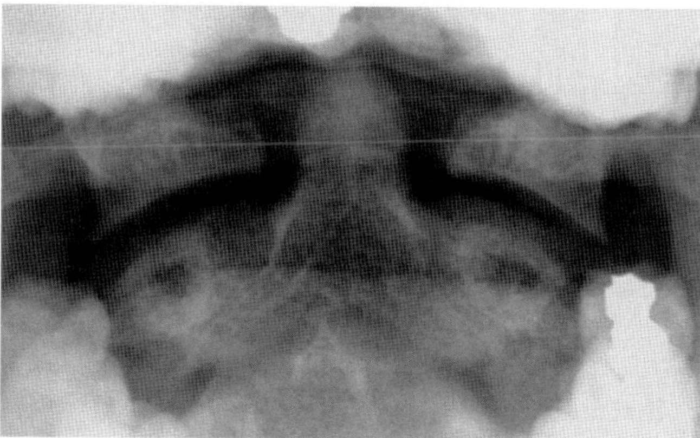

Figure 5.5

Mach line (Figure 5.5). Open mouth view of the cervical spine shows a lucency at the base of the dens from the overlying shadow of the occiput base, indicating an artifact.

► Os odontoideum: The etiology is uncertain but os odontoideum may be a sequela of an odontoid synchondral fracture prior to union at age 5–7. Hypertrophy or sclerosis of the anterior arch and hypoplasia of the posterior arch of C1 can be observed as a sign of compensation of increased stress on C1. The level of mobility is below the level of the transverse atlantal ligament, which can result in atlantoaxial instability and spinal cord compression.

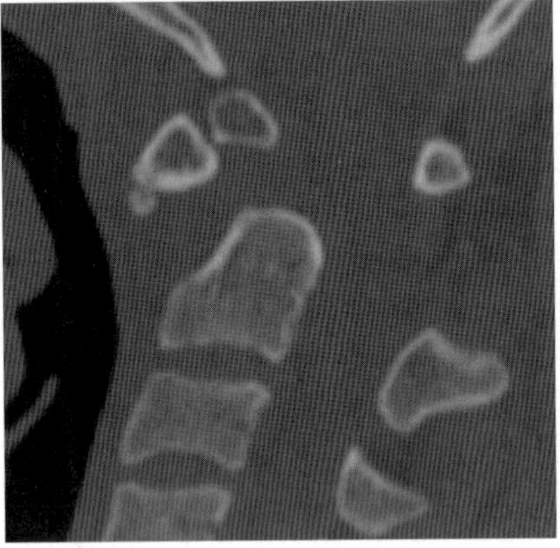

Figure 5.6

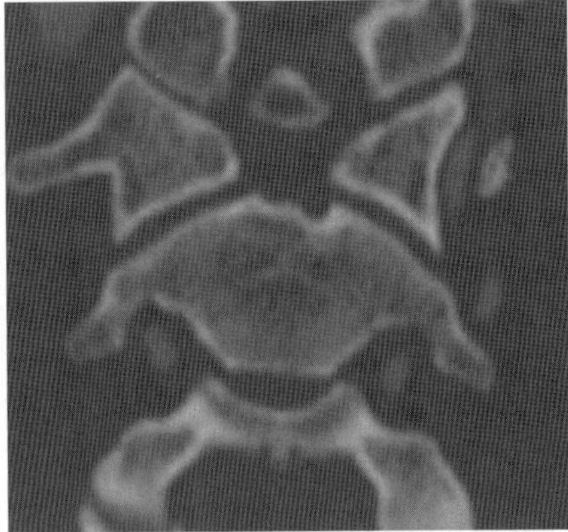

Figure 5.7

Sagittal and coronal CT reformatted images (Figures 5.6 and 5.7) show an os odontoideum with an anteriorly displaced os.

► Persistent ossiculum terminale (also known as Bergmann's ossicle or ossiculum terminale of Bergmann) refers to the failure of the secondary ossification center by age 12. It is considered a normal anatomical variant of the axis and is stable as it lies above the transverse alar ligament and is rarely symptomatic.

Discussion

Dens fractures (also known as an odontoid or peg fracture) are the most common upper cervical spine fractures resulting from flexion loading. A commonly used classification proposed by Anderson and D'Alonzo in 1974 divides dens fractures into three categories.

► Type I (<5%) (**Figures 5.8 and 5.9**): avulsion fracture of the tip due to avulsion of the alar ligament; it is usually stable but potentially unstable in association with occipitoatlantal dislocation.

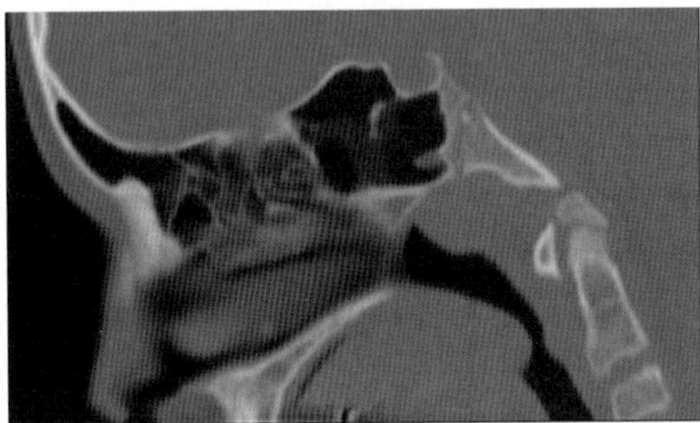

Figure 5.8

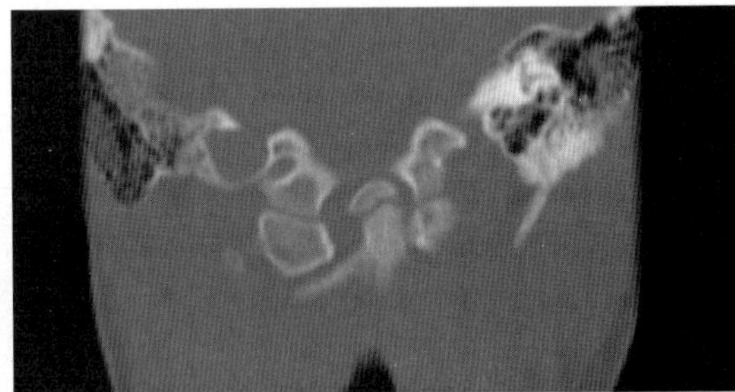

Figure 5.9

Type I dens fracture (Figures 5.8 and 5.9). Sagittal and coronal CT reformatted images show an old, healed Type I dens fracture without significant displacement.

► Type II (>60%): the most common type of dens fracture (**Figures 5.10 and 5.11**) involving the base; it is considered unstable with a high risk of nonunion; age greater than 50 years was found to be a highly significant risk factor (21 times higher) for failure of halo immobilization due to nonunion (especially Type II fractures in elderly patients with limited vascular supply).

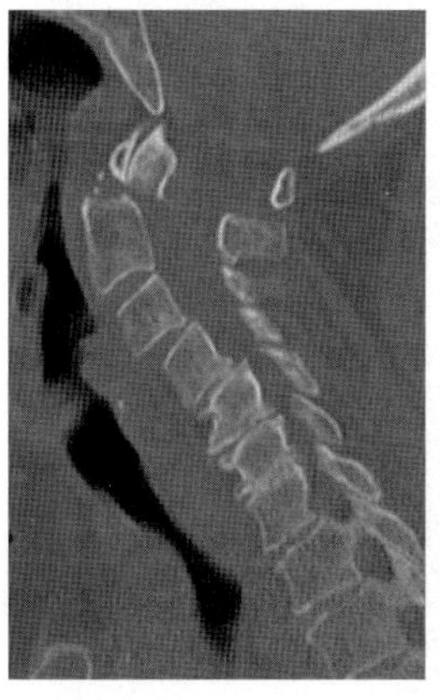
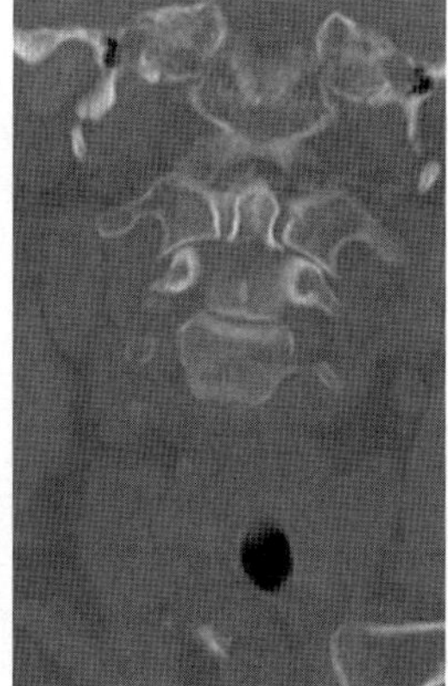

Figure 5.10   Figure 5.11

Type II dens fracture (Figures 5.10 and 5.11). Sagittal and coronal CT reformatted images demonstrate a Type II dens fracture with anteriorly displaced body.

▶ Type III (~30%): subdentate fracture through the C2 body; mechanically unstable as it allows the atlas and the occiput to move as a unit but carries the best prognosis because of the larger surface area for healing (Figures 5.12, 5.13, and 5.14).

Radiological Evaluation

Plain films are easily available and are typically used first, but CT demonstrates the presence of fractures better and MR helps to evaluate underlying ligamentous, disc, spinal cord, and soft tissue injuries. Potential pitfalls of plain films include a mach line (Figure 5.5) in which an artifactual lucency from a superimposed occiput base traverses the base of the dens on the open mouth, which is not present on lateral views.

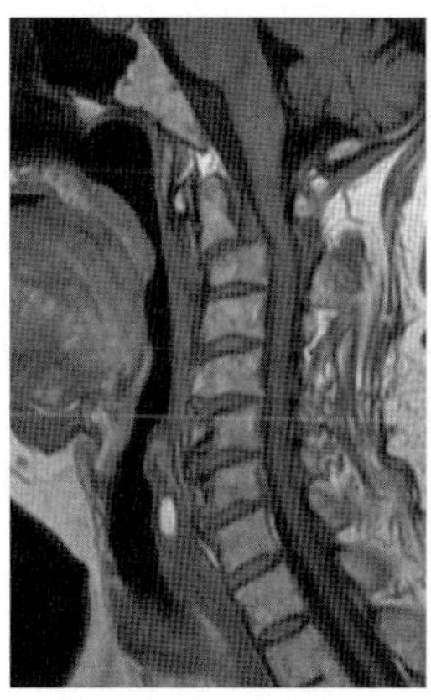
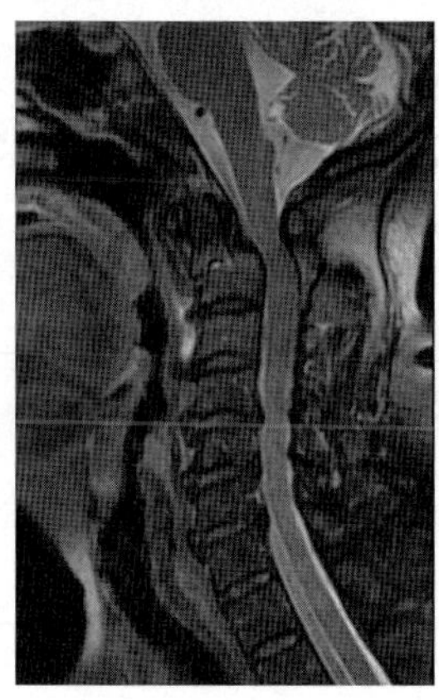
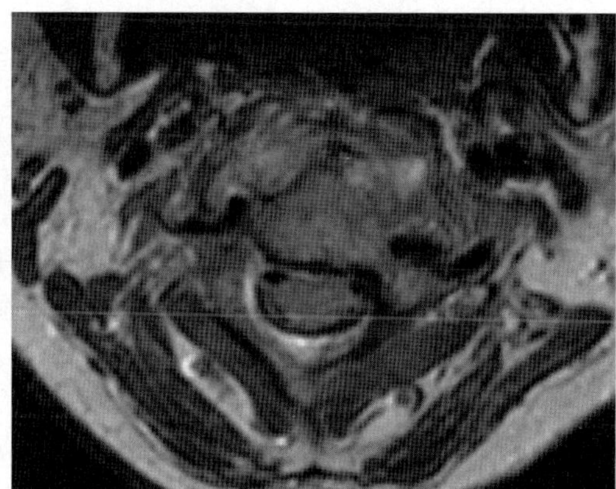

Figure 5.12   Figure 5.13   Figure 5.14

Type III dens fracture (Figures 5.12, 5.13, and 5.14). Sagittal T1 (Figure 5.12), fat-suppressed sagittal T2 (Figure 5.13), and axial T2-weighted (Figure 5.14) MR demonstrate a Type III dens fracture resulting in spinal canal stenosis and associated compression and edema of the cervical cord.

Management

A Type I fracture is typically treated with a hard or semirigid collar for 6–8 weeks. Treatment of Type II fractures is controversial due to the poor potential for fracture healing in elderly patients and morbidity associated with prolonged halo brace placement. With only mild displacement, these fractures can often heal with a fibrous nonunion, which is typically asymptomatic. Relative indications for surgical treatment of Type II fractures include more than 5-mm fracture displacement, more than 10-degree angulation, and failed attempts at closed reduction. A Type III fracture can be treated with 12 weeks of immobilization with a halo-vest to allow healing by bony union. Surgical intervention, however, may be necessary (**Figures 5.15, 5.16, 5.17, 5.18, 5.19, and 5.20**). Complications vary based on the age of the patient and amount of displacement and include nonunion, malunion, and pseudoarthrosis.

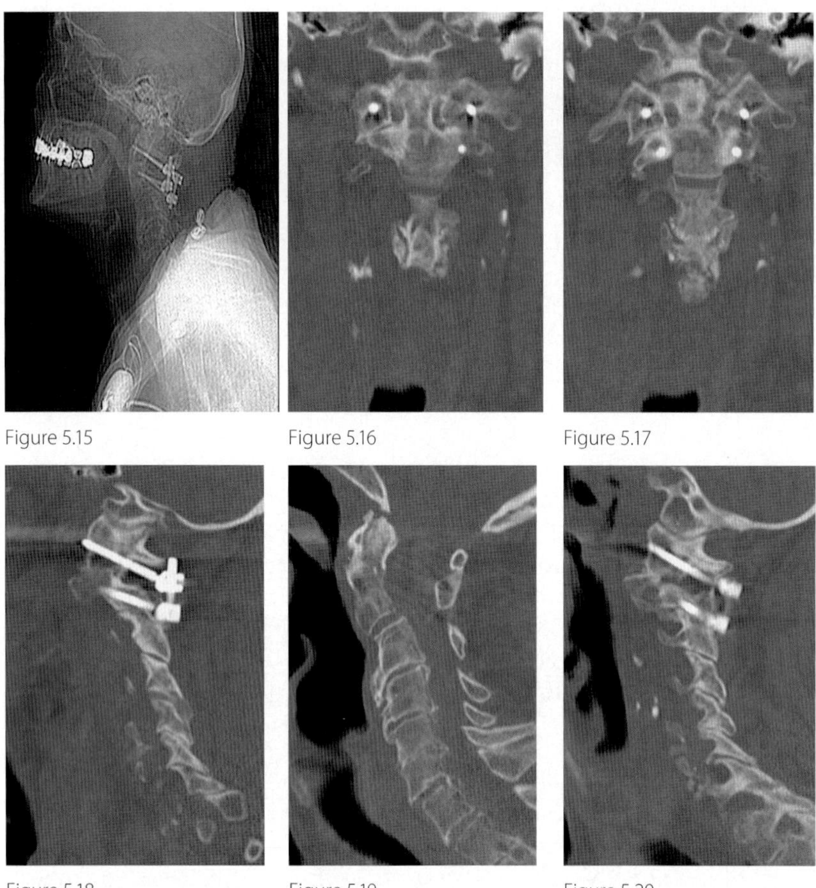

Figure 5.15 Figure 5.16 Figure 5.17

Figure 5.18 Figure 5.19 Figure 5.20

Postoperative appearance of a Type II dens fracture (Figures 5.15, 5.16, 5.17, 5.18, 5.19, and 5.20). Scout lateral view (Figure 5.15), coronal (Figures 5.16 and 5.17), and sagittal (Figures 5.18, 5.19, and 5.20) CT reconstructions demonstrate uncomplicated postsurgical changes from bilateral C1–C2 posterior fusion of a Type II dens fracture. The dens fracture demonstrates healing and union.

Teaching Points

- ► Dens fracture is the most common type of upper cervical spine fracture.
- ► CT demonstrates the presence of fractures better than the radiographs and MRI helps to evaluate underlying ligamentous, disc, spinal cord, and soft tissue injuries.
- ► Complications include nonunion, malunion, pseudoarthrosis, and spinal cord contusion. They depend on the patient's age and the degree of displacement of the fracture.

Further Reading

1. Anderson LD and D'Alonzo RT. Fractures of the odontoid process of the axis. J Bone Joint Surg Am 1974;56(8):1663–1674.
2. Lennarson PJ, Mostafavi H, Traynelis VC, and Walters BC. Management of type II dens fractures: A case-control study. Spine 2000;25(10):1234–1237.
3. Daffner RH. Pseudofracture of the dens: Mach bands. AJR Am J Roentgenol 1977;128(4):607–612.
4. Dunn ME and Seljeskog EL. Experience in the management of odontoid process injuries: An analysis of 128 cases. Neurosurgery 1986;18(3):306–310.
5. Clark CR and White AA. 3rd Fractures of the dens. A multicenter study. J Bone Joint Surg Am 1985;67(9):1340–1348.

Chapter 6

Bruce Lehnert, Brad Currier, and Arjun Sebastian

History

► A 32-year-old intoxicated female presents to the emergency department after a fall from a height of 20 feet (**Figures 6.1, 6.2, and 6.3**).

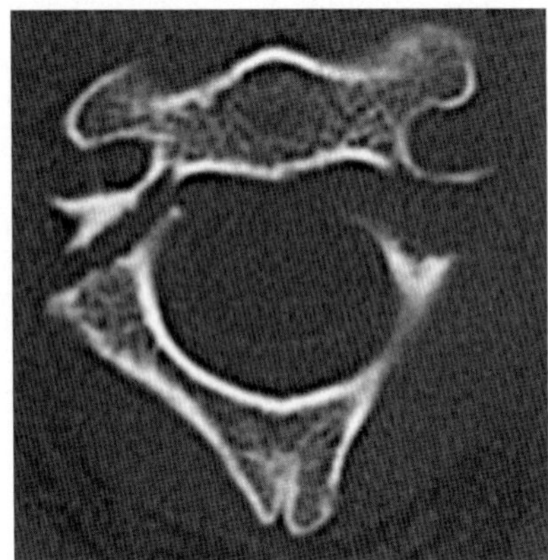

Figure 6.1

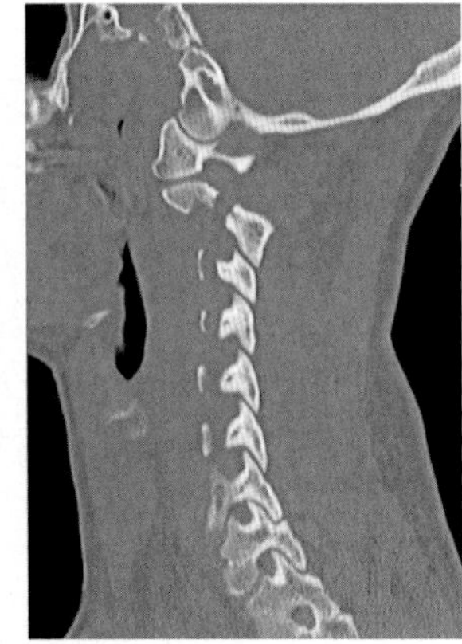

Figure 6.2

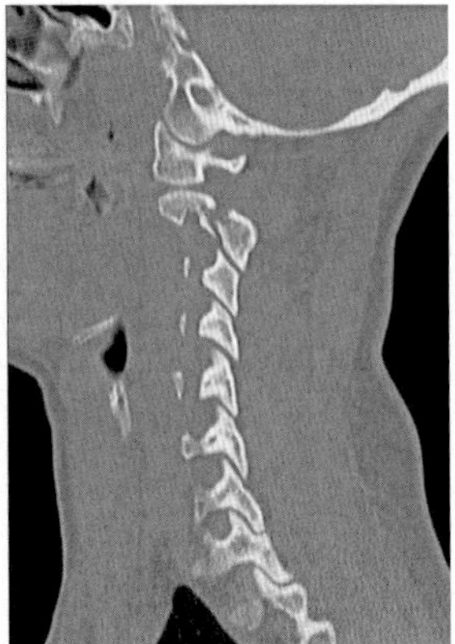

Figure 6.3

Findings

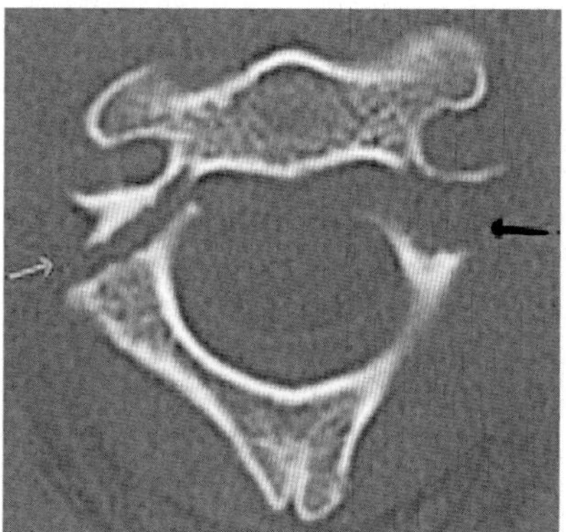

Figure 6.4

Hangman fracture on CT. An axial CT image (**Figure 6.4**) demonstrates a Type IIa fracture through the bilateral pars interarticularis. This is consistent with a Type IIa Hangman fracture. Parasagittal CT images (**Figures 6.5 and 6.6**) demonstrate displacement through the pars fracture on the left and right, respectively. A midsagittal CT image (**Figures 6.7 and 6.8**) demonstrates 15.1 degrees of angulation and mild grade 1 anterolisthesis of C2 on C3 with approximately 2.5 mm of displacement.

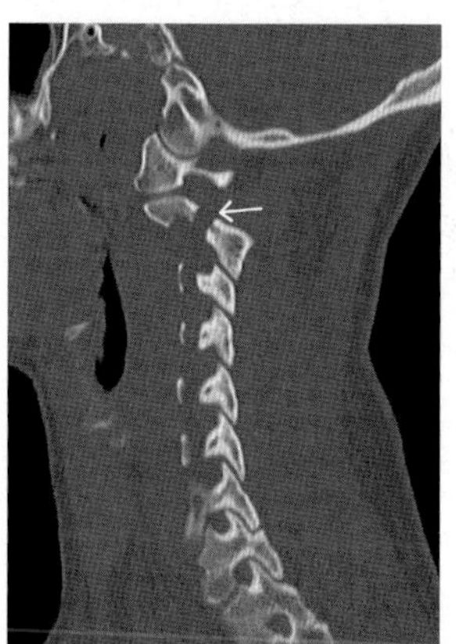

Figure 6.5

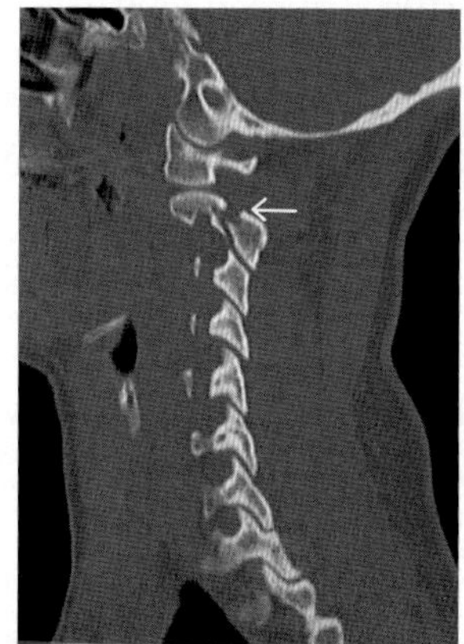

Figure 6.6

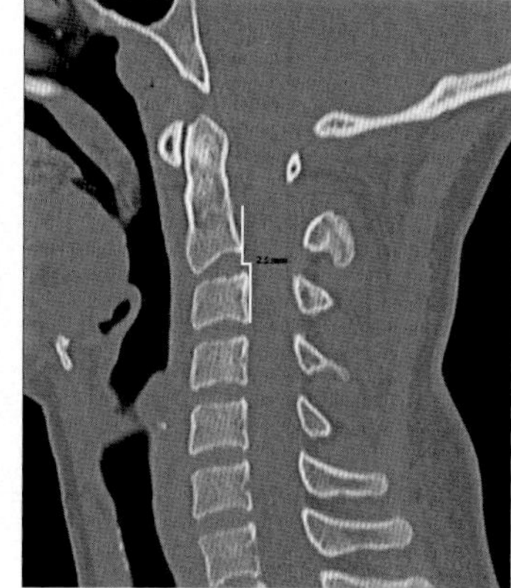

Figure 6.7

Figure 6.8

Discussion

A hangman fracture is a fracture involving both pars interarticularis at C2. The term "hangman" was coined after this fracture pattern was observed following judicial hangings. The mechanism of injury typically involves hyperextension and distraction.

Radiological Evaluation

Hangman fractures can be classified using the Levine and Edwards classification. Accurate classification using this system requires proper assessment of fracture angulation, defined as the angle between the inferior endplates of C2 and C3 (**Figure 6.7**), as well as anterior translation, defined as the distance between the posterior vertebral body margins of C2 and C3 at the level of the disc space (**Figure 6.8**).

▶ **Type I:** Minimally displaced fracture with minimal angulation and less than 3 mm of displacement.

▶ **Type II:** Fracture with both significant angulation and displacement.

▶ **Type IIa:** Disc injury with severe angulation and minimal displacement.

▶ **Type III:** Fracture with bilateral facet dislocation.

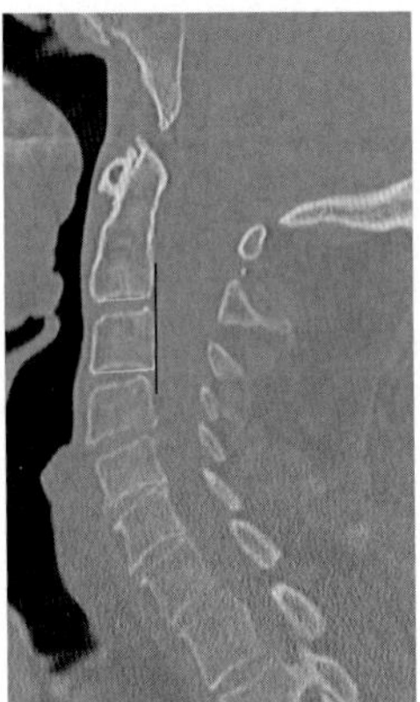
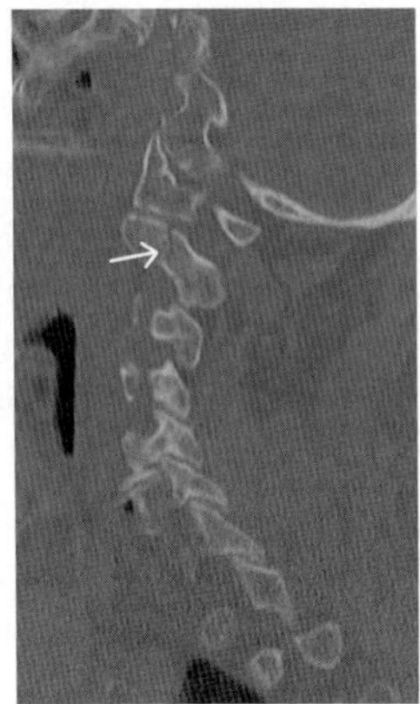

Figure 6.9   Figure 6.10

Type 1 Hangman fracture (**Figures 6.9 and 6.10**). Midsagittal and parasagittal CT imaging showing a Type I fracture without any evidence of displacement or angulation.

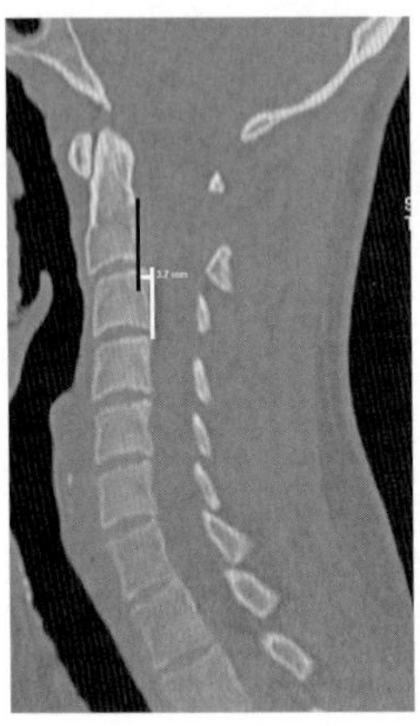
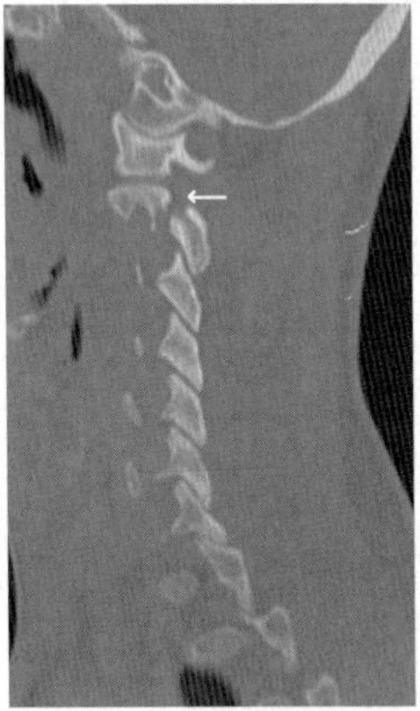

Figure 6.11   Figure 6.12

Type II Hangman fracture (**Figures 6.11 and 6.12**). Midsagittal and parasagittal CT images showing a Type II fracture with greater than 3 mm of anterior translation

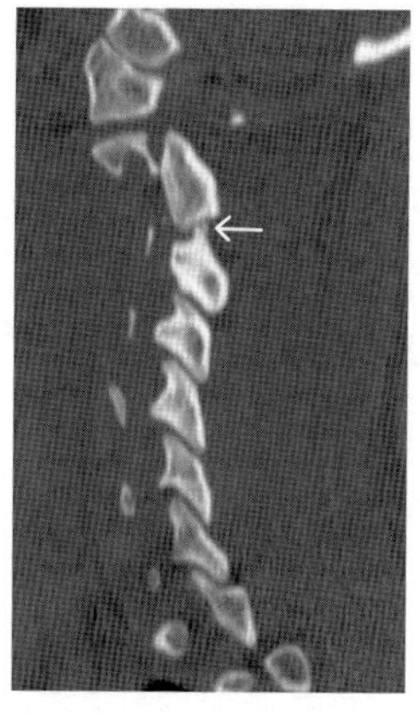 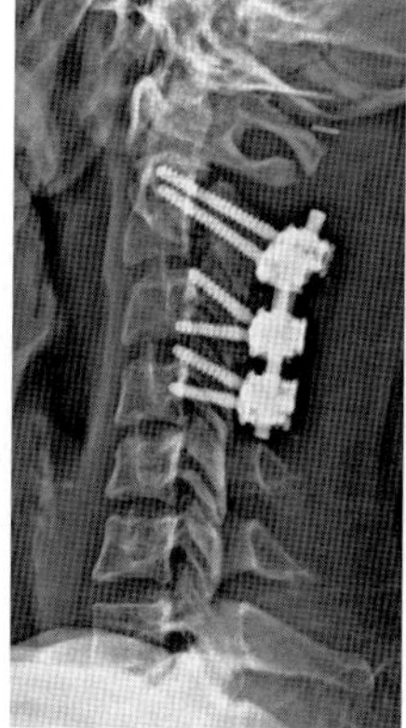

Figure 6.13
Figure 6.14

Type III Hangman fracture (**Figures 6.13 and 6.14**). Parasagittal CT (**Figure 6.13**) of a Type III fracture dislocation with spinal cord injury. A sagittal radiograph (**Figure 6.14**) demonstrates the reduction, C2 pars repair, and C2–C4 fusion performed for stabilization.

Although the Levine and Edwards classification was originally assessed utilizing plain lateral radiographs, sagittal CT images can be used as well to classify fracture patterns. Regardless of the imaging modality, anterolisthesis C2 on C3 and ventral angulation of C2 relative to C3 should raise suspicion for a hangman fracture. Although most hangman fractures have an expansive effect on the spinal canal, atypical patterns (in which the fracture extends through the posterior aspect of the vertebral body leading to potential cord compression) have been described. MRI is useful in patients with a neurological deficit to assess for spinal cord injury.

Management

Accurate classification of fracture patterns can help guide the treatment options. Type I fractures are usually well treated in a hard cervical collar. Type II fractures are often treated with gentle traction and halo immobilization. Given the disc disruption seen in Type IIa fractures, the use of traction in these patients is typically avoided as this may risk spinal cord injury due to distraction. Instead, Type IIa fractures should be reduced and immobilized with halo fixation. If gentle closed reduction is not possible, operative reduction with fixation is sometimes required. Type III fractures require reduction of the dislocation followed by operative stabilization with either anterior interbody fusion, posterior fusion, or direct C2 pars repair.

Teaching Points

► Hangman fractures are bilateral pars interarticularis fractures involving C2.
► Fractures are classified into Types I, II, IIa, and III based on angulation, translation, and facet joint integrity.
► Avoid traction in Type IIa fractures.

Further Reading

1. Levine AM and Edwards CC. The management of traumatic spondylolisthesis of the axis. J Bone Joint Surg Am 1985;67:217–226.
2. Li XF. A systematic review of the management of hangman's fractures. Eur Spine J 2006;15(3):257–269.
3. Starr JK and Eismont FJ. Atypical hangman's fractures. Spine 1993;18(14):1954–1957.

Chapter 7 Jumped Facets

Bruce Lehnert, Brad Currier, and Emily Nguyen

History

► A 24-year-old male presents with neck pain and acute tetraplegia status post-high-speed motor vehicle crash (**Figure 7.1**).

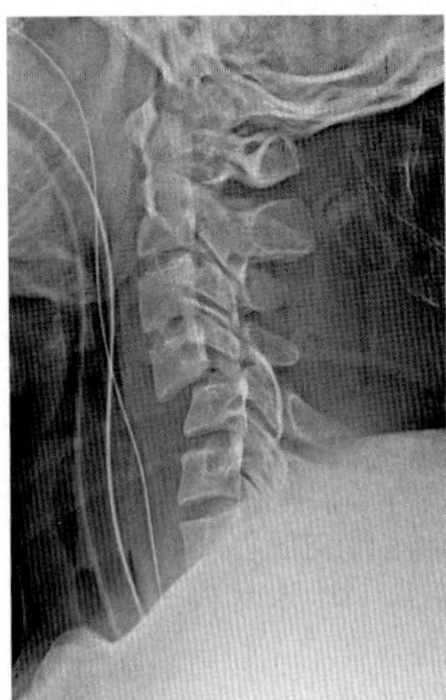

Figure 7.1

Findings

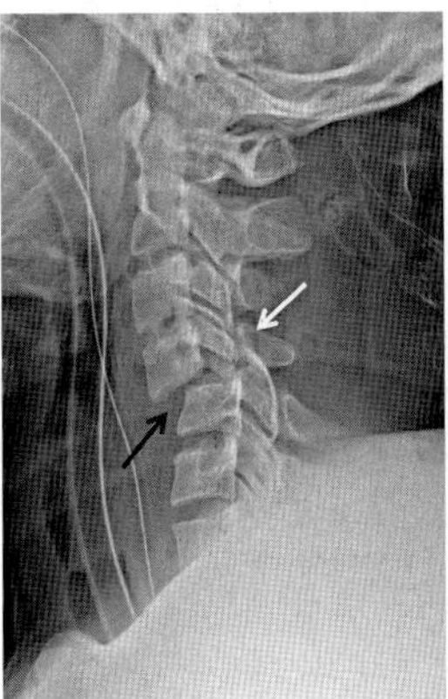

Figure 7.2

Jumped facet (Figure 7.2). A lateral cervical spine radiograph obtained during resuscitation demonstrates gross malalignment of the cervical spine with greater than 50% anterolisthesis of C4 on C5 (black arrow) and anterior dislocation of the C4/C5 facets (white arrow).

Differential Diagnosis

► Unilateral/bilateral facet subluxation or perched facets (with or without fracture and/or disc herniation)
► Unilateral/bilateral facet dislocation or jumped facets (with or without fracture and/or disc herniation)

Discussion

Jumped facets are often a devastating injury frequently resulting in tetraplegia when occurring in the cervical spine. The mechanism of injury typically involves flexion distraction with or without rotation. The posterior ligamentous complex is always disrupted, and disc disruption and/or herniation often occur.

Important complications include spinal cord injury (especially in the setting of underlying preexisiting degenerative disease/central canal stenosis) and vertebral artery injury.

Radiological Evaluation

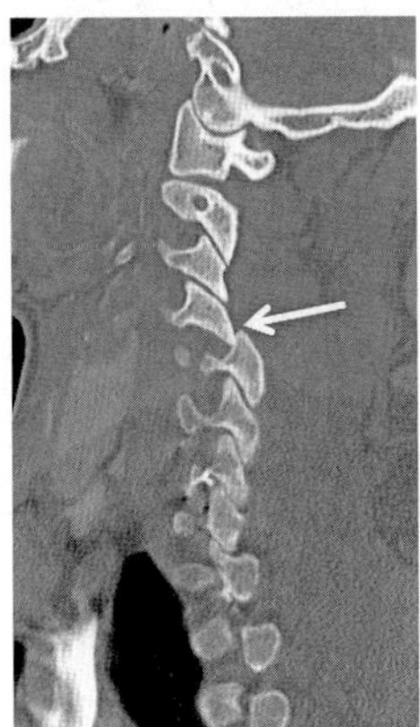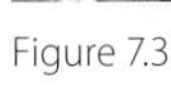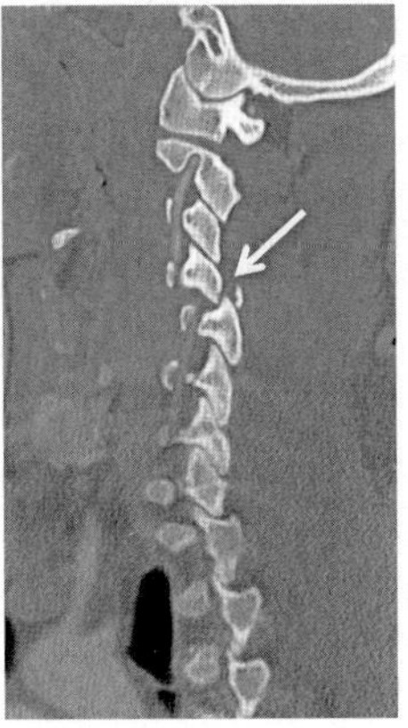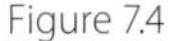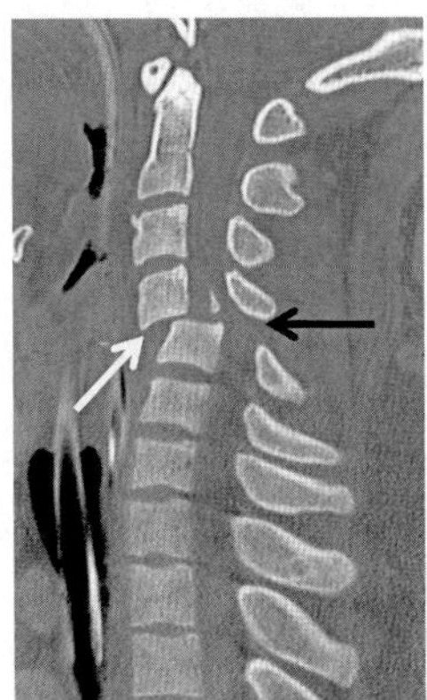

Figure 7.3   Figure 7.4   Figure 7.5

Sagittal CT reformats (Figures 7.3 and 7.4) demonstrate anterior and cephalad dislocation of the C4 facet on C5 with no apposition of articular surfaces (white arrows). Sagittal CT reformat at the midline (Figure 7.5) demonstrates greater than 50% anterior displacement of the C4 vertebral body on C5 with focal kyphosis (white arrow) with associated severe narrowing of the spinal canal (black arrow).

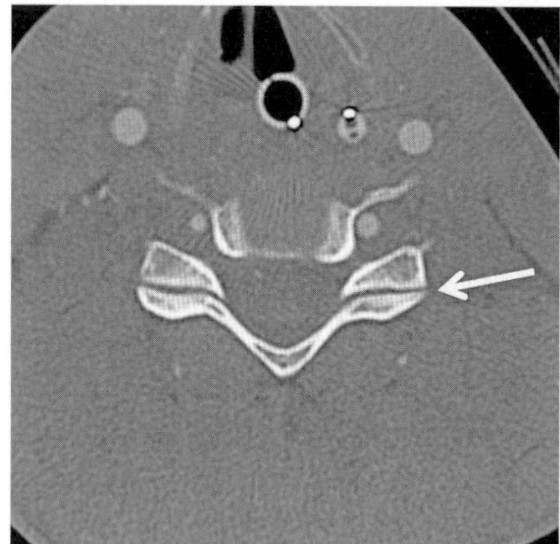

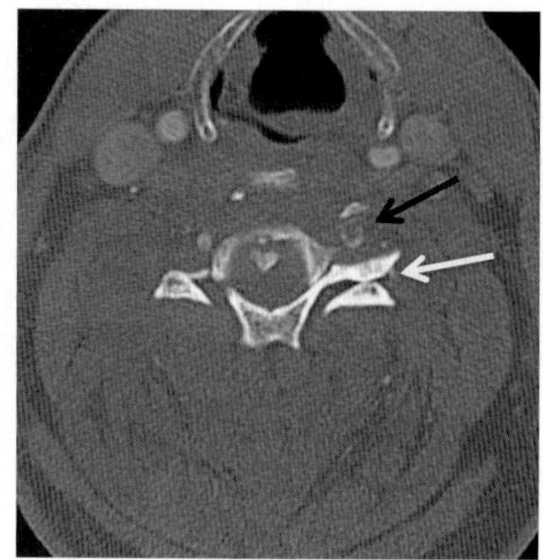

Figure 7.6

Figure 7.7

Axial CT image of the cervical spine (Figure 7.6) demonstrates normal facet alignment, often described as the "hamburger bun" sign, with the opposed facets forming the top and bottom buns of a hamburger (white arrow). Figure 7.7 demonstrates the "reverse hamburger bun" sign seen in facet dislocation (white arrow). Incidental note is made of thrombus in the left vertebral artery, indicating associated vascular injury (black arrow).

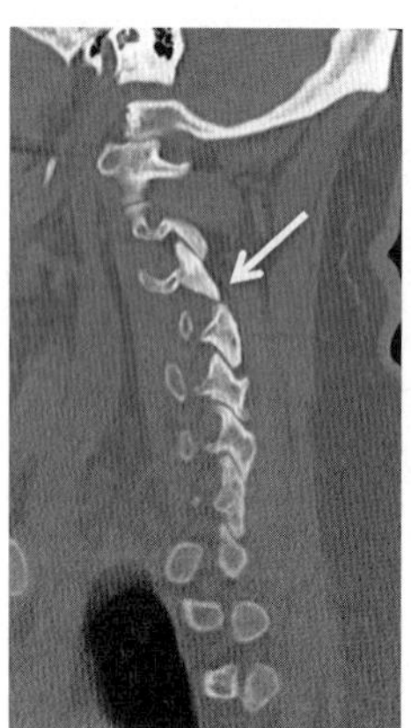

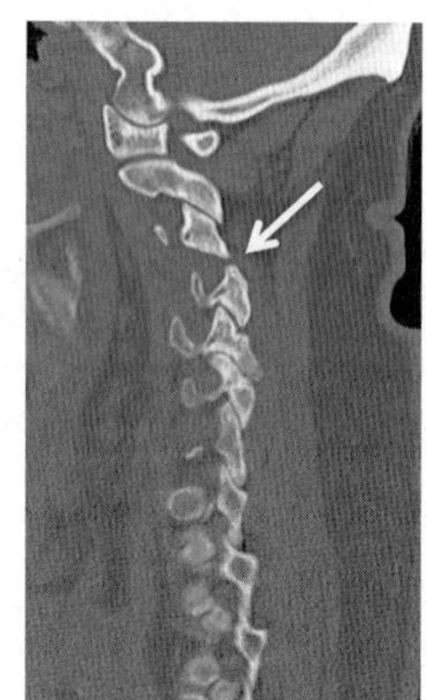

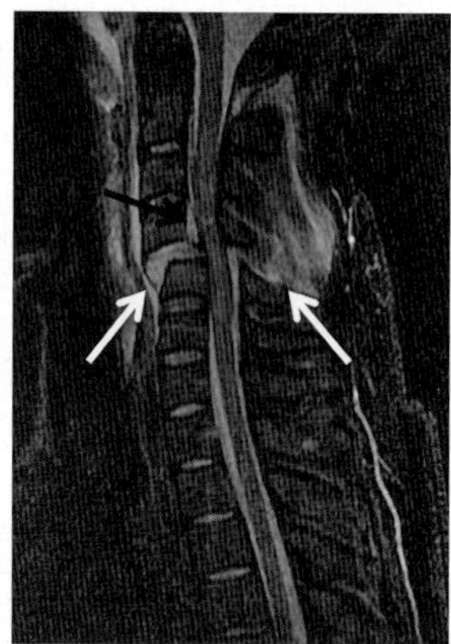

Figure 7.8

Figure 7.9

Figure 7.10

The imaging evaluation of jumped facets included radiographs, CT, and MRI (**Figures 7.8, 7.9, and 7.10**). Bilateral cervical facet injuries are classified based on their degree of ligamentous disruption resulting in an injury spectrum from facet subluxations to facet dislocations or jumped facets. In jumped facets, the inferior articular process translates cephalad and anterior to the superior articular process of the caudad level (Figure 7.8). Perched facets occur when the tip of the inferior articular process abuts the superior articular process representing less than full apposition of the articular facets and may qualify as a dislocation if there is no articular surface apposition.

MRI will show disruption of the interspinous and supraspinous ligaments, facet capsules, possible fracture, often a torn ligamentum flavum, and partial disruption of the posterior annulus or a disc herniation/extrusion (Figure 7.7). CT angiography is often indicated to evaluate the integrity of the vertebral arteries.

Sagittal CT reformats (**Figures 7.8 and 7.9**) from a different patient demonstrate perched bilateral facets with the tip of the inferior C3 facet subluxed anteriorly and abutting the cranial tip of the C4 superior articular process (white arrows).

Sagittal Short T1 Inversion Recover (SITR) MRI (**Figure 7.10**) demonstrates an abnormal signal and widening of the C4/C5 disk, consistent with disruption, as well as an extensive abnormal signal in the posterior ligaments, consistent with injury (white arrows). An abnormal signal is present in the cervical cord at this level, consistent with severe contusion and partial transection (black arrow).

Management

Urgent or emergent reduction is critical. Controversy exists regarding the role and timing of MRI to assess for traumatic disc herniation, hematoma, or other space occupying lesions. If the patient is awake, alert, not intoxicated, and reliably cooperates with a neurological examination, closed traction reduction under fluoroscopy may proceed before MRI. However, serial neurological examinations following each additional weight change must be performed to ensure that there is no change in neurological status. Alternatively, an MRI may be obtained prior to any reduction attempt, particularly in the neurologically intact or incomplete patient. If the patient develops any paresthesias or worsening neurological status during the reduction, an MRI is necessary prior to operative reduction/stabilization.

In the obtunded patient or unsuccessful reduction, an MRI followed by open reduction is necessary. Final stabilization is often necessary with either a halo or operative fixation (Figure 7.11). The operative approach may be anterior, posterior, or combined anteroposterior depending on the associated pathology.

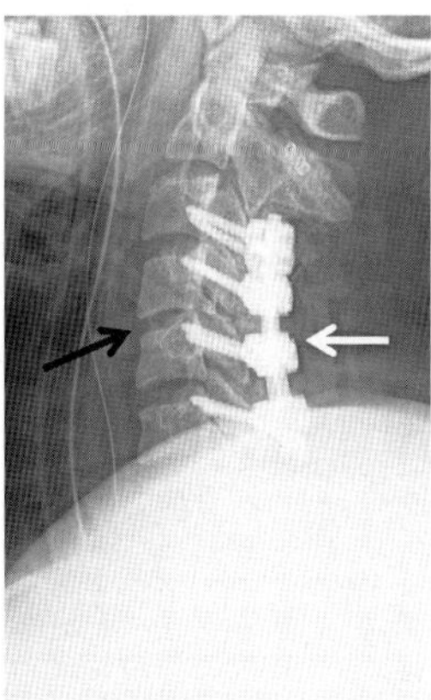

Figure 7.11

Lateral radiograph status post-posterior fixation (white arrow) (**Figure 7.11**) demonstrates complete reduction and anatomic alignment of the cervical spine (black arrow).

Teaching Points

- Bilateral facet dislocation, or jumped facets, is a flexion distraction injury in the subaxial cervical spine that often results in a neurological deficit.
- There is disruption of the interspinous and supraspinous ligaments and facet capsules, often a torn ligamentum flavum, which may be associated with fracture.
- There is often a partial disruption of the posterior annulus of the involved disc or even a disc herniation/extrusion.
- In the awake, alert, and cooperative patient, emergent reduction without MRI or MRI before any attempt at reduction is an acceptable method of treatment provided repeat neurological examinations are performed at each step during the reduction.
- In the obtunded patient or failed closed reduction, an MRI must be performed prior to operative treatment.

Further Reading

1. Bono CM, Schoenfeld A, Gupta G, et al. Reliability and reproducibility of subaxial cervical injury description system. Spine 2011;36:1140–1144.
2. Vaccaro AR, Madigan L, Schweitzer ME, et al. Magnetic resonance imaging analysis of soft tissue disruption after flexion-distraction injuries of the subaxial cervical spine. Spine 2001;26:1866–1872.
3. Zigler JE, Eismont FJ, et al. *Spine Trauma*, 2nd ed. Rosemont, IL: American Academy of Orthopaedic Surgeons, 2011.

Chapter 8

Bruce Lehnert, Yazeed Gussous, and Ahmad Nassr

History

▶ A 28-year-old polytrauma patient following a motor vehicle accident presents with an intact neurological examination. In addition, the patient has bilateral pneumothoraces treated with chest tubes (**Figures 8.1, 8.2, and 8.3**).

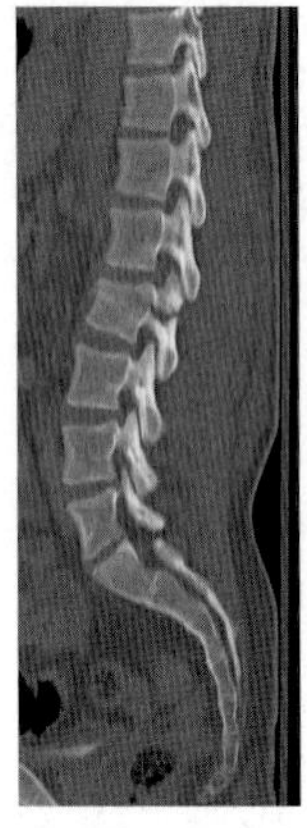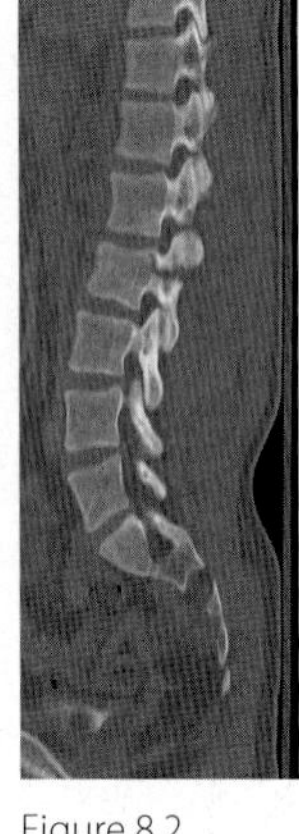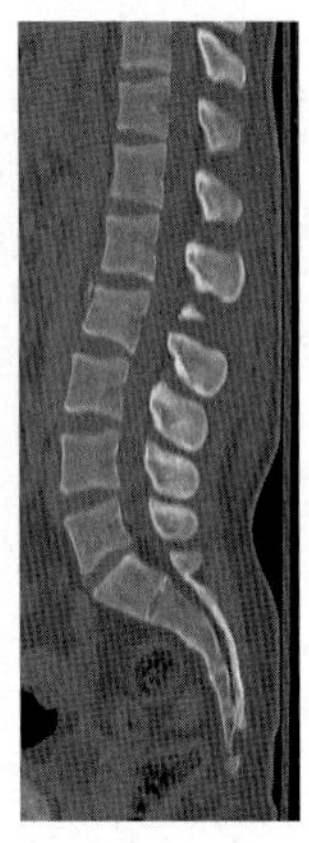

Figure 8.1   Figure 8.2   Figure 8.3

Findings

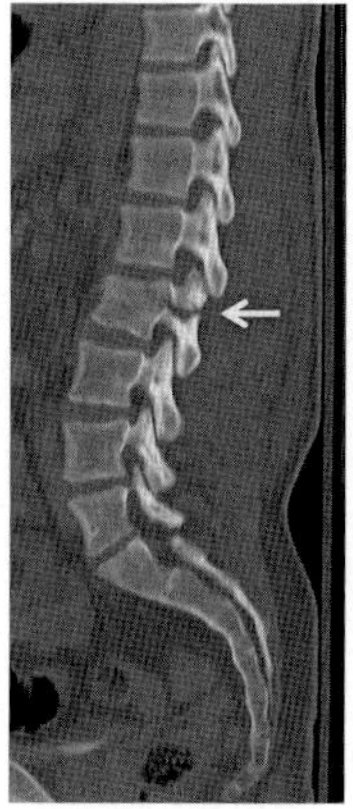 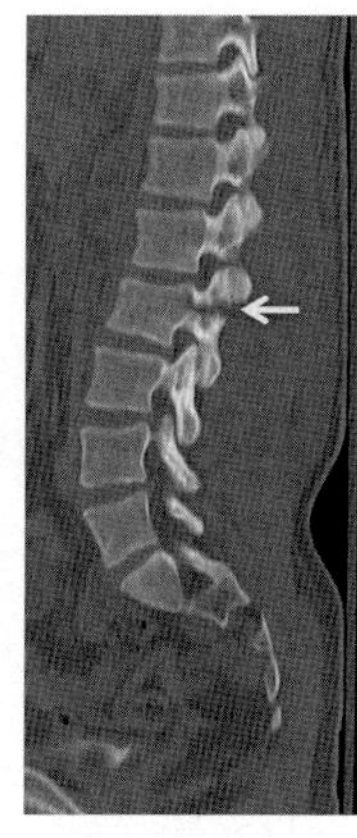 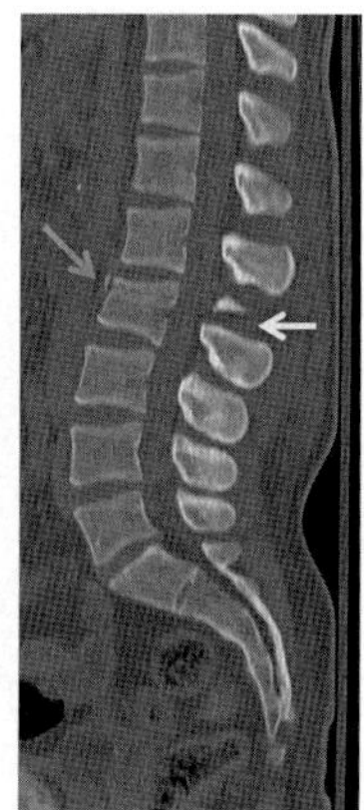

Figure 8.4   Figure 8.5   Figure 8.6

Chance fracture on CT. Sagittal CT reformats (**Figures 8.4 and 8.5**) demonstrate transverse fractures through the pedicles of L2 bilaterally with asymmetric widening of the fracture posteriorly, consistent with distraction (white arrows). **Figure 8.6** demonstrates a distracted fracture of the L2 spinous process (white arrow) as well as minimal L2 superior endplate compression (grey arrow).

Differential Diagnosis

► Flexion distraction injury without bony involvement

Discussion

Chance fracture is an eponym for a bony flexion distraction injury typically of the thoracolumbar spine. The mechanism usually involves forced flexion across a lap belt during a motor vehicle crash (MVC), resulting in a distracting force in the posterior spine. This manifests as a transverse fracture through posterior elements, pedicles, and the posterior aspect of the affected vertebral body. There may be some degree of anterior compression. Intraabdominal pressure increases with this mechanism and this injury is maybe associated with abdominal injuries in 50% of the cases.

Radiological Evaluation

Plan radiographs and CT scan will delineate the bony involvement, and MRI will demonstrate ligamentous injury on Short TI Inversion Recovery (STIR) sequence the best (**Figures 8.7, 8.8, 8.9, 8.10, 8.11, and 8.12**).

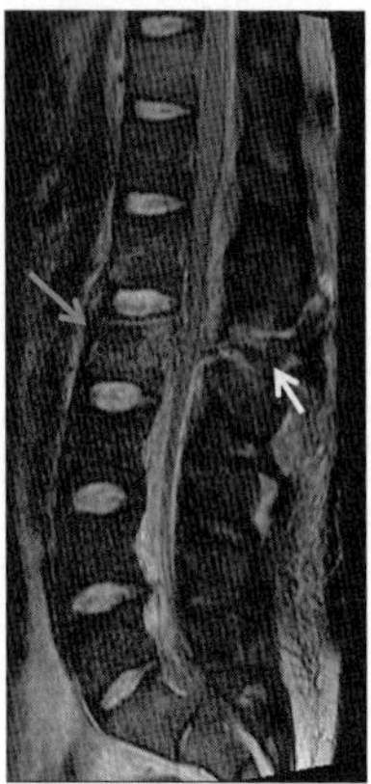

Figure 8.7

Sagittal STIR MRI (**Figure 8.7**) demonstrates heterogeneous signal at the location of the spinous process fracture, consistent with edema and hemorrhage (white arrow). Increased signal is present in the L2 vertebral body (grey arrow) related to superior endplate compression and extension of the transverse pedicle fracture through the posterior vertebral body.

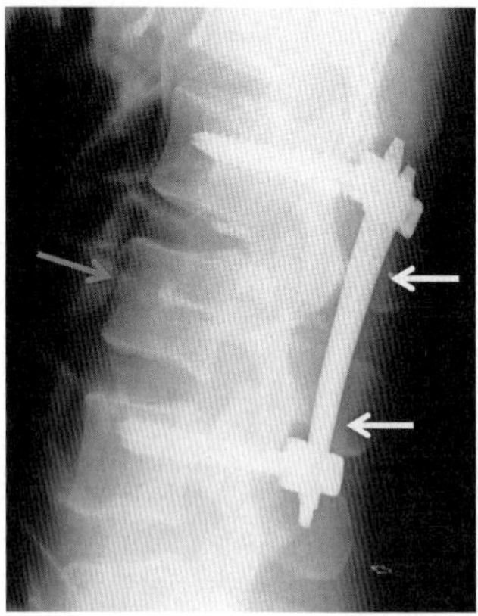

Figure 8.8

The patient underwent posterior fixation with pedicle screws and rods (white arrows) (**Figure 8.8**). There is preservation of vertebral body height and alignment (grey arrow).

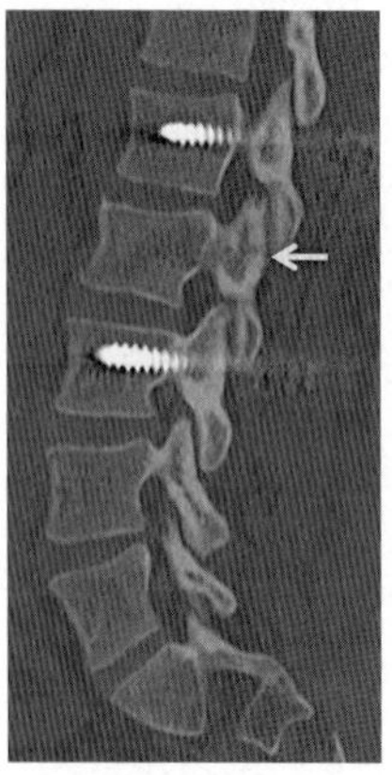

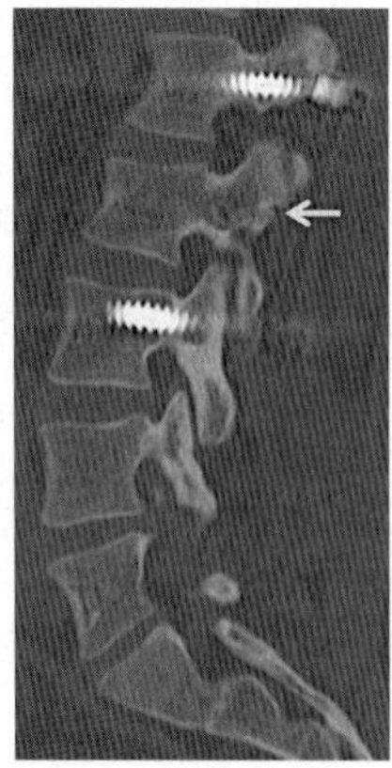

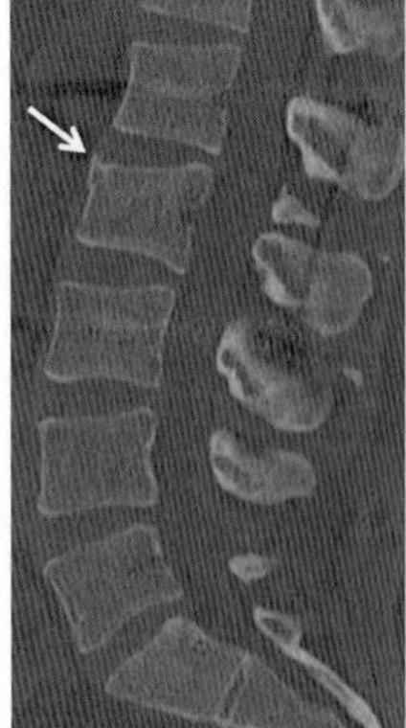

Figure 8.9   Figure 8.10   Figure 8.11

Sagittal CT reformats (Figures 8.9 and 8.10) 1 year postinstrumentation demonstrate healed pedicle fractures (white arrows). There is also a healed compression deformity at the superior L2 endplate (white arrow) with no additional loss of vertebral body height (Figure 8.11).

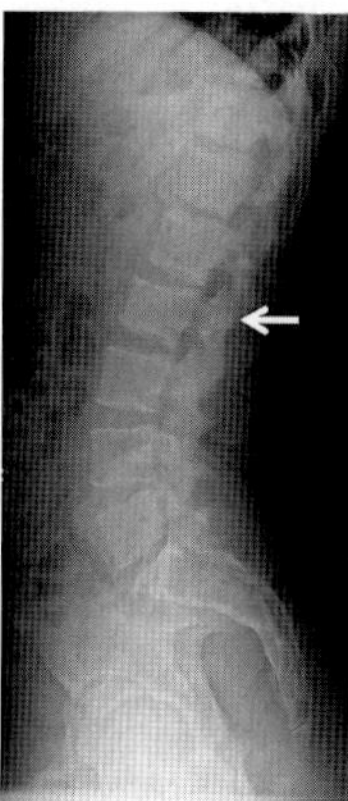

Figure 8.12

Lateral radiograph 2 years postinjury and after instrumentation removal demonstrates persistent but unchanged mild L2 endplate compression deformity but otherwise normal spinal alignment (white arrow) (Figure 8.12).

Management

A patient with a Chance fracture, by definition, has a bony fracture through the pedicles. This injury pattern is amenable to healing with a hyperextension cast or brace. Our patient had bilateral pneumothoraces that impeded his placement in a cast and thus percutaneous fixation of the fracture was elected. Instrumentation was removed a year after radiographic evidence of healing and follow-up radiographs at 2 years show a good outcome with preserved vertebral body height and alignment.

Teaching Points

► Chance fracture is by definition a bony injury that should be differentiated from flexion distraction variants through discoligamentous structures.
► While the bony injury is amenable to treatment in hyperextension immobilization, specific patient condition including other associated systemic injuries needs to be considered when planning treatment.

Further Reading

1. Chance GQ. Note a type of flexion fracture of the spine. Br Radiol 1948;21(249):452.
2. Sutter S, et al. Operative treatment of Chance injuries in the paediatric population. Eur Spine J 2013;22(3):510–514.
3. Mulpuri K, et al. The spectrum of abdominal injuries associated with Chance fractures in pediatric patients. Eur J Pediatr Surg 2007;17(5):322–327.

Chapter 9

H. Kate Lee

History

▶ A 43-year-old female presents with weakness and decreased range of motion in the upper extremity after diving into a pool (**Figures 9.1, 9.2, and 9.3**).

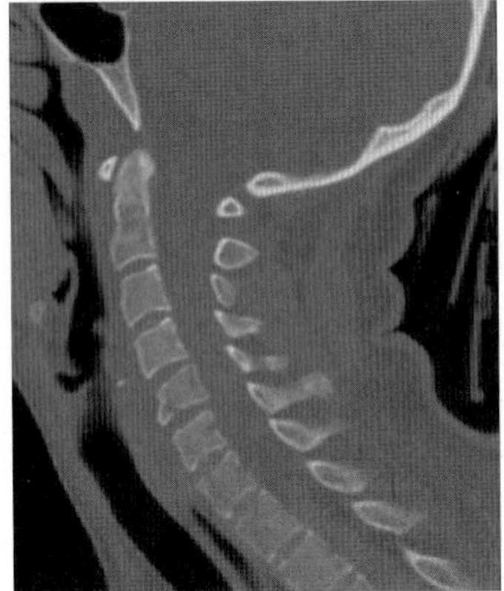

Figure 9.1

Figure 9.2

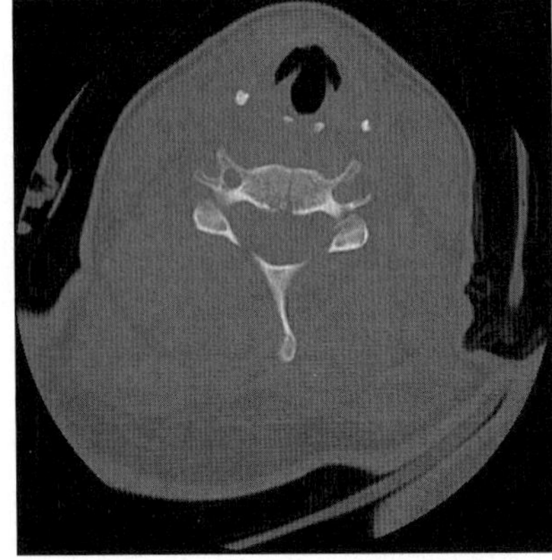

Figure 9.3

Findings

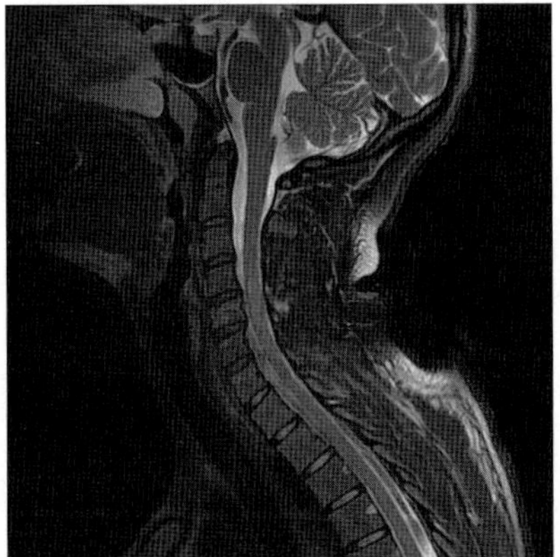

Figure 9.4

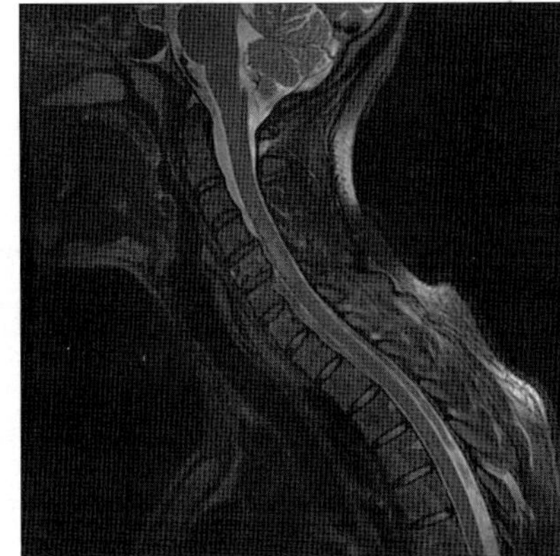

Figure 9.5

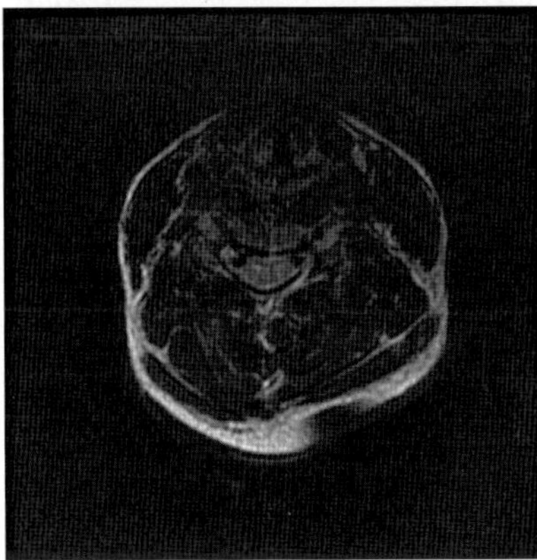

Figure 9.6

Hyperextension injury to the cervical spine (**Figures 9.1, 9.2, 9.3, 9.4, 9.5, and 9.6**). Sagittal (**Figure 9.1 and Figure 9.2**) and axial (**Figure 9.3**) CT reconstruction images show a minimally displaced fracture at the anterior inferior corner of the C5 vertebral body that extends to the posterior cortex (**Figure 9.3**). **Figure 9.2** better demonstrates an additional fracture at C7. Fat-suppressed sagittal T2-weighted MR images (**Figure 9.4 and Figure 9.5**) and non-fat-suppressed axial T2-weighted MR images (**Figure 9.6**) demonstrate bone marrow edema surrounding the C5 and C7 fractures as well as near the C6 superior endplate. T2 hyperintense signal abnormality in the expanded C4–C6 cord indicates cord edema or contusion.

Differential Diagnosis
- ► Hyperflexion injury
- ► Cervical spondylosis
- ► If trauma history is unknown, additional considerations include
  - Infection
  - Demyelination/inflammation
  - Neoplasm

Discussion

Hyperextension cervical injuries result from sudden, forced extension of the neck and account for up to 38% of blunt traumatic injuries of the cervical spine. They may result from either a direct contact mechanism or a noncontact mechanism (i.e., whiplash injuries). Though they are not as severe as flexion teardrop injuries, patients can present with serious injuries with devastating neurological sequelae. They encompass the following.

▶ Avulsion fractures of the anterior arch of C1.
▶ Vertical fracture through the posterior arch of the atlas as a result of compression.
▶ Fracture of the dens.
▶ Hangman fracture of C2 (traumatic spondylolisthesis of C2).
▶ Hyperextension teardrop fracture.
▶ Hyperextension dislocation.
▶ Laminar fractures.
▶ Central cord syndrome.

A subgroup of patients is at substantial risk for devastating hyperextension spine injury--patients with diffuse idiopathic skeletal hyperostosis (DISH) or ankylosing spondylitis (AS). After a minor trauma these patients may need to undergo MR despite having no identifiable fractures on standard imaging.

Hyperextension teardrop fracture is commonly seen in diving accidents. Younger patients will have avulsion most commonly in the lower cervical spine, with extensive soft tissue swelling and spinal cord injury, reflecting a greater degree of traumatic force required to produce this injury. In elderly osteoporotic patients, the fracture typically involves C2 due to fusion deformities in the lower cervical spine and little force can produce this injury in an underlying weak spine, with little or no soft tissue swelling and no neurological impairment. If neurologically impaired, up to 80% of patients may present with central cord syndrome due to buckling of the ligamentum flavum into the spinal canal. This injury is stable in flexion but unstable in extension.

Radiological Evaluation

This case illustrates a hyperextension teardrop fracture at C5 on CT (**Figure 9.1, Figure 9.2, and Figure 9.3**). MR images reveal a T2 hyperintense signal in the central cervical cord (**Figure 9.4, Figure 9.5, and Figure 9.6**). Along with the patient's symptoms, a T2 hyperintense signal abnormality in the expanded C4–C6 cord is consistent with cord edema or contusion in central cord syndrome. Prevertebral soft tissue edema is also noted.

Both flexion and extension teardrop fractures manifest as displaced anteroinferior bony fragments; however, extension teardrop fracture is a true avulsion of intact fibers of the anterior longitudinal ligament (ALL) off the anterior inferior corner of the vertebral body because of the sudden hyperextension, while flexion teardrop fracture is caused by compression. The vertical dimension of the fragment is equal to or greater than its transverse dimension, which helps differentiate the avulsed fragment from the fragment seen in the hyperflexion teardrop. A flexion teardrop fracture is a more severe injury compared to an extension teardrop injury (**Figure 9.7, Figure 9.8, and Figure 9.9**).

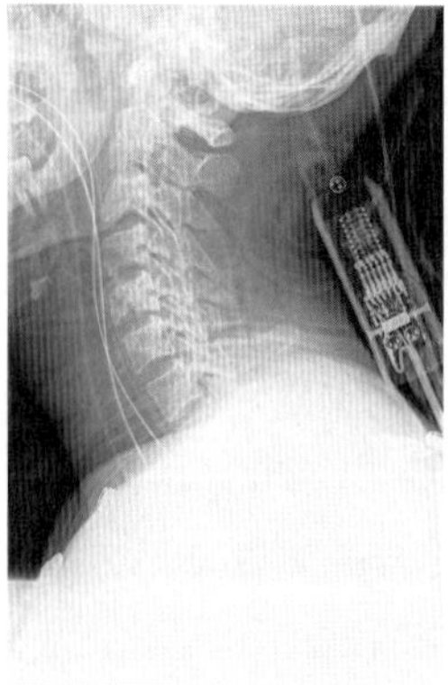

Figure 9.7

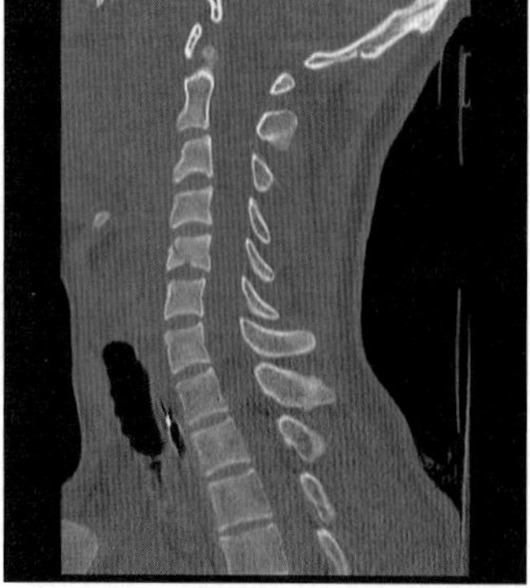

Figure 9.8

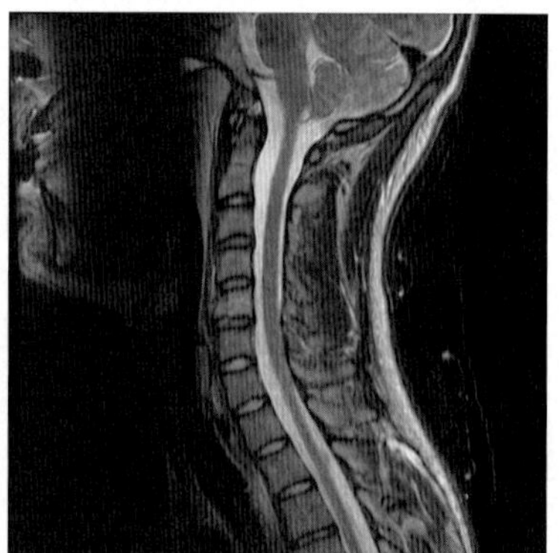

Figure 9.9

Extension teardrop fracture in an 18-year-old male after a motor vehicle crash (MVC). A lateral radiograph of the cervical spine (**Figure 9.7**) demonstrates a nondisplaced fracture at the anteroinferior aspect of C5. A sagittal CT reformat (**Figure 9.8**) again depicts this fracture and shows normal cervical alignment. The interspinous spaces are not widened. Bone marrow edema is seen associated with the fracture on a sagittal T2-weighted image (**Figure 9.9**).

Management

Hyperextension injuries are typically managed by immobilization in a rigid cervical collar and activity restriction for 4–6 weeks. The neurological status for patients with cord or nerve root dysfunction is carefully monitored. A subgroup of patients prone to hyperextension injury (DISH or AS) may need operative stabilization or halo-vest immobilization as this injury in those patients can be highly unstable and conservative measures are less likely to be successful than in other patients.

Teaching Points

- ▶ Hyperextension cervical injuries are not uncommon.
- ▶ Hyperextension either by a direct contact mechanism or a noncontact mechanism can manifest as a multiple pattern of injuries.
- ▶ Immobilization of the cervical spine is the mainstay of management of hyperextension injuries although a subset of patients vulnerable to hyperextension injuries may require surgical stabilization.

Further Reading

1. Berquist TH and Cabanela ME. The spine. In *Imaging of Orthopedic Trauma and Surgery* (Berquist TH, ed.). Philadelphia, PA: Saunders, 1986, pp. 91–180.
2. Rao SK, Wasyliw C, and Nunez DB. Spectrum of imaging findings in hyperextension injuries of the neck. RadioGraphics 2005;25:1239–1254.
3. Torretti JA and Sengupta DK. Cervical spine trauma. Indian J Orthop 2007;41(4):255–267.
4. Lee JS, Harris JH Jr, and Mueller CF. The significance of prevertebral soft tissue swelling in extension teardrop fracture of the cervical spine. Emerg Radiol 1997;4(3):132–139.
5. Marcon RM, Cristante AF, Teixeira WJ, Narasaki DK, Oliveira RP, and de Barros Filho TE. Fractures of the cervical spine. Clinics (Sao Paulo) 2013;68(11):1455–1461.
6. Watanabe M, Sakai D, Yamamoto Y, Sato M, and Mochida J. Clinical features of the extension teardrop fracture of the axis: Review of 13 cases. J Neurosurg Spine 2011;14(6):710–714.
7. Bernstein M and Baxter A. Cervical spine trauma: Pearls and pitfalls. In *Pitfalls in Clinical Imaging* (Anderson S, ed.). ARRS Categorical Course Syllabus, 2012.
8. Daffner R and Daffner S. Vertebral injuries: Detection and implications. Eur J Radiol 2002;42:100–116.

Chapter 10

Bruce Lehnert

History

▶ A 21-year-old female presenting with acute quadriplegia status post-motor vehicle crash (MVC) (**Figure 10.1**).

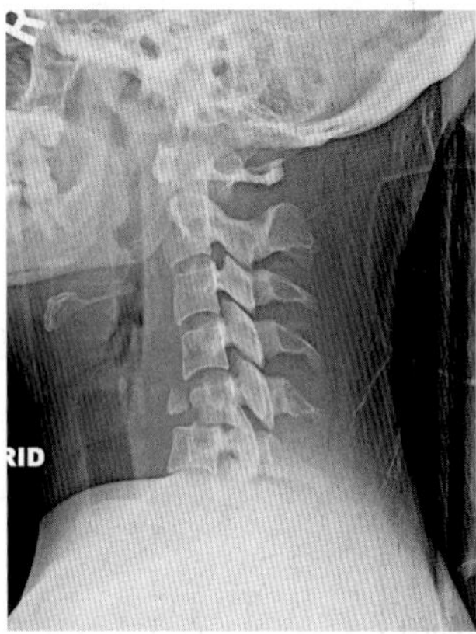

Figure 10.1

Findings

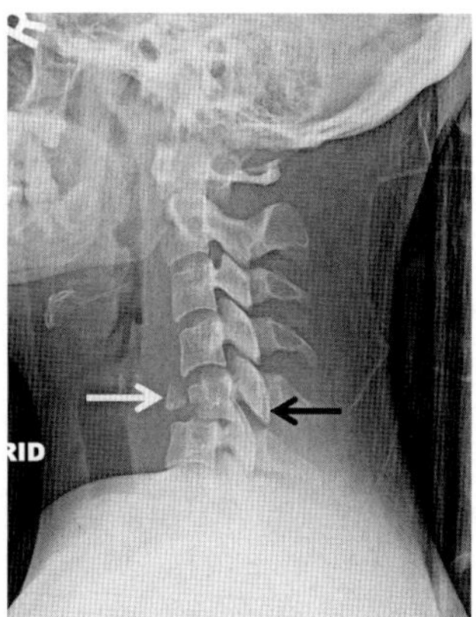

Figure 10.2

Lateral radiograph of the cervical spine obtained during resuscitation (**Figure 10.2**) demonstrates focal kyphosis at an anterior triangular fracture fragment from the inferior C5 vertebral body (white arrow) with retropulsion of the remainder of C5 and bilateral facet joint widening (black arrow), consistent with a flexion teardrop fracture.

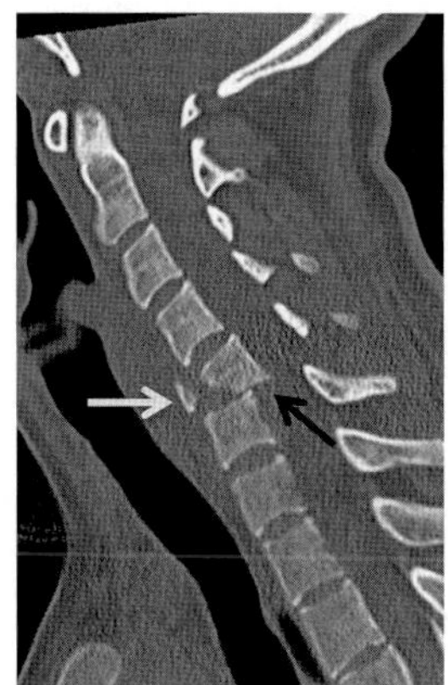

Figure 10.3

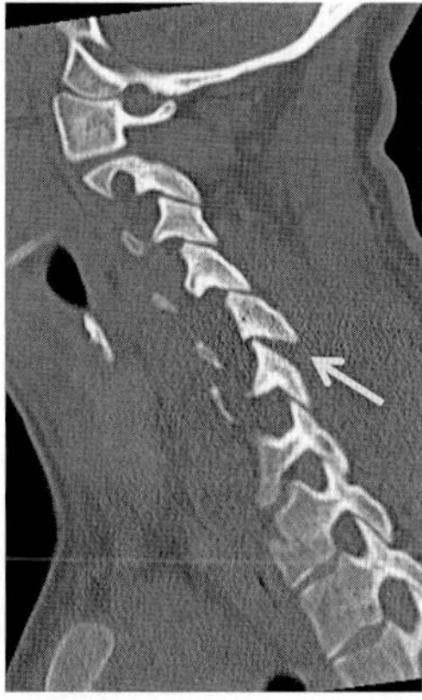

Figure 10.4

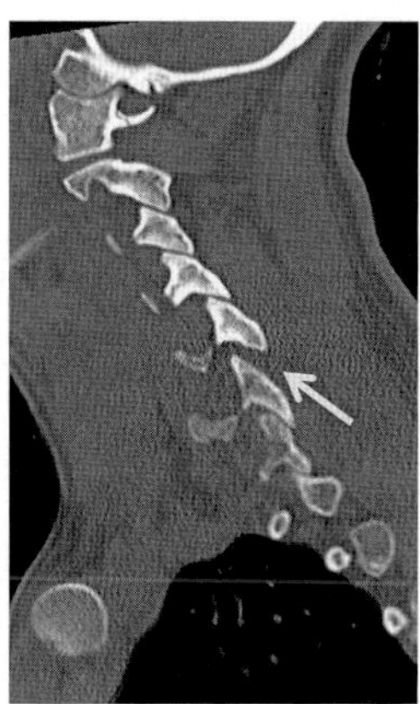

Figure 10.5

Sagittal CT reformats at the midline (**Figure 10.3**) better demonstrate the typical anterior inferior vertebral body teardrop fracture (white arrow) and retropulsion of the C5 vertebral body into the central canal (black arrow).

Sagittal CT reformats through the facets (**Figures 10.4 and 10.5**) demonstrate facet joint widening and subluxation (white arrows), indicating disruption of the posterior joint capsules and ligamentous structures.

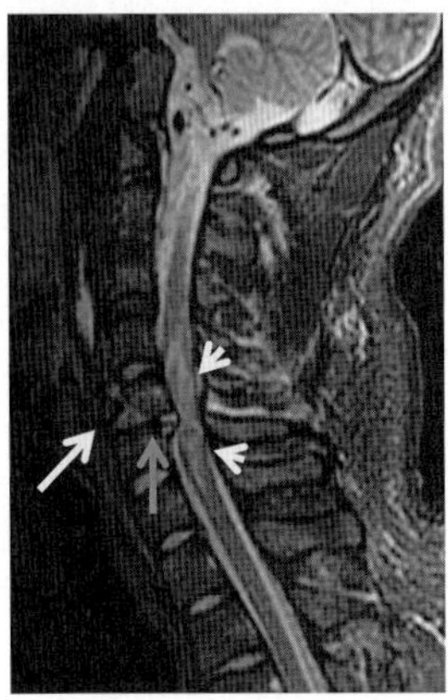

Figure 10.6

Sagittal short T1 inversion recover (STIR) MRI at the midline (**Figure 10.6**) again demonstrates the flexion teardrop fracture (white arrow) and bony retropulsion (grey arrow) with disruption of the anterior longitudinal ligament and stripping of the posterior longitudinal ligament from the subjacent vertebral body. There is abnormal signal in the adjacent cervical cord indicating edema and hemorrhage (white arrowheads).

Discussion

Hyperflexion injuries can range in severity from a mild sprain to the very unstable flexion teardrop fracture with associated spinal cord injury and quadriplegia. Hyperflexion injuries occur when there is some degree of posterior ligamentous complex disruption.

Radiological Evaluation

A diagnosis of hyperflexion injury may be made with conventional radiographs or CT of the cervical spine. MRI is useful to demonstrate the extent of ligamentous injury and to evaluate for spinal cord injury.

In a hyperflexion sprain, the lateral view of the cervical spine demonstrates a focal kyphotic deformity, widening of the interspinous distance at the level of injury, and partial superior facet joint uncovering at the vertebral body immediately below the kyphotic deformity. There may be slight (1–3 mm) anterior vertebral body displacement and/or slight anterior superior endplate compression of the vertebral body below the lesion.

Signs of an unstable anterior subluxation injury include more than 3.5 mm anterolisthesis, focal kyphosis greater than 11 degrees, and subluxation of the articular facets at the affected level.

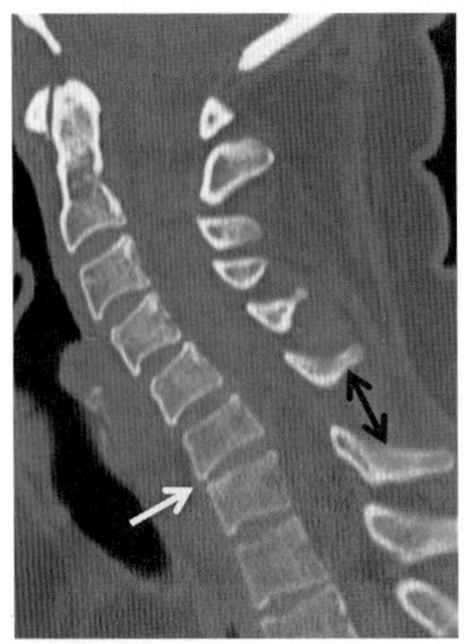

Figure 10.7

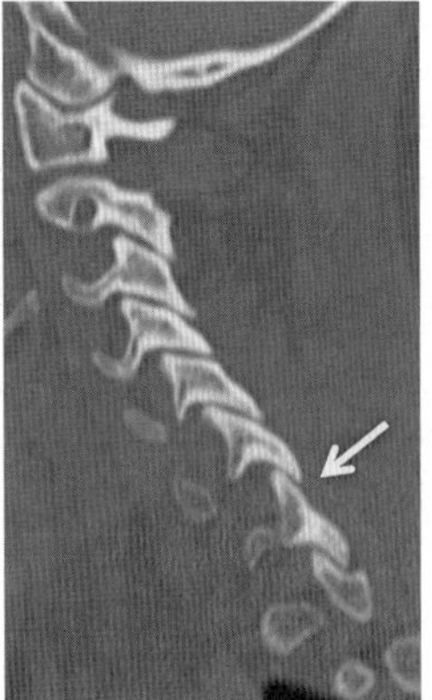

Figure 10.8

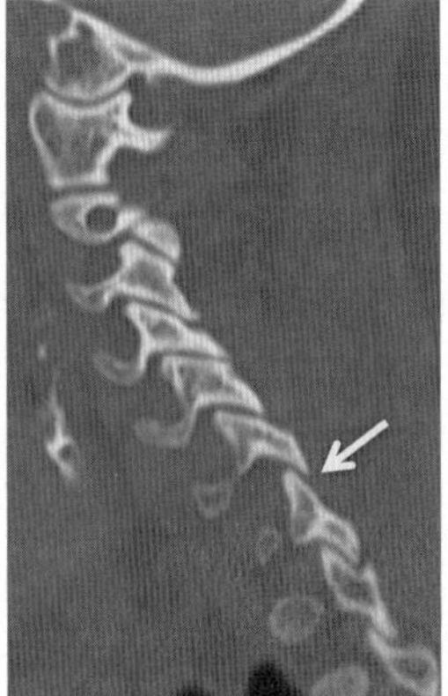

Figure 10.9

Sagittal CT reformats at the midline in a different patient suspected of having a hyperflexion injury (**Figure 10.7**) demonstrate anterior disk space loss at C6/C7 (white arrow), mild superior CT endplate compression, focal kyphosis, and abnormal widening of the spinous processes at this level (black arrow).

Sagittal CT reformats through the facets (**Figures 10.8 and 10.9**) demonstrate bilateral facet joint subluxation (white arrows), consistent with an unstable hyperflexion sprain injury.

The most severe hyperflexion injury in the cervical spine is the flexion teardrop fracture. This injury typically results in a comminuted vertebral body fracture with a triangular fragment at the anterior inferior vertebral body (the "teardrop"), retropulsion of the posterior vertebral body fragments into the central canal, and a sagittal fracture through the posterior arch. There is associated complete disruption of the posterior ligamentous structures and of the anterior longitudinal ligament, making this injury extremely unstable.

Management

Hyperflexion injuries without significant vertebral body subluxation or kyphosis, such as sprain injuries, may be managed conservatively. Unstable hyperflexion injuries with posterior ligamentous disruption and the severe flexion teardrop injuries generally require internal stabilization. Anterior, posterior, or combined anterior and posterior fixation may be considered, depending on the type and severity of the injury.

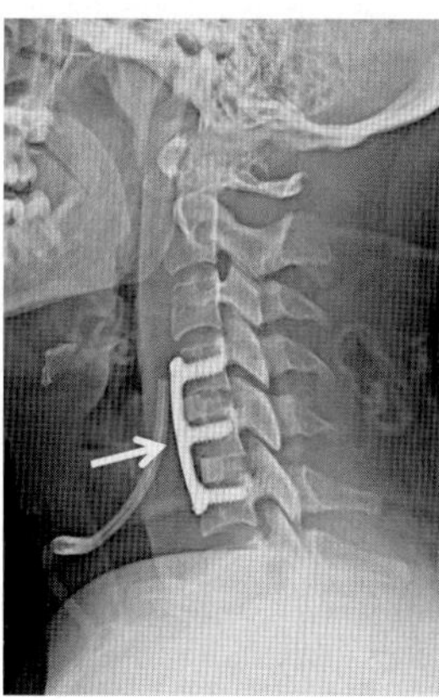

Figure 10.10

Lateral radiograph of the cervical spine demonstrates reduction to anatomic alignment of the flexion teardrop injury status post-anterior fixation (white arrow) (**Figure 10.10**).

Teaching Points

▶ Hyperflexion injuries of the cervical spine represent a spectrum of injuries from the stable hyperflexion "sprain" to the highly unstable flexion teardrop fracture.

▶ The diagnosis may be initially made with radiographs while CT is useful for more detailed evaluation of bony injuries and alignment. MRI is helpful in delineating the extent of soft tissue, ligamentous, and spinal cord involvement.

▶ Stable hyperflexion "sprain" injuries may be managed conservatively. Unstable injuries are typically managed with internal stabilization.

Further Reading

1. Dvorak MF, Fisher CG, Fehlings MG, et al. The surgical approach to subaxial cervical spine injuries: An evidence-based algorithm based on the SLIC classification system. Spine 2007;32(23):2620–2629.
2. Gelb DE, Aarabi B, Dhall SS, et al. Treatment of subaxial cervical spinal injuries. Neurosurgery 2013;72(Suppl 2):187–194.
3. Greenspan A. *Orthopedic Imaging: A Practical Approach*. Philadelphia, PA: Lippincott Williams & Wilkins, 2004.
4. Schwartz ED and Flanders AE. 2007. Spinal trauma : imaging, diagnosis, and management. Philadelphia: Lippincott Williams & Wilkins

Chapter 11

Francesco D'Amore, Chia-Shang J. Liu, and Mark S. Shiroishi

History

► Status post-motor vehicle accident (**Figures 11.1 and 11.2**).

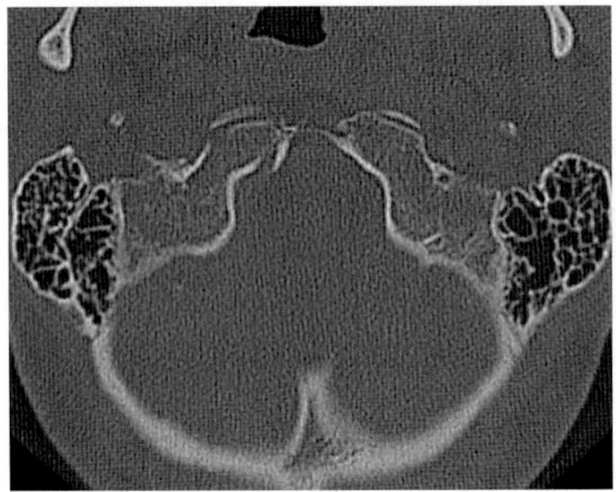

Figure 11.1

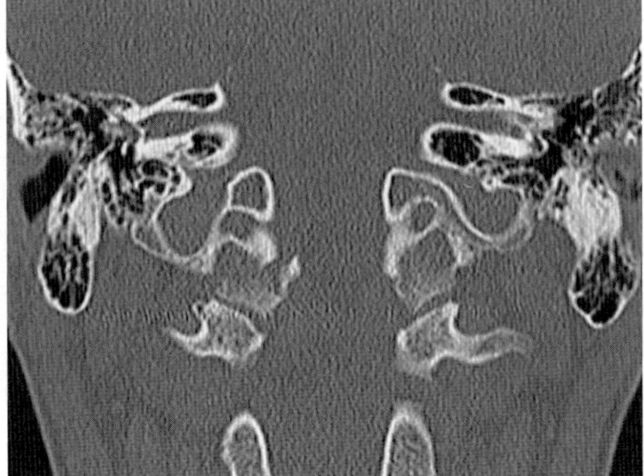

Figure 11.2

Findings

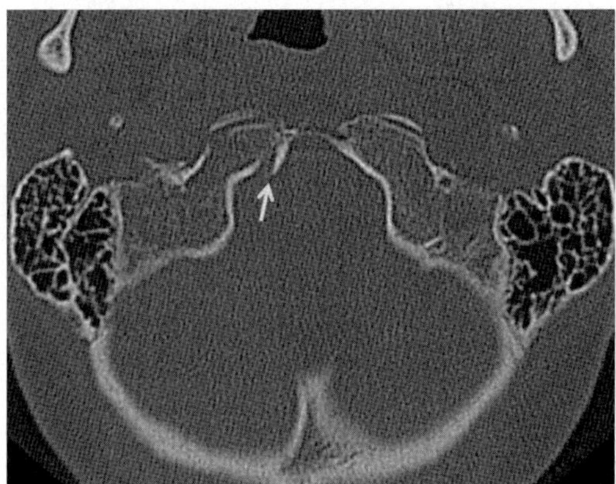
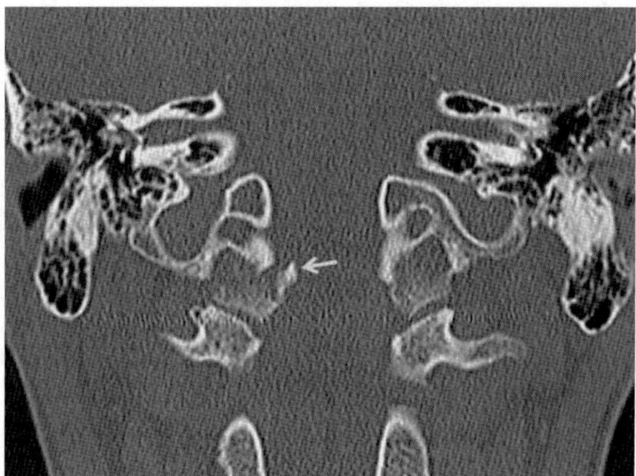

Figure 11.3

Figure 11.4

Occipital condyle fracture (OCF) (**Figures 11.3 and 11.4**). Axial (Figure 11.3) and coronal (Figure 11.4) CT demonstrate a mildly displaced avulsion fracture (white arrow) of the right inferomedial occipital condyle, compatible with a Type 3 Anderson and Montesano OCF.

Differential Diagnosis

The differential diagnosis includes vascular channel/nutrient foramen, pathological fracture from underlying osseous metastasis, and technical artifact.

Discussion

OCFs typically result from high-energy blunt trauma and can be frequently missed on imaging exams. OCFs have been reported in 4% of traffic accident deaths. Another study estimated the frequency of OCF to be between one and two fractures per 1000 trauma patients.

As a diagnostic tool, CT imaging has taken over the role of conventional radiography, whose limitations due to osseous superimpositions have resulted in an underestimation of its occurrence during the pre-CT era.

MRI has a role in the evaluation of the surrounding soft tissue, ligaments, and spinal cord. Most importantly, compared to CT, it can better display the anatomic relationship between the bone fragments and structures such as the brainstem, subarachnoid spaces, and neurovascular structures.

Radiological Evaluation

In 1988, Anderson and Montesano classified OCFs depending on the vector of the injuring force. This is the most commonly used classification system and divided OCFs into three types. A Type 1 OCF is a comminuted fracture of the occipital condyle due to impaction. It is generally stable because the tectorial membrane and contralateral alar ligament remain intact; however, if both condyles are involved, it may be unstable.

A Type 2 OCF is a basilar skull fracture with extension into one or both occipital condyles. This type is also considered a stable fracture because the alar ligament and tectorial membrane are usually spared (**Figures 11.5 and 11.6**).

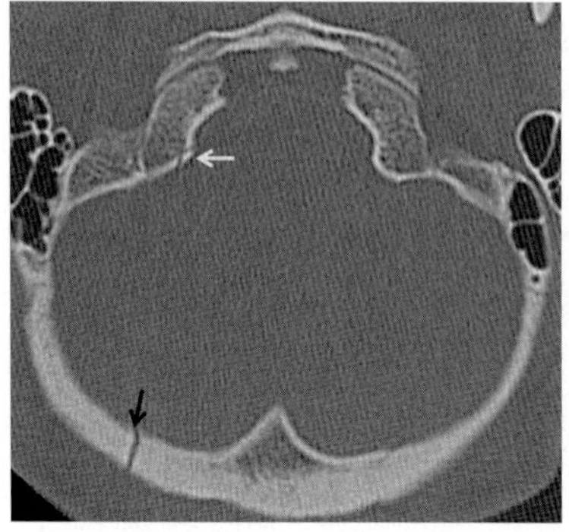
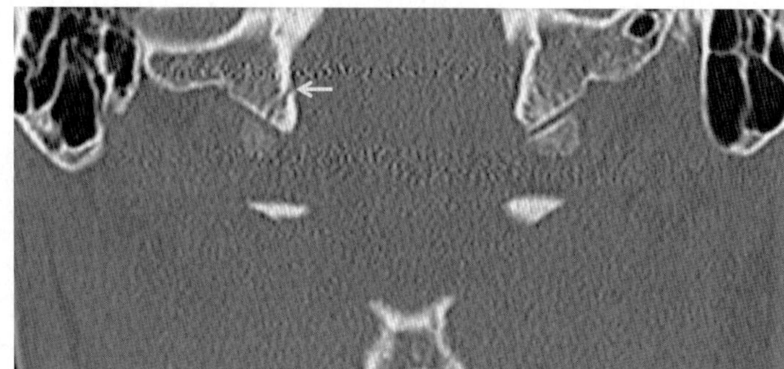

Figure 11.5

Figure 11.6

Type 2 OCF (Figures 11.5 and 11.6). Axial (Figure 11.5) and coronal (Figure 11.6) CT demonstrate a nondisplaced right occipital bone fracture (black arrow, Figure 11.5) that extends to the right occipital condyle (white arrow, Figure 11.6), compatible with a Type 2 Anderson and Montesano right OCF.

A Type 3 OCF is an avulsion fracture of the inferomedial condyle at the alar ligament attachment that is due to a forced rotation in conjunction with lateral bending. This is the most common type of OCF and it may result in a partial or complete tear of the contralateral alar ligament and tectorial membrane. Thus, a Type 3 fracture is potentially unstable (Figures 11.1 and 11.2). Involvement of the inferior clivus may also be apparent.

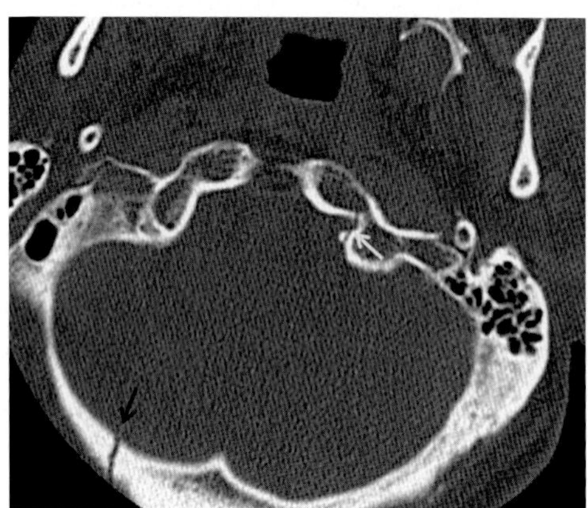
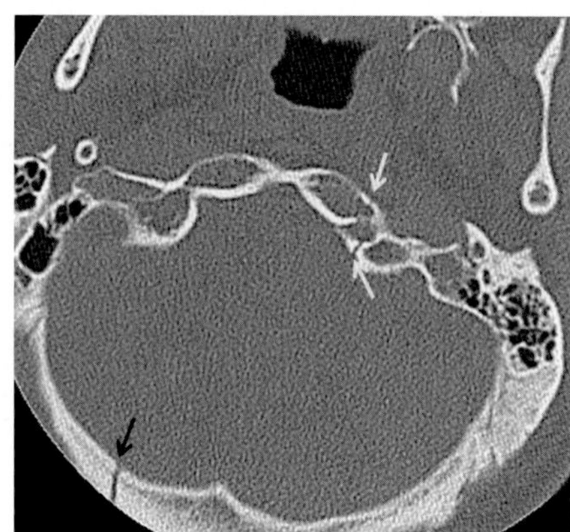

Figure 11.7

Figure 11.8

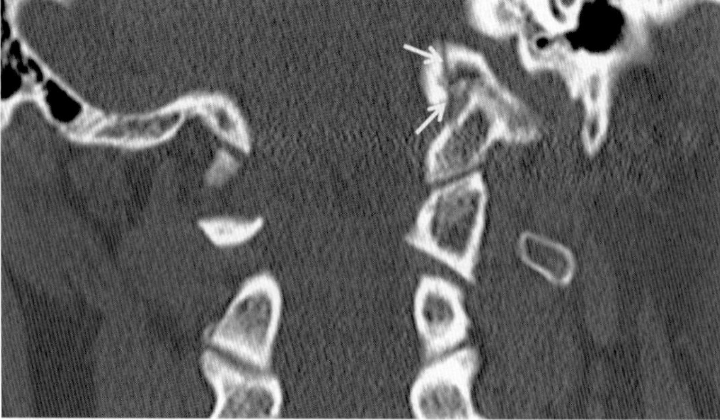

Figure 11.9

Type 2 OCF (**Figures 11.7, 11.8, and 11.9**). Axial (Figures 11.7 and 11.8) and coronal (Figure 11.9) CT demonstrate another nondisplaced Type 2 Anderson and Montesano also with a right occipital bone skull base fracture (black arrows, Figures 11.7 and 11.8). The fracture extends to the left occipital condyle (white arrows, Figures 11.7, 11.8, and 11.9) across the hypoglossal canal. The hypoglossal canal contains the hypoglossal nerve, an emissary vein, and a meningeal branch of the ascending pharyngeal artery. Thus, any of these structures can be injured by a fracture through the canal.

The Tuli classification was introduced in 1997 and divided OCFs into two major types, depending on whether a displacement of fragments was detectable and as well as on an assessment of craniocervical junction stability. In the 2001, the Hanson classification subdivided the Type 3 Anderson and Montesano OCFs into stable and unstable types.

The clinical presentation of OCFs is variable. Most neurological deficits can be traced to the severity of intracranial injury rather than OCF itself. Vascular and brainstem lesions are rarely encountered because they are usually fatal. The most common neurological deficits are lower cranial nerve palsies from OCFs involving the jugular foramen and hypoglossal canal (Figures **11.7, 11.8, and 11.9**). Symptoms may be immediate or delayed until months after injury.

Management

Optimal management of OCFs is still unclear given the small number of cases in the literature. In general, rigid or semirigid collars are used in stable fractures while rigid collar, halo traction vest, or surgical fixation is used in unstable injuries. Surgical stabilization involves occipital-cervical fixation.

Teaching Points

▶ OCFs result from high-energy blunt trauma and they can be easily missed in a severely injured patient. CT is the imaging modality of choice because of its multiplanar capabilities and MRI is helpful for the evaluation of soft tissue, ligamentous, and cord injury.
▶ The most commonly used classification system for OCFs is the three type Anderson and Montesano classification system. Type 3 OCFs are potentially unstable due to injuries to the contralateral alar ligament and tectorial membrane.

Further Reading

1. Tuli S, Tator CH, Fehlilngs MG, and Mackay M. Occipital condyle fractures. Neurosurgery 1997;41(2):368–376; discussion 376–377.
2. Hanson JA, Deliganis AV, Baxter AB, et al. Radiological and clinical spectrum of occipital condyle fracture: Retrospective review of 107 consecutive fractures in 95 patients. Am J Roentgenol 2002;178:1261–1268.
3. Leone A and Cerase A. Occipital condylar fractures: A review. Radiology 2000;216(3):635–644.
4. Clayman DA, Sykes CH, and Vines FS. Occipital condyle fractures: Clinical presentation and radiologic detection. AJNR 1994;15:1309–1315.
5. Schrödel MH, Kestlmeier R, and Trappe AE. Bilateral occipital condyle fracture: Report of two cases. Skull Base 2002;12(2):93–96.
6. Anderson PA and Montesano PX. Morphology and treatment of occipital condyle fractures. Spine 1988;13(7):731–736.
7. Noble ER and Smoker WR. The forgotten condyle: The appearance, morphology, and classification of occipital condyle fractures. AJNR Am J Neuroradiol 1996;17(3):507–513.
8. Maserati MB and Stephens B. Occipital condyle fractures: Clinical decision rule and surgical management. J Neurosurg Spine 2009;11(4):388–395.
9. Mueller FJ, Fuechtmeier B, Kinner B, et al. Occipital condyle fractures. Prospective follow-up of 31 cases within 5 years at a level 1 trauma centre. Eur Spine J 2012;21:289–294.

Chapter 12

Bruce Lehnert

History

▶ The status of a 31-year-old male post-motorcycle crash is evaluated (**Figures 12.1 and 12.2**).

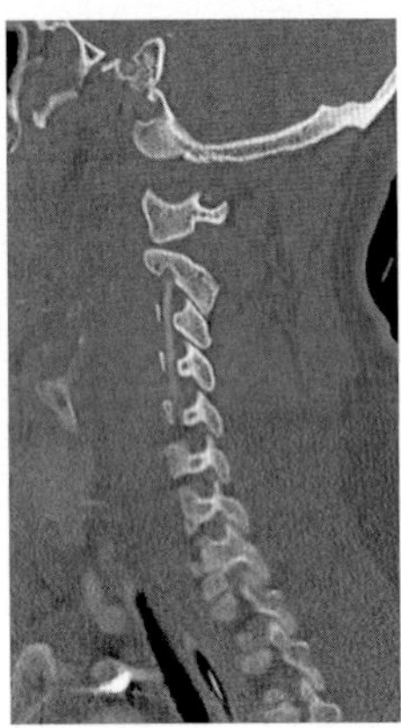

Figure 12.1

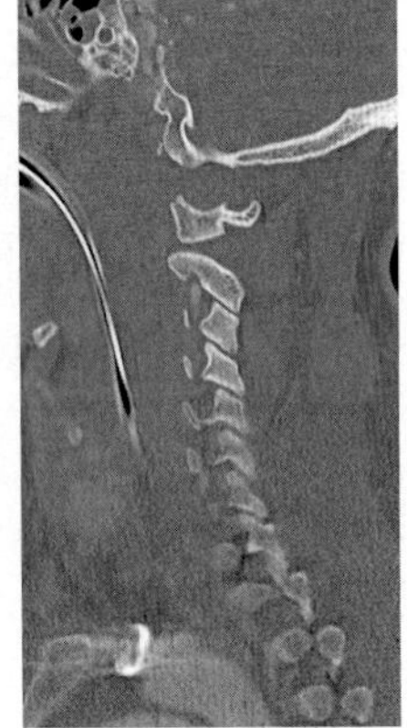

Figure 12.2

Findings

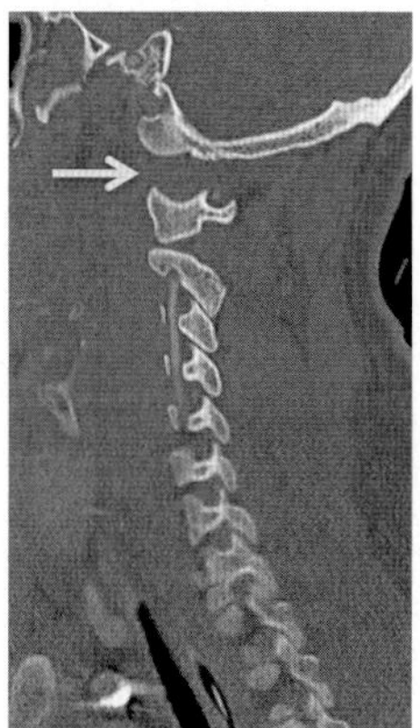

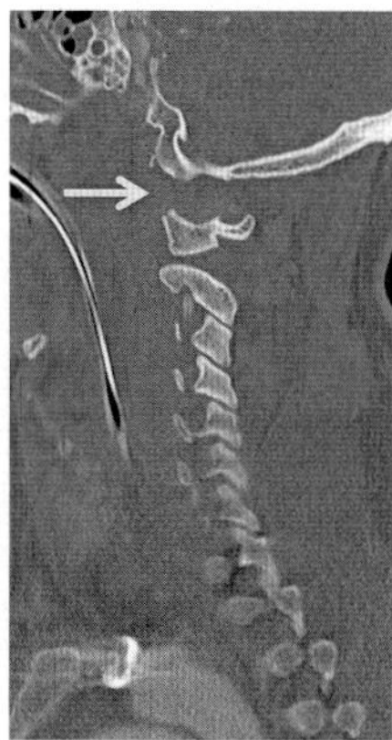

Figure 12.3   Figure 12.4

Craniocervical dissociation on CT (**Figures 12.3 and 12.4**). Sagittal CT reformats demonstrate marked widening of the C0–C1 joints bilaterally (white arrow). A coronal CT reformat (**Figure 12.5**) again demonstrates marked abnormal widening of the C0–C1 articulations bilaterally (white arrow).

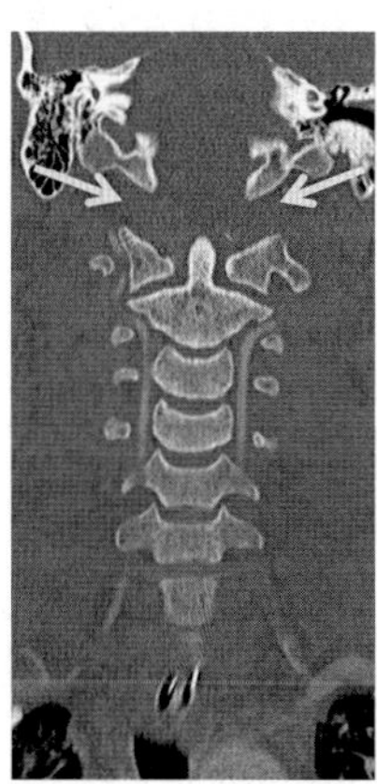

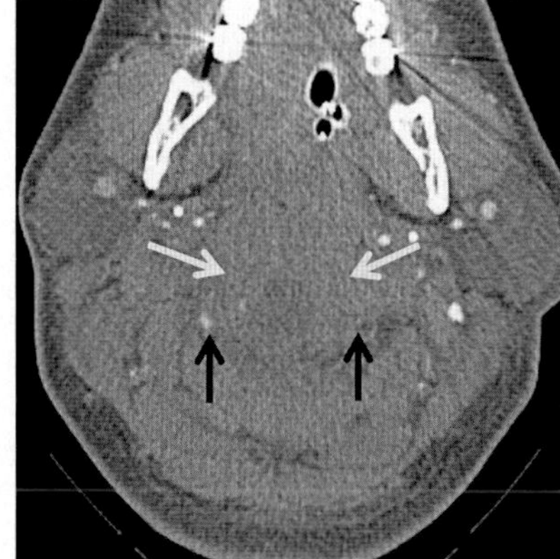

Figure 12.5   Figure 12.6

An axial CT image (**Figure 12.6**) through the expected location of the craniocervical junction (white arrows) demonstrates no osseous structures, consistent with a severe distraction injury. There is associated traumatic occlusion of the vertebral arteries bilaterally (black arrows).

Discussion

Craniocervical dissociation is an uncommon and frequently fatal injury, likely resulting from high-energy hyperflexion or hyperextension with distraction and extensive ligamentous and soft tissue injury. Injuries may involve the atlantooccipital articulation, the atlantoaxial articulation (AAD), or both.

There are three principal injury patterns as described by Traynelis et al. The most common is anterior and superior displacement of the cranium relative to the cervical spine. The second is superior displacement without anterior or posterior displacement. The least common is superior and posterior displacement of the cranium.

Radiological Evaluation

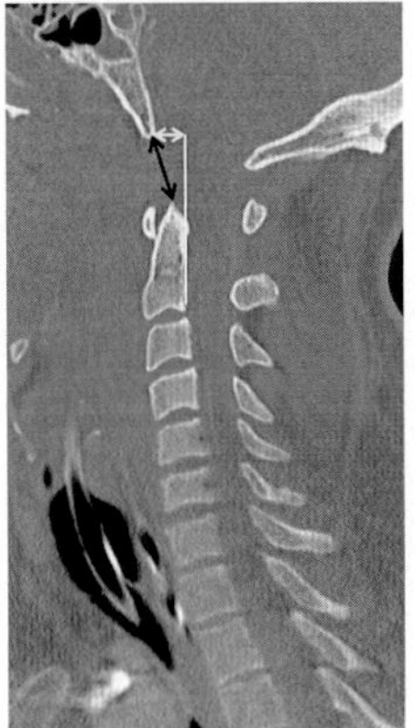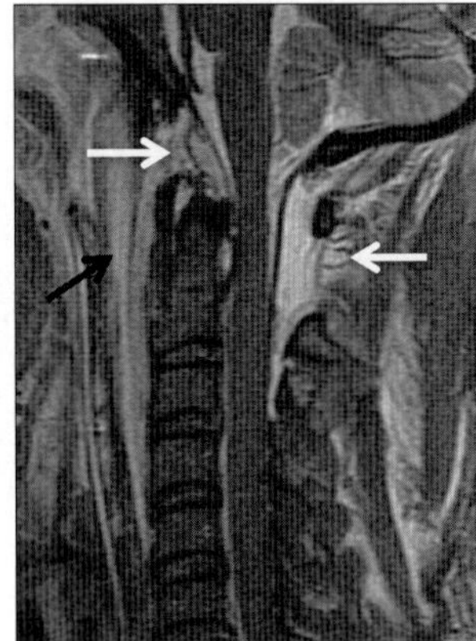

Figure 12.7   Figure 12.8

Patients with CCD present to the emergency department after high-energy trauma. Radiographs and CT remain the mainstay for diagnosis, which both depend on recognition of an abnormal craniocervical relationship. Radiographs are often limited to a lateral view of the cervical spine during resuscitation where as many as 50% of cases may be missed. CT of the cervical spine is critical for delineating the alignment of the craniocervical junction, in addition to determining the presence of underlying associated fractures. CT is also useful in the evaluation of postoperative patients (Figure 12.7). MRI is important to assess the degree of soft tissue damage and to evaluate for spinal cord injury (**Figure 12.8**).

While no single imaging measurement is perfect for demonstrating an abnormal craniocervical relationship, the basion dens interval (BDI) and the basion axial interval (BAI) are the most reliable and reproducible (**Figure 12.7**). The BDI is measured from the basion to the tip of the odontoid process and should not be greater than 12 mm. The BAI is determined by measuring the distance of the basion from a line drawn along the posterior cortex of the C2 body and extended superiorly. The basion should be less than 12 mm anterior or 4 mm posterior to this line. The presence of upper cervical spine prevertebral soft tissue swelling should also raise suspicion for CCD.

Sagittal CT reformat at the midline (**Figure 12.7**) demonstrates an abnormal BDI measuring >12 mm (black arrow), consistent with CCD. The BAI is normal in this case, measuring <12 mm (white arrow).

Sagittal short T1 inversion recovery (STIR) MRI (**Figure 12.8**) demonstrates a markedly abnormal signal about the craniocervical junction (white arrows), consistent with severe ligamentous and soft tissue injury. There is associated upper cervical spine prevertebral edema (black arrow).

Management

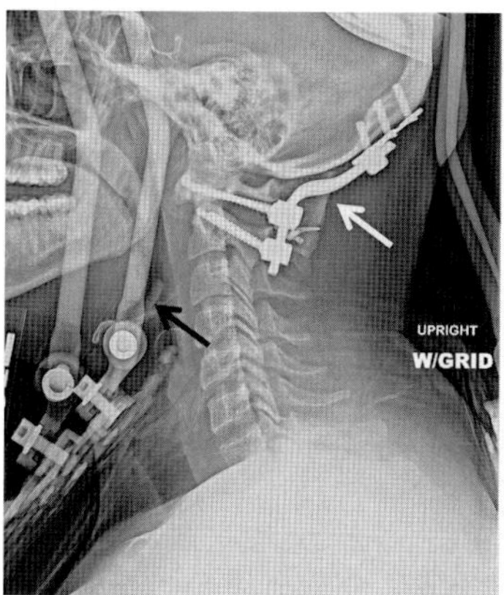

Figure 12.9

A lateral radiograph of a different patient (**Figure 12.9**) demonstrates post-occiput to C2 fixation (white arrow) with an external halo immobilizer in place (black arrow).

Patients may initially be externally immobilized in a halo device, allowing reduction and stabilization of the injury prior to surgical fixation. Internal fixation involving occipitocervical stabilization is the definitive treatment. Mortality is high following these injuries.

Teaching Points

► Craniocervical dissociation is a severe, frequently fatal ligamentous and soft tissue injury resulting in separation of the cranium from the cervical spine.
► The BDI and BAI are the most reliable and reproducible measurements of craniocervical relationships to diagnose craniocervical dissociation.
► Management may involve external halo immobilization followed by internal occipitocervical fusion.

Further Reading

1. Deliganis AV, Baxter AB, Hanson JA, et al. Radiologic spectrum of craniocervical distraction injuries. Radiographics 2000;20(Spec No):S237–250.
2. Harris JH Jr, Carson GC, Wagner LK, and Kerr N. Radiologic diagnosis of traumatic occipitovertebral dissociation: 2. Comparison of three methods of detecting occipitovertebral relationships on lateral radiographs of supine subjects. AJR. Am J Roentgenol 1994;162(4):887–892.
3. Schwartz ED and Flanders AE. *Spinal Trauma: Imaging, Diagnosis, and Management*. Philadelphia, PA: Lippincott, Williams & Wilkins, 2007.
4. Traynelis VC, Marano GD, Dunker RO, and Kaufman HH. Traumatic atlanto-occipital dislocation. Case report. J Neurosurg 1986;65(6):863–870.

Chapter 13

Keith A. Cauley and Christopher G. Filippi

History

► A 75-year-old male is evaluated following a high-speed motor vehicle collision (MVC) (**Figures 13.1 and 13.2**).

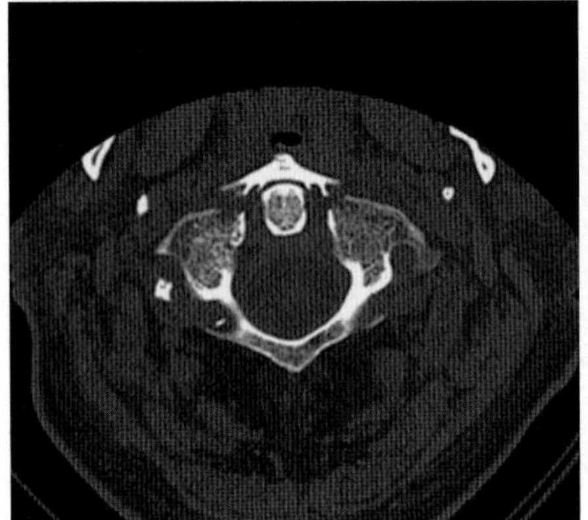

Figure 13.1

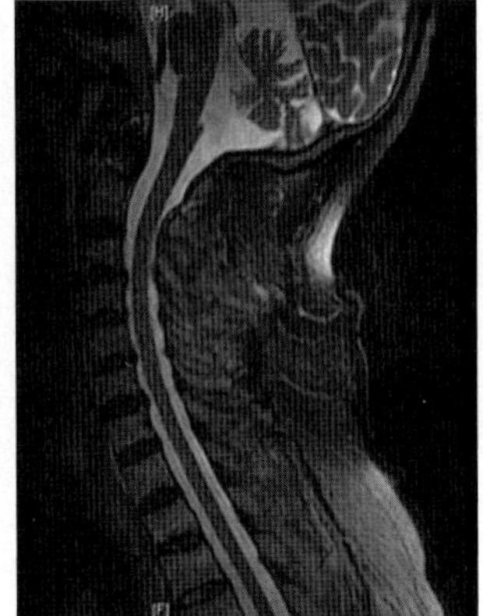

Figure 13.2

Findings

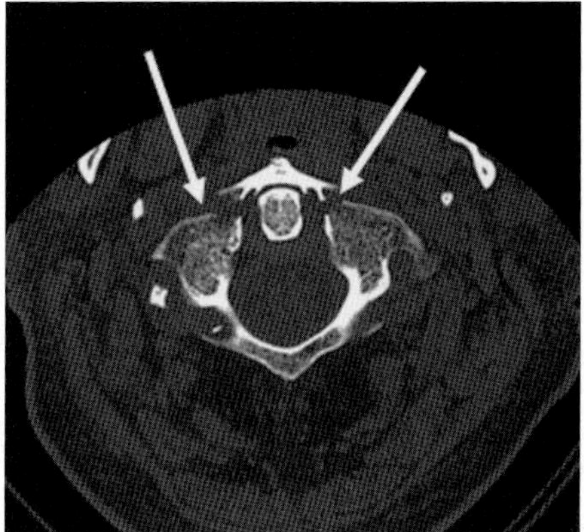

Figure 13.3

Jefferson fracture (C1 fracture) (**Figure 13.3**). An axial CT image (Figure 13.3) demonstrates symmetric fractures through the anterior ring of C1. A T2-weighted, fat-suppressed sagittal MR image (Figure 13.2) appears essentially normal.

Discussion

C1 fractures are not uncommon and result from axial loading or hyperextension, such as from a diving accident. As a burst fracture, they typically do not result in canal narrowing or direct cord compression and are often managed without surgery.

Radiological Evaluation

Classically, the Jefferson fracture is a burst fracture of the C1 vertebrae caused by an axial loading injury, with ring fractures through both anterior and posterior vertebral arches. However, there are three general types of Jefferson fractures:

1. Bilateral single arch (anterior or posterior). Our case shows a Type I Jefferson fracture.
2. Concurrent anterior and posterior arch fractures (classical four-point fracture).
3. Lateral mass fracture.

C1 fractures can be stable or unstable; to determine the stability of a C1 injury requires assessment of
▶ the configuration of the bony fracture and
▶ the integrity of the transverse atlantal ligament.

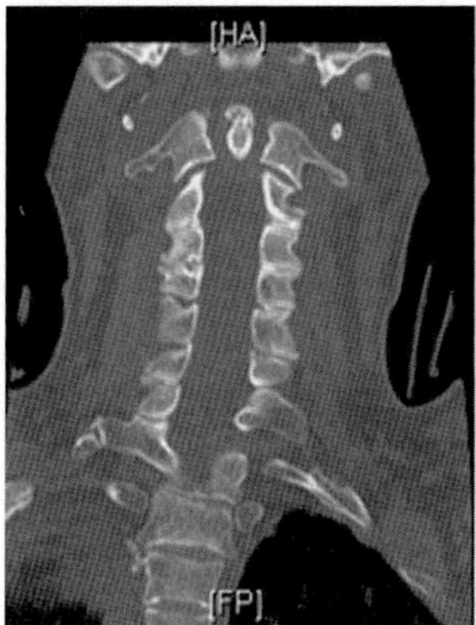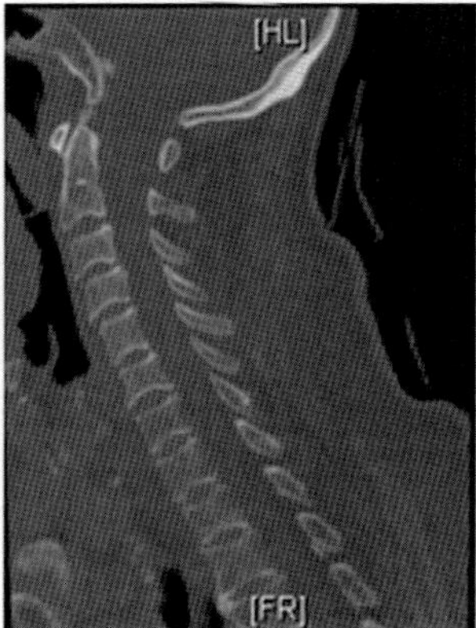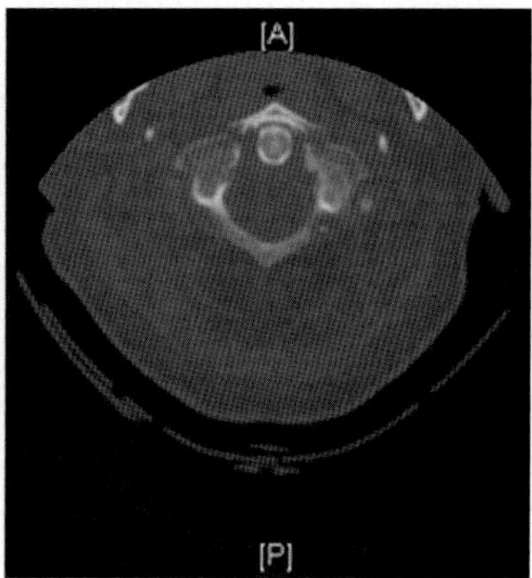

Figure 13.4

Jefferson fracture seen on CT (**Figure 13.4**). Coronal, sagittal, and axial CT images are shown. A fracture through the anterior arch of C1 (Jefferson fracture) is best seen on axial images, thereby stressing the importance of reviewing images in all planes.

Fractures of C1 can be difficult to detect by radiography. Plain films can appear negative, without abnormal soft tissue thickening or malalignment of the spinal lines. Multiplanar CT is essential, and fracture may not be evident on single imaging planes (**Figure 13.4**). Jefferson fractures are associated with other fractures, most commonly C2 fractures.

Abnormal relationships of the C1 lateral masses on open-mouth radiographs or abnormal widening of the atlantodental interval offer indirect evidence of injury to the transverse ligament (**Figure 13.5**), but are not sensitive for ligamentous injury. If such injury is suspected, further evaluation with CT or MRI is required.

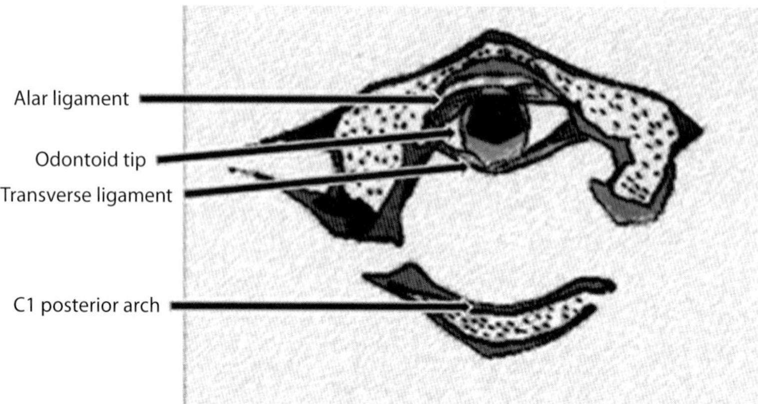

Figure 13.5

Schematic of axial CT images of C1 (Figure 13.5) shows the transverse atlantal ligament located behind the dens.

Management

Jefferson fractures may be treated conservatively with a rigid cervical collar. Ligamentous disruption may require more extensive treatment such as traction, halo immobilization, or surgical stabilization. The long-term prognosis for these injuries is generally good.

Teaching Points

▶ Jefferson fractures are burst fractures of C1, typically the result of an axial loading injury.
▶ These fractures may go undetected with plain film study and require multiplanar CT.
▶ Associated ligamentous injury may be identified with CT or MRI study.

Further Reading

1. Kesterson L, Benzel E, Orrison W, and Coleman J. Evaluation and treatment of atlas burst fractures (Jefferson fractures). J. Neurosurg 1991;75(2):213–220.
2. Lee C and Woodring JH. Unstable Jefferson variant atlas fractures: An unrecognized cervical injury. AJNR Am J Neuroradiol 1991;12(6):1105–1110.
3. Dundamadappa SK and Cauley KA. MR imaging of acute cervical spinal ligamentous and soft tissue trauma. Emerg Radiol 2012;19:277–286.

Section 2   Tumors

Nima Jadidi and Sylvie Destian

History

▶ A 43-year-old female presents with gradual onset lower back pain (**Figures 14.1, 14.2, 14.3, and 14.4**).

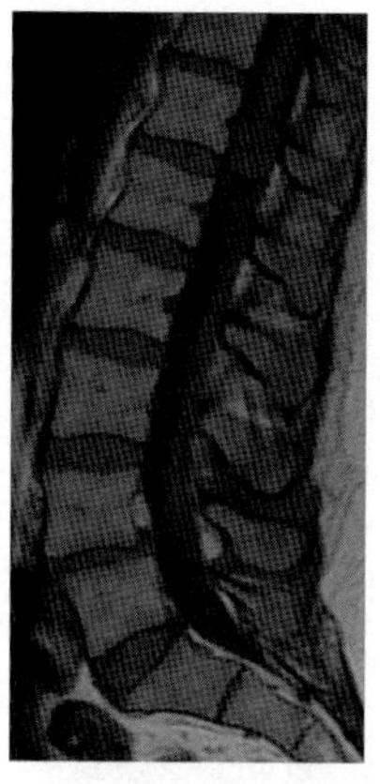

Figure 14.1

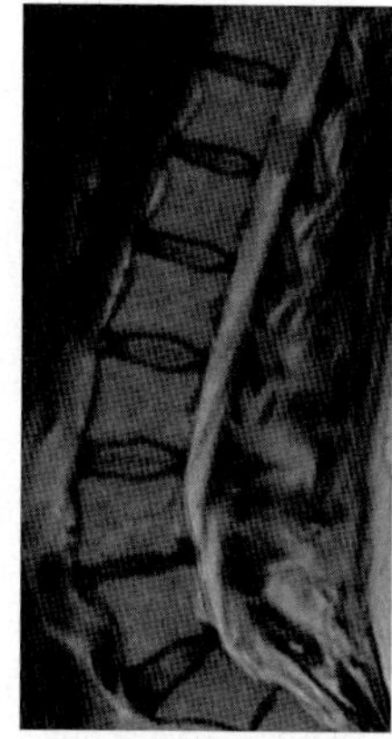

Figure 14.2

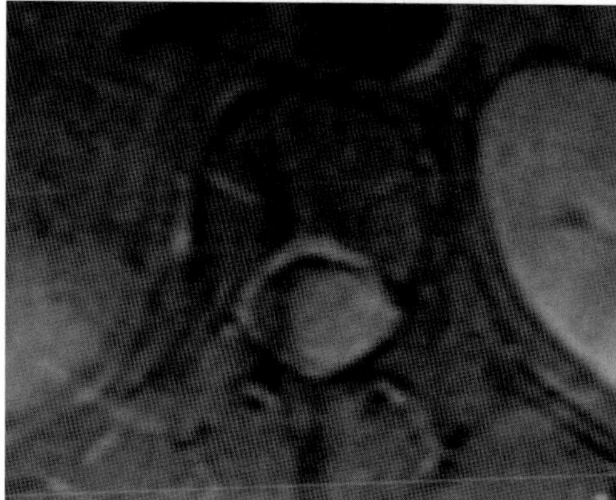

Figure 14.3

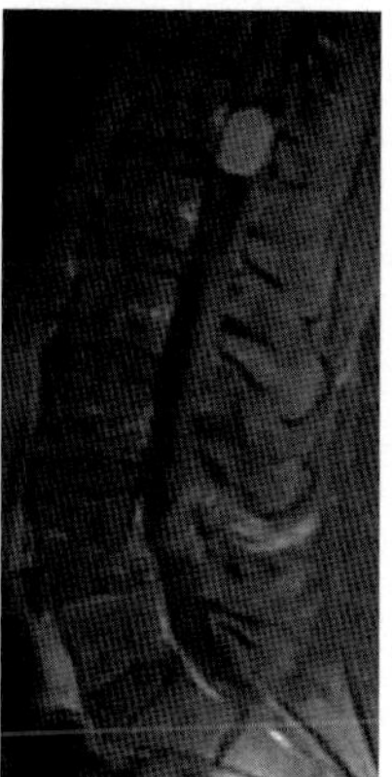

Figure 14.4

Chapter 14 **Meningioma**

Findings

Thoracolumbar meningioma (**Figures 14.1, 14.2, 14.3, and 14.4**). Sagittal T1 (Figure 14.1) demonstrates a well-circumscribed mass within the spinal canal that has an isointense signal relative to the spinal cord. On sagittal T2-weighted imaging (Figure 14.2), the lesion is also intense to the signal of the adjacent cord. Axial (Figure 14.3) and sagittal (Figure 14.4) postcontrast T1-weighted images demonstrate homogeneous enhancement of this extramedullary, intradural mass. This was a pathologically proven meningioma.

Differential Diagnosis

▶ Neurofibroma
▶ Schwannoma

Discussion

Meningiomas arise from meningothelial cells such as those found in arachnoid "cap" cells and from dural fibroblasts. The WHO organization categorizes meningiomas into subtypes depending on their radiographic features and how aggressive they are. Spinal meningiomas comprise a small percentage of all meningiomas. About a quarter of spinal meningiomas occur in the intradural extramedullary space. The protoypical patient is a middle aged woman.

Radiological Evaluation

Spinal meningiomas occur most commonly in the thoracic spine. They can also occur in the cervical region from the clivus to C2. Although most spinal meningiomas occur in the posterior and lateral intradural extramedullary space, they can occur rarely in the extradural space or in both the extradural and intradural space, appearing dumbbell shaped, as more commonly seen within schwannomas. When they arise from the clivus, they have a fan-like appearance and extend into the upper cervical canal resulting in compression of the brainstem and upper cervical cord.

Meningiomas are also more likely solitary lesions compared to nerve sheath tumors. On MRI, meningiomas are isointense to slightly hypointense on T1WI and isointense to slightly hyperintense on T2WI compared to the spinal cord signal. They usually enhance homogeneously. Additional features that are not always present include bone remodeling, dural thickening, and a dural "tail."

Management

Although the majority of meningiomas are benign, neurological symptoms from cord and nerve root compression at the time of presentation may require surgical intervention. Because these lesions typically have well-defined margins and are located posterior to the spinal cord, complete excision following posterior laminectomies usually has an excellent prognosis.

Teaching Points

▶ Spinal meningiomas most commonly occur in the posterior and lateral intradural extramedullary space of the thoracic spine.
▶ Patients present with neurological symptoms from cord and nerve root compression due to mass effect.

Further Reading

1. Gottfried ON, Gluf W, Quinones-Hinojosa A, et al. Spinal meningiomas: Surgical management and outcome. Neurosurg Focus 2003;14:e2.
2. Grossman RI and Yousem DM. *Neuroradiology, the Requisites.* St. Louis, MO: Mosby, 2003, p. 819.

Nima Jadidi and Sylvie Destian

History

► A 45-year-old female presents with lower back pain and a tingling sensation in her right lower extremity (**Figures 15.1, 1.2, and 15.3**).

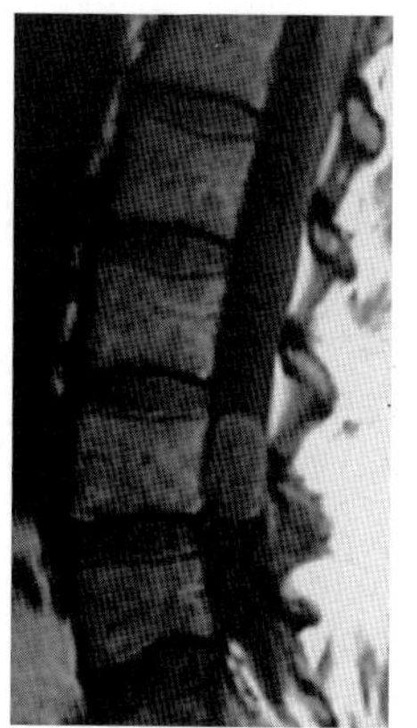

Figure 15.1

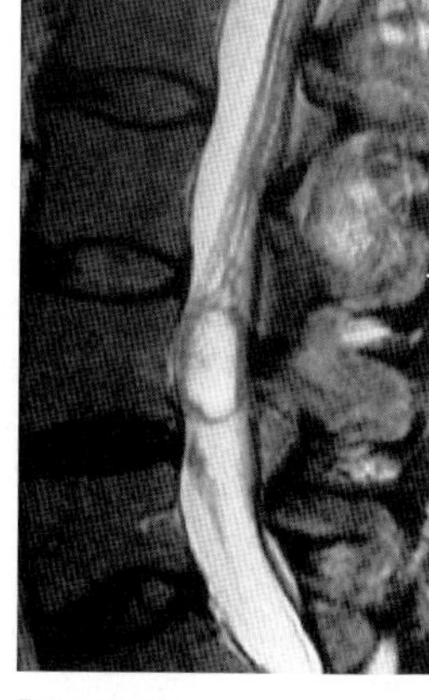

Figure 15.2

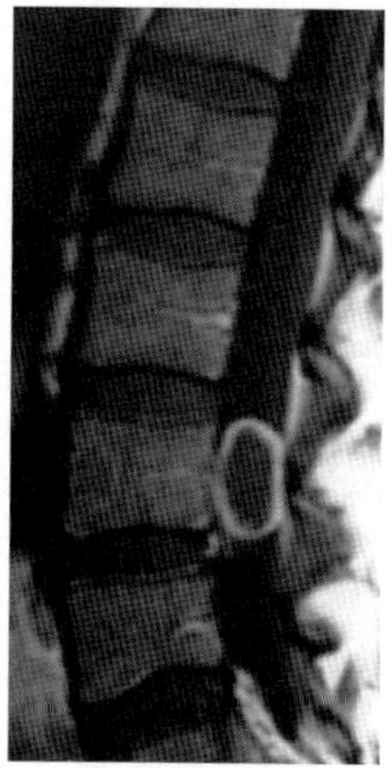

Figure 15.3

Chapter 15 **Schwannoma**

Findings

Nerve sheath tumor (**Figures 15.1, 15.2, and 15.3**). A sagittal T1WI precontrast image (Figure 15.1) demonstrates the isointense signal of this mass relative to the cauda equina nerve roots. This lesion is well-circumscribed and hyperintense on sagittal T2WI (Figure 15.2). Notice the displacement of the cauda equina nerve roots. A sagittal T1WI postcontrast image (Figure 15.3) demonstrates peripheral enhancement of a well-circumscribed extramedullary intradural mass in the mid lumber spine. The peripheral enhancement indicates cystic degeneration.

Differential Diagnosis

▶ Meningioma
▶ Neurofibroma

Discussion

A schwannoma is a benign slowing growing nerve sheath tumor, historiographically distinct, yet radiologically similar to another nerve sheath tumor, neurofibroma. Schwannomas do not have a gender predilection and tend to occur in the fourth through sixth decade of life. Although both nerve sheath tumors arise due to proliferation of Schwann cells, schwannomas have a fibrous capsule while neurofibromas do not. Another distinguishing feature of schwannomas, in contradistinction to neurofibromas, is their propensity to hemorrhage or undergo degeneration. Schwannomas have an association with neurofibromatosis type 2.

Radiological Evaluation

Schwannomas are commonly found in the intradural and extramedullary space, giving them a dumbbell-shaped appearance. Like meningiomas, they can less commonly be found outside the dura. Schwannomas are well-circumscribed lesions that usually avidly enhance following contrast administration on CT unless they have undergone cystic degeneration. Schwannomas can cause remodeling of the adjacent bone (**Figures 15.4 and 15.5**). MR imaging findings include an isointense signal on T1WI, a hyperintense signal on T2WI, and almost always enhancement with contrast. Heterogeneity in the appearance may indicate hemorrhage or cystic degeneration (Figures 15.1 and 15.3).

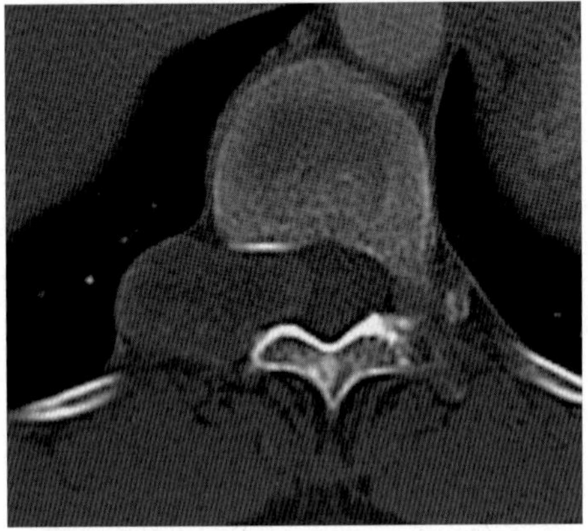

Figure 15.4

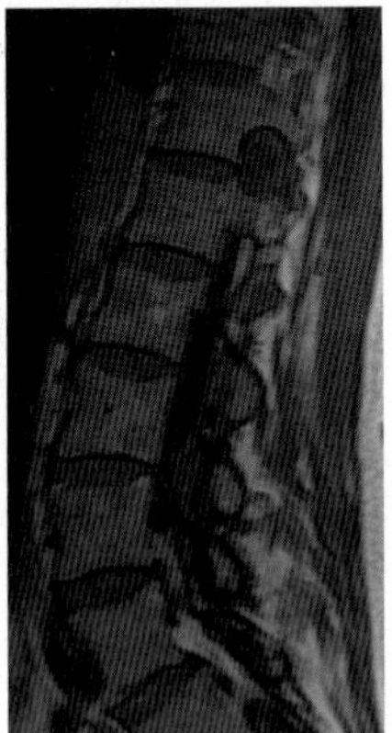

Figure 15.5

Osseous remodeling secondary to a nerve sheath tumor (Figures 15.4 and 15.5). An axial CT image demonstrates a well-circumscribed mass situated in the right aspect of the spinal canal and extending through the right neural foramen into the right paraspinal soft tissues. The intraspinal and extraspinal canal components give this mass a characteristic dumbbell-shaped appearance. Notice the osseous remodeling compared to the normal left side. Sagittal T1WI without contrast (Figure 15.5) shows this same mass in the lower thoracic spine widening the neural foramen.

Management

Although schwannomas are slow growing and benign tumors, they can become very large and will invariably cause compression of the spinal cord or nerve roots. Treatment is typically resection of the tumor in symptomatic patients.

Teaching Points

- ▶ Typically intradural and extramedullary.
- ▶ Radiographically difficult to distinguish from neurofibromas, although schwannomas have a higher propensity to hemorrhage or undergo cystic degeneration.

Further Reading

1. Friedman DP, Tartaglino LM, and Flanders AE. Intradural schwannomas of the spine: MR findings with emphasis on contrast-enhancement characteristics. AJR Am J Roentgenol 1992;158(6):1347–1350.
2. Grossman RI and Yousem DM. *Neuroradiology, the Requisites*. St. Louis, MO: Mosby, 2003, pp. 820–821.

Chapter 16

Martin Arrigan, Manraj Kanwal Singh Heran, and Paul Celestre

History

▶ A 61-year-old female presents with back pain. She has a history of a right-sided, grade 2, T1 renal cell carcinoma, treated with a right sided nephrectomy without chemotherapy or radiotherapy 5 years prior (**Figures 16.1, 16.2, 16.3, 16.4, and 16.5**).

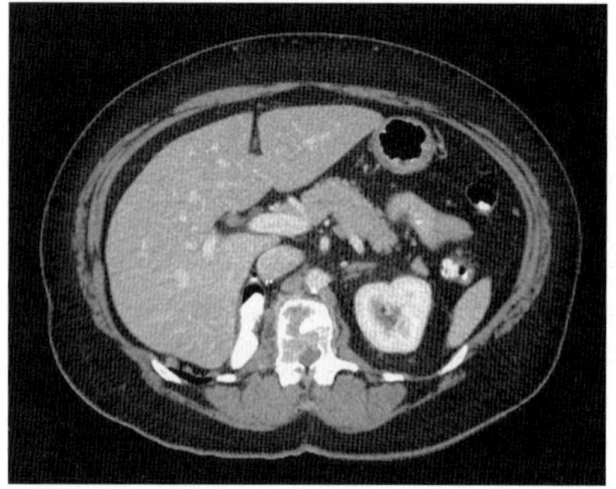

Figure 16.1

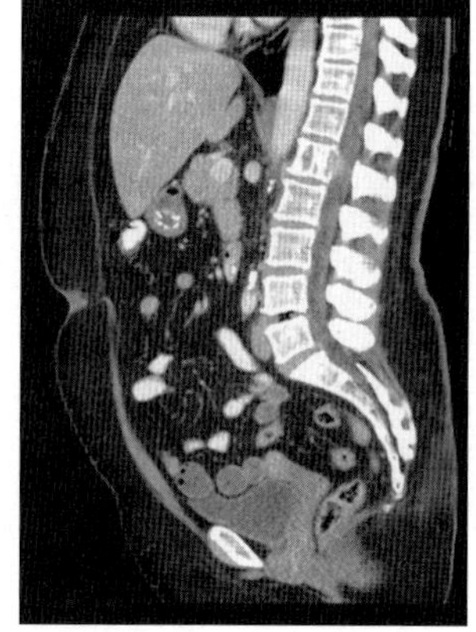

Figure 16.2

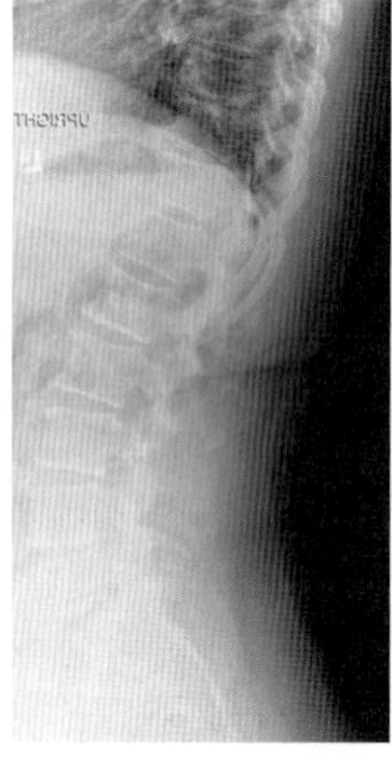

Figure 16.3

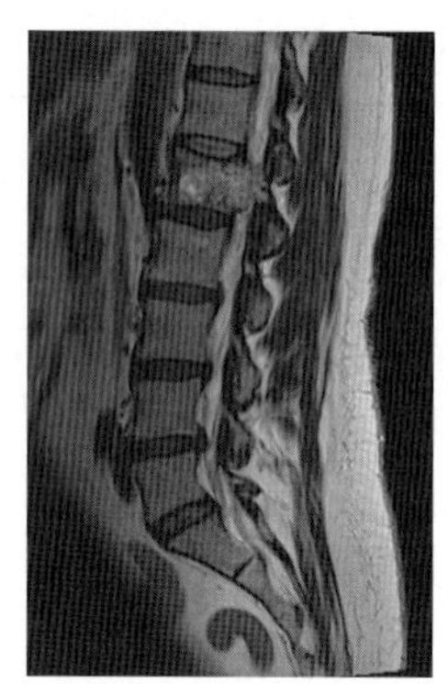

Figure 16.4

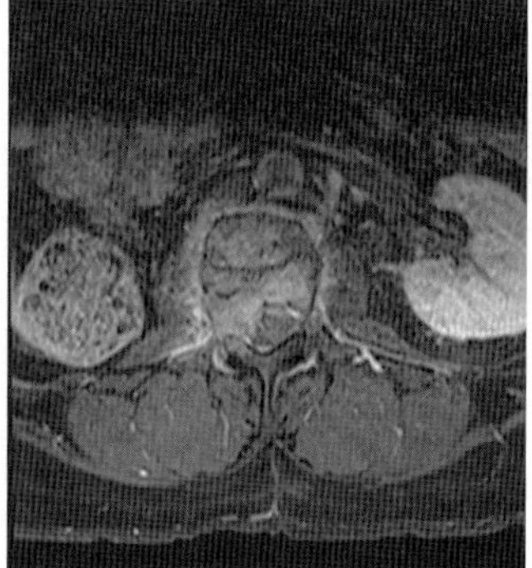

Figure 16.5

Findings

Metastatic disease secondary to renal cell carcinoma (Figures 16.1, 16.2, 16.3, 16.4, and 16.5). Axial CT with sagittal reformats (Figure 16.1 and Figure 16.2) demonstrates a destructive soft tissue lesion in the body and right pedicle of L1, extending through the posterior cortex of the L1 vertebra with mild spinal canal narrowing. The L1 vertebra is of normal height with no evidence of pathological fracture. Standing lateral radiograph of the lumbar spine 3 weeks later (Figure 16.3) demonstrates a mixed lytic-sclerotic lesion in L1 with a slight loss of the superior endplate and poor definition of the pedicle. Sagittal T2 MRI (Figure 16.4) demonstrates the L1 lesion with intralesional flow voids. Postcontrast axial imaging (Figure 16.5) demonstrates avid enhancement of the lesion with peritumoral enhancement.

Differential Diagnosis

The differential diagnosis for bony metastasis is wide, and includes benign and malignant primary bone lesions. The list can be narrowed when taking into consideration patient age, gender, history, and the radiological characteristics of the lesion. Common lesions that mimic metastasis typically include multiple myeloma and lymphoma.

Discussion

Metastasis is the most commonly encountered malignant lesion in the spine. Moreover, the spine is the most common location for skeletal metastatic disease, and is the third most common site of metastasis after the lung and liver. Symptomatic spinal metastasis is the initial presentation in up to 20% of malignancies, with pain being the most common clinical feature.

Radiological Evaluation

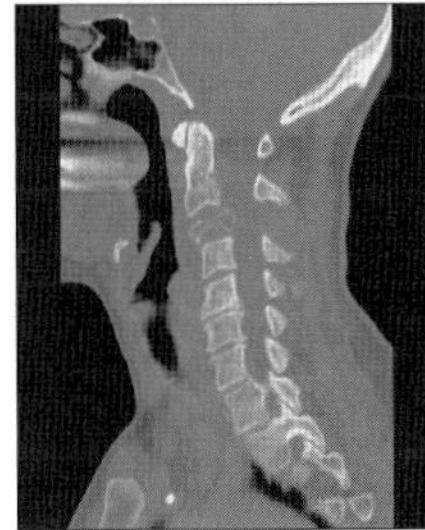

Figure 16.6

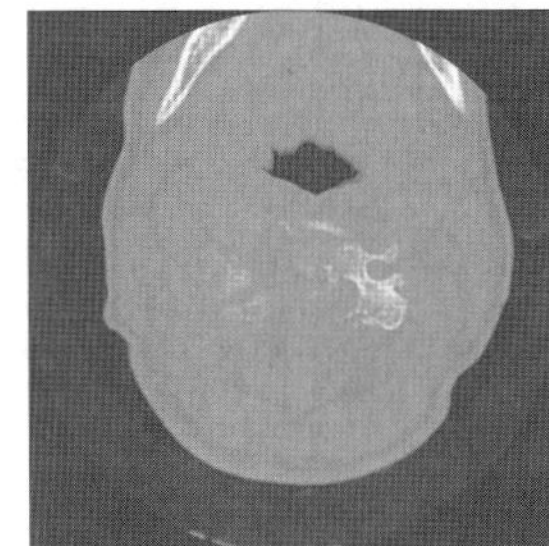

Figure 16.7

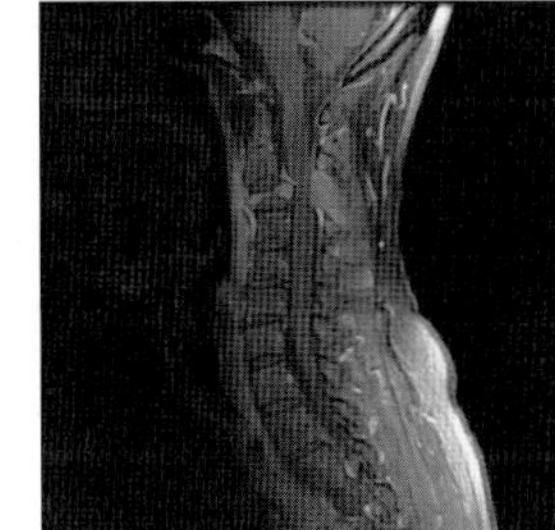

Figure 16.8

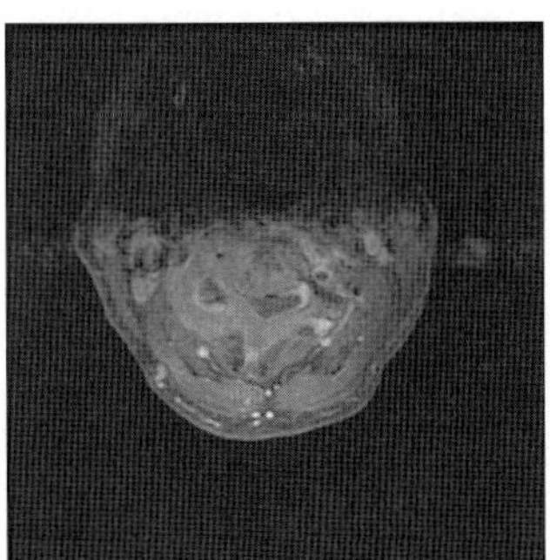

Figure 16.9

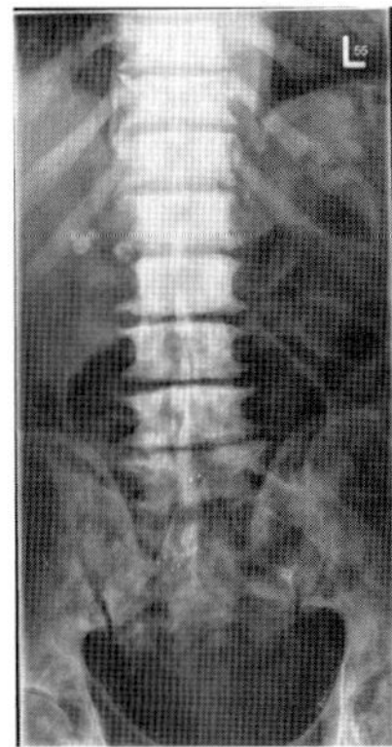

Figure 16.10

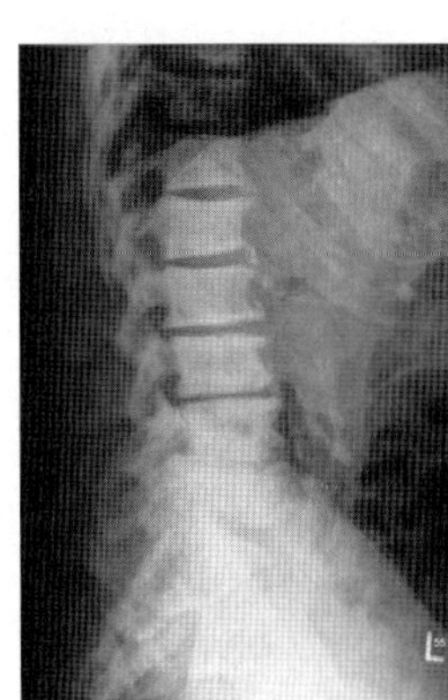

Figure 16.11

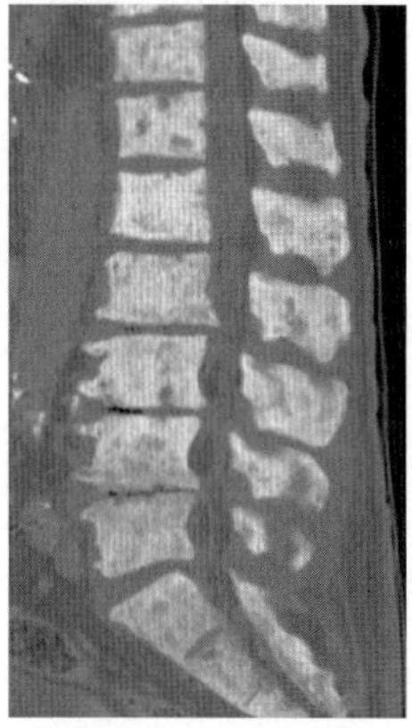

Figure 16.12

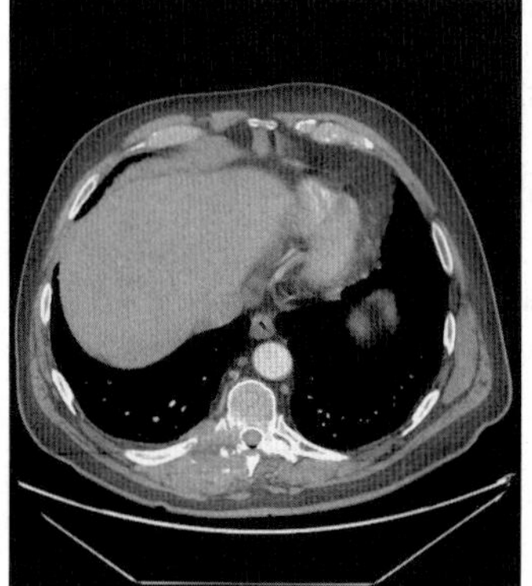

Figure 16.13

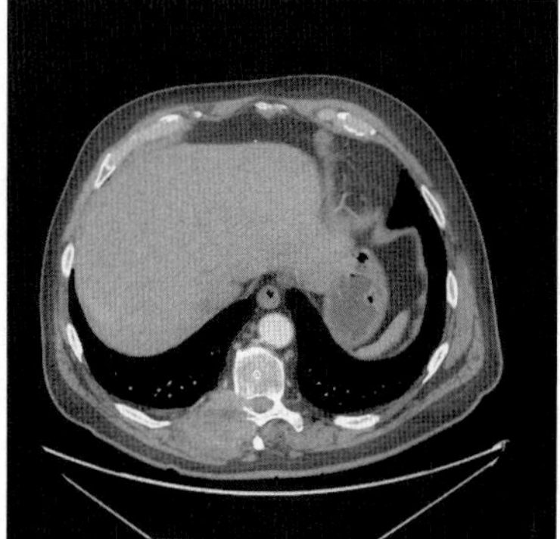

Figure 16.14

Figure 16.15

Table 16.1. Characterization of Spinal Metastasis

Osteolytic	*Osteoblastic*	*Mixed*
Lung	Prostate	Breast
Gastrointestinal	Medullary thyroid	Lymphoma
Renal cell carcinoma	Osteosarcoma	Urothelial
Melanoma		
Multiple myeloma		

Table 16.2. Vascularity of Spinal Metastatic Disease Based on Primary Site

Hypervascular (large accessible feeding arteries)	*Hypovascular*
Renal cell carcinoma	Breast
Thyroid (follicular type)	Lung
Sarcoma	Colon
Hepatocellular carcinoma	
Germ cell	
Neuroendocrine	

*Hypervascular metastases from melanoma and multiple myeloma are often supplied via a fine capillary network and are not always accessible intravascularly.

Metastatic lesions have a wide variety of imaging features and should be included in the differential diagnosis of a bony spinal lesion in patients older than 40 years of age. All imaging modalities play a role in the evaluation of spinal metastatic disease. Metastases can be lytic, sclerotic, or mixed in appearance, and can vary from indolent to aggressive on imaging (**Figures 16.6, 16.7, 16.8, and 16.9**). Metastases can be characterized by an osteolytic or osteoblastic appearance (**Table 16.1; Figures 16.10, 16.11, 16.12, 16.13, 16.14, and 16.15**). Characterization is also possible by tumor vascularity, with hypervascularity predicted on MRI by avid contrast enhancement, prominent intratumoral flow voids, and enlarged feeding arteries (**Table 16.2**). The absence of these findings, however, does not exclude a hypervascular lesion, and tumor histology alone can be an important predictor for consideration for preoperative embolization. MRI is especially useful in detecting subtle marrow changes (**Figures 16.16 and 16.17**). Postcontrast MR images are also excellent in depicting spinal leptomeningeal disease (**Figure 16.18**).

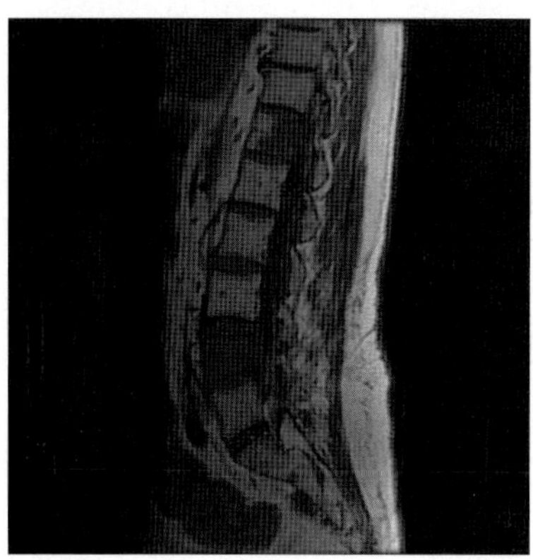

Figure 16.16

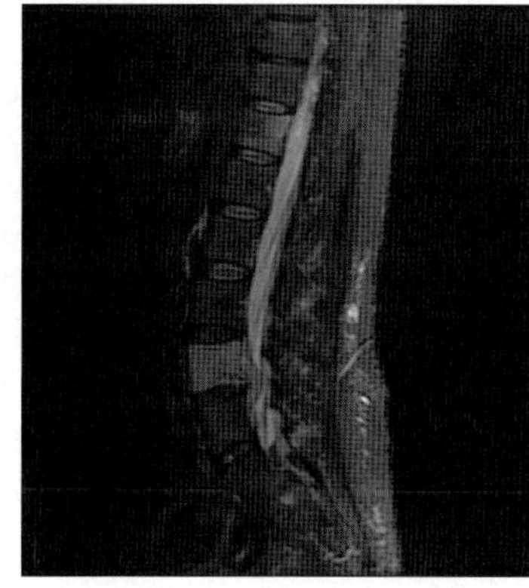

Figure 16.17

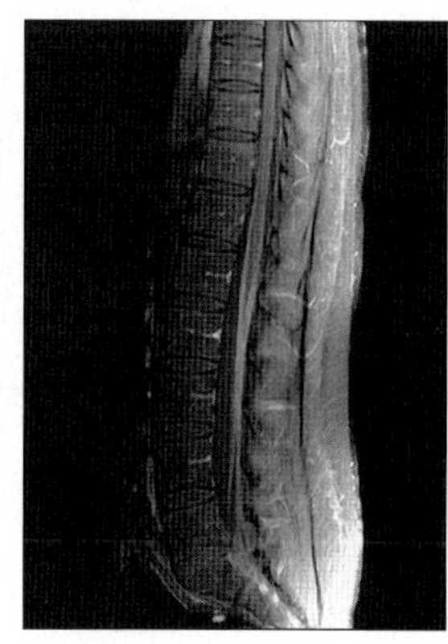

Figure 16.18

Metastatic breast cancer in a 56-year-old female (Figures 16.6, 16.7, 16.8, and 16.9). Sagittal and axial (Figures 16.6 and 16.7) CT images demonstrate a lytic, destructive lesion centered at C3 involving both the vertebral body and posterior elements. The degree of soft tissue involvement is best shown on MRI. Postcontrast sagittal and axial T1-weighted images (Figures 16.8 and 16.9) demonstrate abnormal enhancing soft tissue that extends into the paravertebral and paraspinal soft tissues. A subsequent biopsy demonstrated metastatic breast cancer.

Diffuse osteoblastic metastatic disease secondary to prostate cancer in a 76-year-old male (Figures 16.10, 16.11, 16.12, and 16.13). Extensive osteoblastic metastases are visualized on frontal and lateral radiographs (Figures 16.10 and 16.11) as well as sagittal and axial CT images (Figures 16.12 and 16.13).

Metastatic renal cell carcinoma (Figures 16.14 and 16.15). In a different patient with renal cell carcinoma, there is a lytic metastatic lesion at the right T11 vertebral body, involving the lamina, pedicle, and transverse process. The lesion has a large soft tissue component and also involves the right 11th rib. The patient had additional metastatic lesions to the lungs and bone (not shown).

Metastatic prostate cancer in a 58-year-old male (Figures 16.16 and 16.17). Sagittal T1 and T2 weighted images (Figures 16.16 and 16.17) demonstrate focal lesions in the vertebral bodies, easily distinguished against the normal marrow signal.

Leptomeningeal disease (Figure 16.18). In this 21-year-old male with a history of lymphoma, this sagittal T1-weighted postcontrast image demonstrates abnormal leptomeningeal enhancement including enhancement of the cauda equina.

Management

Management of spinal metastasis is aimed at pain control, management of instability, and preservation of neurological function. There is currently no treatment that increases life expectancy. Radiotherapy is the most common mode of management. Medical options include the use of nonsteroidal medications, high dose steroids, and other agents, including newer tumor immunomodulating or antiangiogenesis medications.

The main indications for surgery are spinal instability or spinal cord compression/cauda equina syndrome. A life expectancy of greater than 3 months is typically required for surgical consideration. Preoperative embolization of hypervascular lesions has been shown to improve surgical visualization, resection margins, with a reduction in associated surgical morbidity and operative time.

Teaching Points

► Vertebral metastasis is the most common malignant lesion in the spine and has a wide variety of imaging appearances.
► Advanced imaging has an important role in assessing underlying spinal stability and lesion vascularity, and can aid in guiding appropriate intervention and management.

Further Reading

1. Heran KSM. Preoperative embolization of spinal metastatic disease: Rational and technical considerations. Semin Musculoskel Radiol 2011;15(2):135–142.
2. White AP, Kwon BK, Lindskog DM, et al. Metastatic disease of the spine. J Am Acad Orthop Surg 2006;14(11):587–598.

Bita Ameri and Shivani Gupta

History

▶ A 59-year-old patient presents with fatigue and bone pain (**Figures 17.1, 17.2, 17.3, 17.4, and 17.5**).

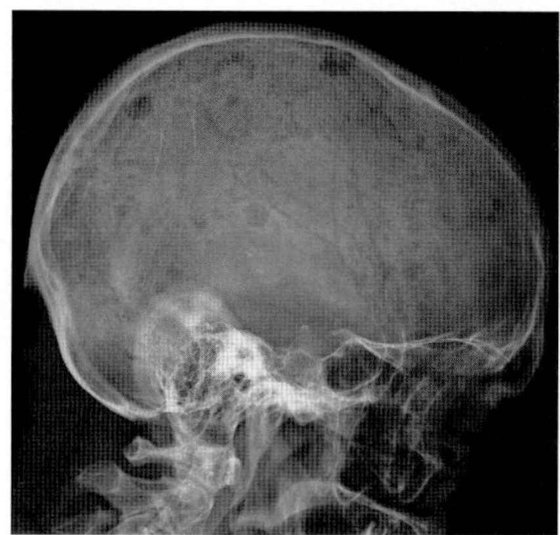

Figure 17.1

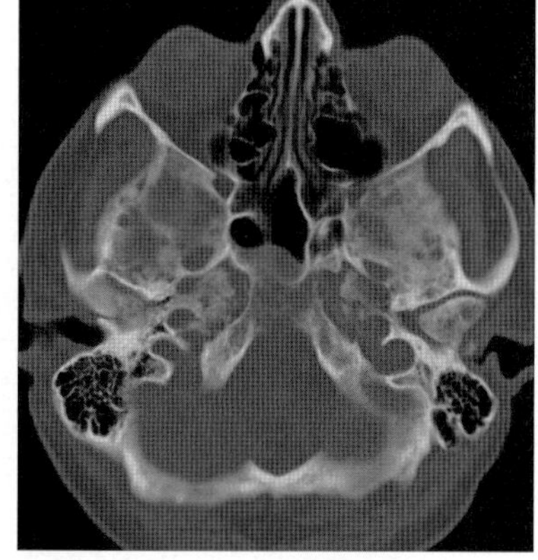

Figure 17.2

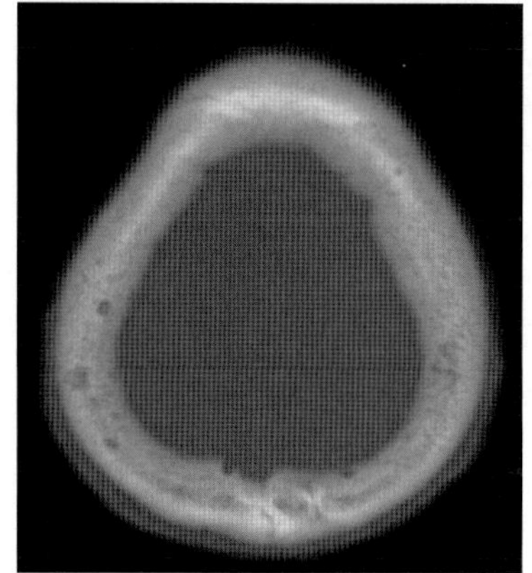

Figure 17.3

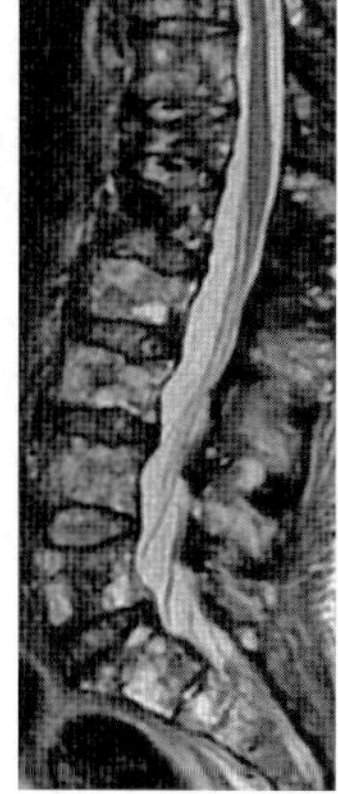

Figure 17.4

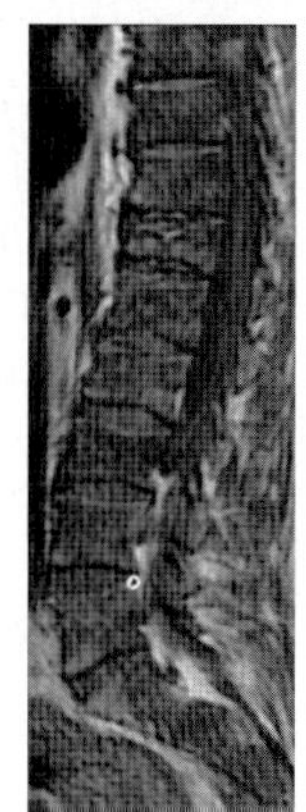

Figure 17.5

Chapter 17 Multiple Myeloma

Findings

Multiple myeloma. A lateral radiograph of the skull (Figure 17.1) demonstrates multifocal "punched out" lytic lesions. An axial head CT image shows multifocal lytic lesions throughout the skull base (Figure 17.2) and calvarium (Figure 17.3). A sagittal STIR MR image (Figure 17.4) shows innumerable hyperintense lesions in the vertebral bodies and spinous processes with associated pathological compression fractures. A sagittal T1-weighted MR image (Figure 17.5) shows hypointense lesions throughout the spine.

Differential Diagnosis

▶ Metastatic disease
▶ B cell malignancy

Discussion

Multiple myeloma (MM) is the most common primary bone tumor, typically occurring in the middle aged to elderly population with a median age of 65 years. MM involves the proliferation of malignant monoclonal plasma cells within the red marrow. These neoplastic plasma cells release osteoclast-stimulating factor resulting in characteristic multifocal osteolytic lesions, most commonly involving the axial skeleton. The plasma cells also produce an excessive monoclonal protein, known as M protein, which circulates in the blood, affecting multiple organ systems.

This multisystem disease yields a spectrum of clinical findings including bone pain, hyper**C**alcemia, **R**enal insufficiency, **A**nemia, and **B**one abnormalities (CRAB). The symptomology varies greatly, ranging from asymptomatic to a fatal illness.

The diagnostic workup includes serum and urine electrophoresis demonstrating monoclonal antibody peaks (IgG 60%, IgA 25%) in the serum and Bence Jones proteins (light chain Ig subunit) in the urine, detection of neoplastic plasma cells on bone marrow aspirate or biopsy, and lytic lesions on skeletal survey.

Four types of multiple myeloma have been described:
▶ Solitary plasmacytoma: a single, often expansile, lytic lesion (Figure 17.5)
▶ Multiple myeloma: classic multifocal "punched out" lesions
▶ Diffuse skeletal osteopenia: only osteopenia, predominantly involves the spine and is associated with compression fractures
▶ Sclerosing myeloma: sclerotic lesions associated with **P**olyneuropathy, **O**rganomegaly, **E**ndocrinopathy, **M** protein, **S**kin changes (POEMS syndrome)

Prognosis also varies, with survival ranging from several months to more than 10 years.

Radiological Evaluation

While the diagnosis of multiple myeloma is usually based on clinical and laboratory findings, imaging is instrumental in staging the disease to help tailor therapy.

Staging is done using the Durie/Salmon Plus System, which is based on a combination of clinical and radiographic findings.
▶ IA: Normal skeletal survey or single lesion (plasmacytoma)
▶ IB: <5 focal lesions or mild diffuse spinal disease
▶ IIA, IIB: 5–20 focal lesions or moderate diffuse spinal disease
▶ IIIA, IIIB: >20 focal lesions or severe diffuse spinal disease
▶ Subclasses A and B (A = normal renal function, B = abnormal renal function)

A radiographic skeletal survey is the initial imaging modality used to diagnose and stage multiple myeloma, with up to 75% of patients demonstrating detectable lytic lesions. However, radiography can underestimate the extent of the disease. MRI, due to its superior sensitivity, can be used to better evaluate the extent of bone disease, helping grade disease as mild, moderate, or severe according to the Durie and Salmon Plus System.

Lastly, FDG PET/CT is used to identify extramedullary disease (present in up to 20% of patients) and to monitor the response to treatment.

The differential diagnosis for multiple myeloma includes metastatic disease and B cell malignancies [acute lymphoblastic leukemia (ALL), non-Hodgkin's lymphoma (NHL), chronic lymphocytic leukemia (CLL), Waldenstrom's macroglobulinemia]. A distinguishing feature of metastatic disease and MM is destruction of the pedicle, which is commonly seen in metastatic disease, but not MM. In addition, metastatic disease rarely involves the intervertebral disk and mandible, unlike MM. B cell malignancy can be differentiated from MM due to its diffuse marrow involvement. A plasmacytoma can be hard to distinguish from a metastatic lesion (**Figure 17.6**).

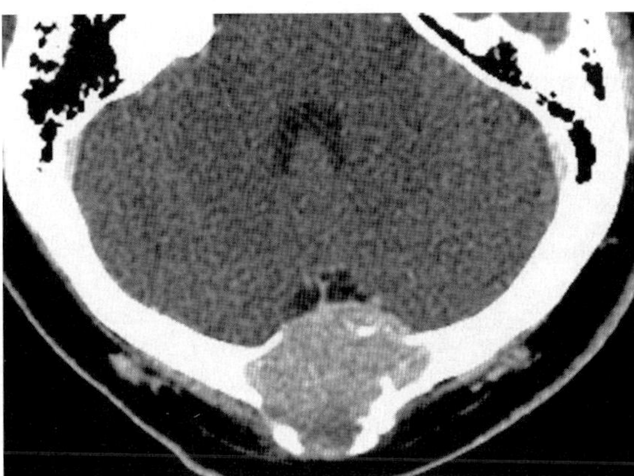

Figure 17.6

Calvarial plasmacytoma. Axial NECT of the skull base (**Figure 17.6**) shows a single expansile lesion within the occipital bone at the midline, consistent with a plasmacytoma (confirmed on pathology). Imaging features, however, are not specific and metastatic disease should also be considered.

Management

The mainstay of therapy is typically an oral regimen of melphalan and prednisone[3]. Autologous stem cell transplantation or kyphoplasty/vertebroplasty can also be considered depending on staging and symptomology, respectively. Open surgical decompression and stabilization are reserved for cases of neurological compression with associated deficit or spinal instability due to bone loss or destruction.

Teaching Points

- ▶ Multiple myeloma is the most common primary bone malignancy.
- ▶ The characteristic imaging finding is multiple "punched out" osteolytic lesions, most commonly affecting the vertebral bodies, often resulting in compression fractures and sometimes cord compression.
- ▶ Staging uses the Durie and Salmon Plus System, which incorporates various clinical and radiographic findings.

Further Reading

1. Mahnken AH, et al. Multidetector CT of the spine in multiple myeloma: Comparison with MR imaging and radiography. Am J Roentgenol 2002;178:1429–1436.
2. Delorme S, et al. Imaging in multiple myeloma. Eur J Radiol 2009;70(3):401–408.
3. Usmani S, et al. Prognostic implications of serial 18-FDG PET/CT in multiple myeloma treated with total therapy 3. Blood 2013;121:1819–1823.
4. Greipp et al. Development of an International Prognostic Index (IPI) for Myeloma: Report of the International Myeloma Working Group. Haematol J. In press, 2003.
5. Bauer et al. Magnetic Resonance Imaging as a Supplement for the Clinical Staging System of Durie and Salmon? Cancer. Vol. 95, No. 6, September 15, 2002; 1334–1345.
6. Durie et al. Whole-body F-FDG PET identifies high-risk myeloma. J Nucl Med. Vol. 43, 2002; 1457–1463.

Chapter 18

Richard Silbergleit and Anant Krishnan

History

► A 51-year-old woman with 1 year of neck stiffness presents with recent onset of neck pain and upper extremity weakness. She was a long distance runner and sought medical attention when she could not keep up with her sisters (**Figures 18.1, 18.2, 18.3, and 18.4**).

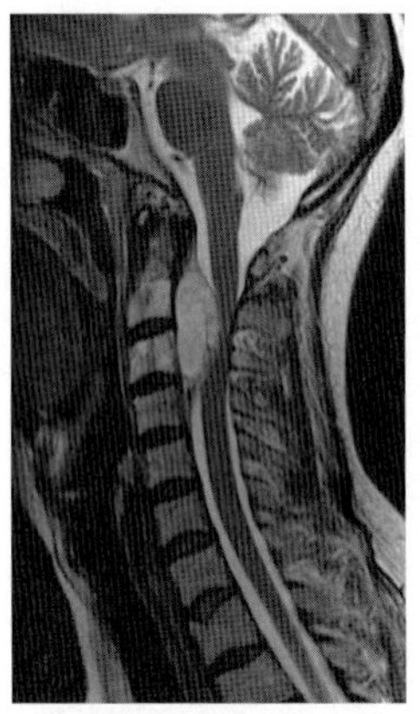

Figure 18.1

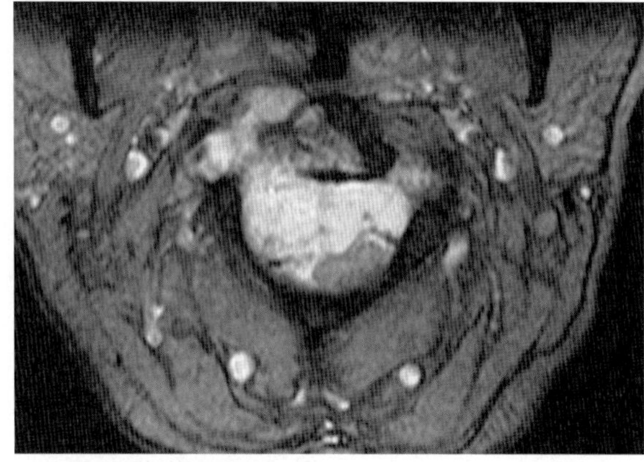

Figure 18.2

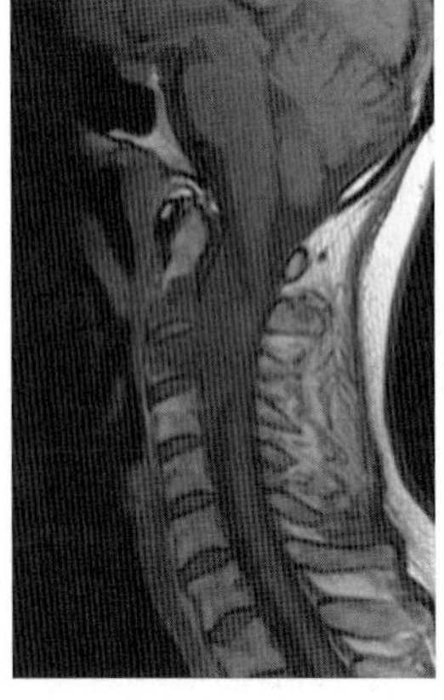

Figure 18.3

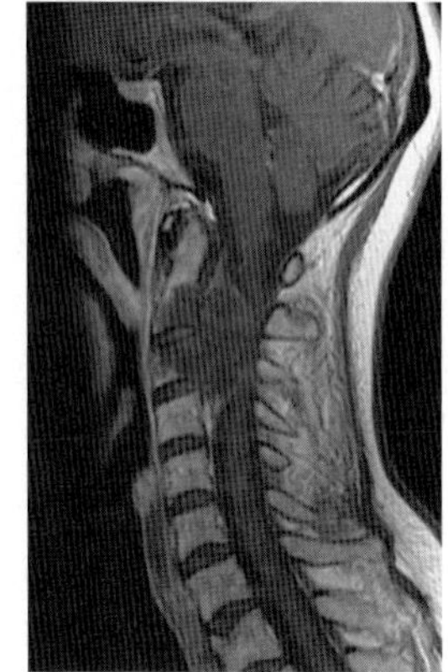

Figure 18.4

Findings

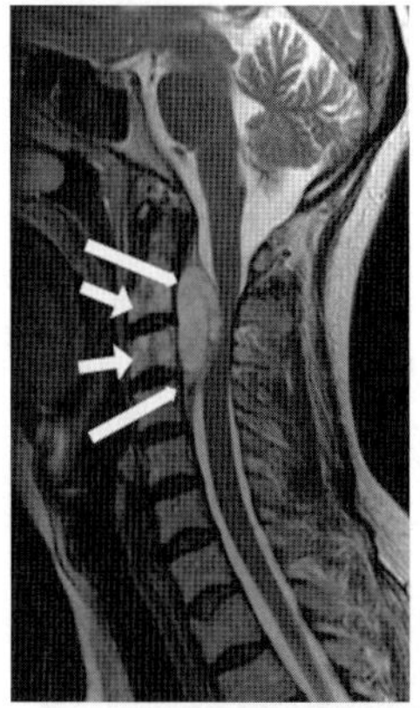

Figure 18.5

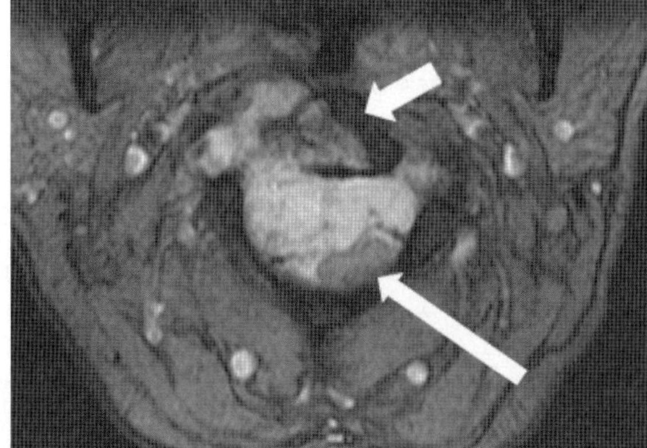

Figure 18.6

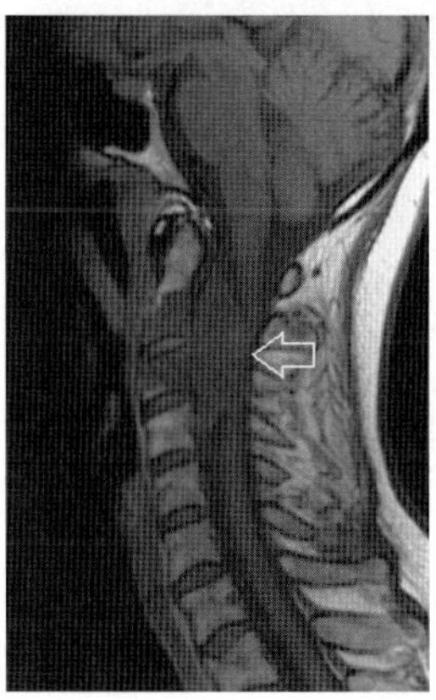

Figure 18.7

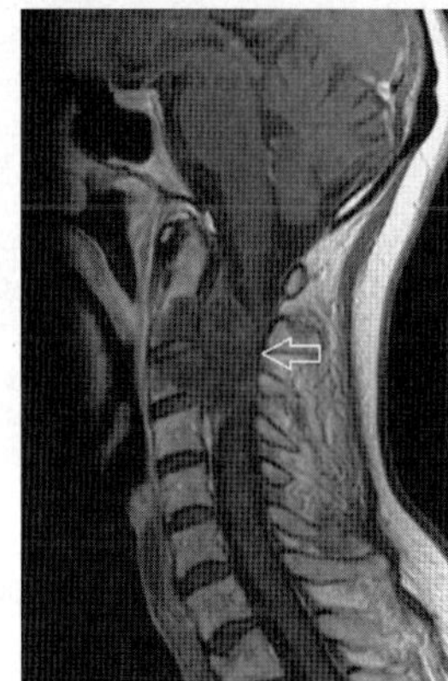

Figure 18.8

Chordoma (**Figures 18.5, 18.6, 18.7, and 18.8**). A sagittal T2-weighted image (Figure 18.5) of the cervical spine demonstrates high signal intensity in the C2 and C3 vertebral bodies (short arrows) and a large contiguous high signal intensity epidural mass (long arrows) compressing the cervical spinal cord. An axial T2*-weighted image (Figure 18.6) demonstrates the high signal intensity in the vertebral body (short arrow) and compression of the cervical spinal cord (long arrow). A sagittal T1-weighted image (Figure 18.7) demonstrates low signal intensity in the involved vertebral bodies and the epidural mass (open arrow). There is minimal enhancement (open arrow) on the sagittal T1-weighted enhanced image (Figure 18.8).

Differential Diagnosis

- ► Chordoma
- ► Multiple myeloma
- ► Metastasis
- ► Lymphoma
- ► Giant cell tumor
- ► Chondrosarcoma

Discussion

Chordomas are low-grade malignant neoplasms that may occur anywhere along the course of the notochord. They are the most common primary tumor of the mobile spine. The sacrococcygeal region is most frequently involved followed by the clivus. The cervical spine is the third most frequent site, then the lumbar spine, with the thoracic spine least commonly involved. Chordomas may be typical with physaliphorous cells causing high signal intensity on T2-weighted images or may be chondroid and not exhibit such marked high signal intensity. Some authors include dedifferentiated as a third type of chordoma.

Radiological Evaluation

Chordomas present as destructive masses in the clivus or spine (Figures 18.9, 18.10, 18.11, and 18.12). Typical chordomas are bright on T2-weighted images and low signal intensity on T1-weighted images. The lesions are frequently calcified. Large soft tissue masses are common, which may be epidural or paravertebral. More than one level may be involved with the intervening disc. Enhancement is quite variable.

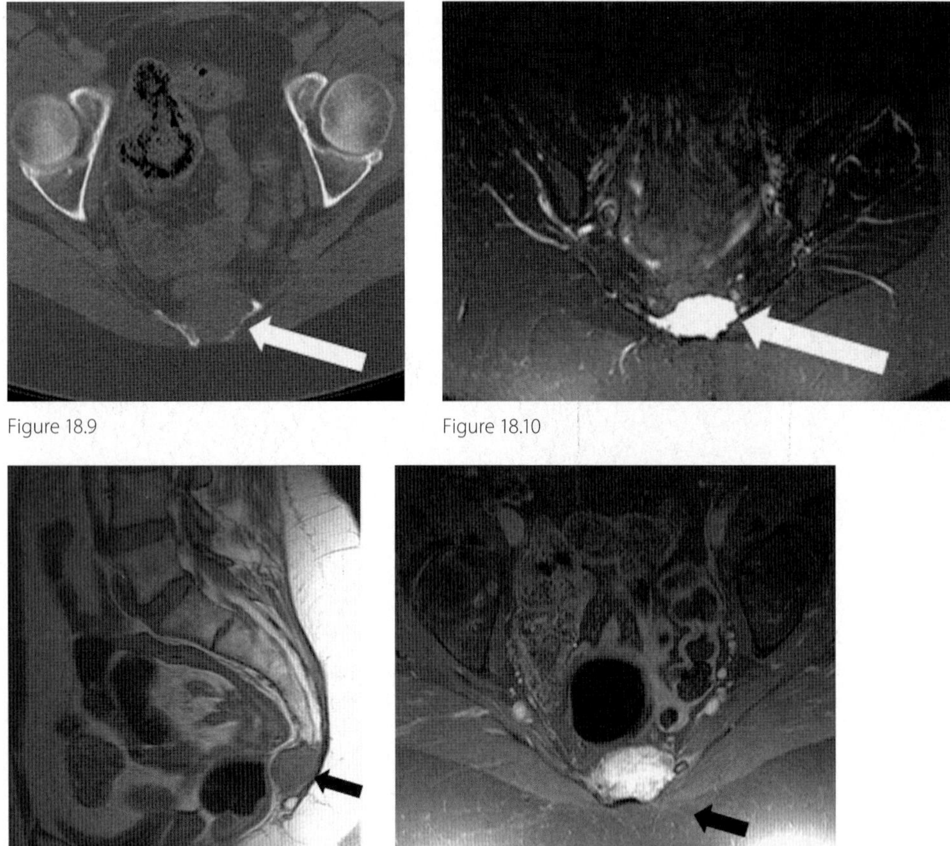

Figure 18.9

Figure 18.10

Figure 18.11

Figure 18.12

Sacral chordoma (**Figures 18.9, 18.10, 18.11, and 18.12**). Noncontrast CT (Figure 18.9) shows a destructive lesion (arrow) in the sacrum. This lesion is not calcified, which is atypical for a sacral chordoma. Oblique coronal STIR (Figure 18.10) demonstrates the typical high signal intensity (arrow). A sagittal T1 image (Figure 18.11) shows a low signal intensity expansile mass (black arrow). A contrast-enhanced fat-suppressed axial image (Figure 18.12) shows intense enhancement (black arrow) in contrast to the cervical spine case above.

Management

When possible, complete surgical excision is the treatment of choice as this is the only treatment associated with being continuously disease free after 5 years. Adjuvant radiation therapy is often used. Recurrence is common since complete surgical resection is difficult given the proximity of neurological and vascular structures.

Teaching Points

- ▶ Chordomas may occur anywhere along the path of the notochord from the clivus through the sacrococcygeal region.
- ▶ The sacrum is the most common location for chordomas.
- ▶ A high T2 signal is characteristic of typical chordomas.
- ▶ Soft tissue masses are common.

Further Reading

1. Boriani S, Bandiera S, Biagini R, et al. Chordoma of the mobile spine: Fifty years of experience. Spine 2006;31:493–503.
2. Rodallec MH, Feydy A, Larousserie F, et al. Diagnostic imaging of solitary tumors of the spine: What to do and say. RadioGraphics 2008;28:1019–1041.
3. Erdem E, Angtuaco EC, Van Hemert R, et al. Comprehensive review of intracranial chordoma. RadioGraphics 2003;23:995–1009.
4. Sciuba DM, Chi JH, Rhines LD, and Gokaslan ZL. Chordoma of the spinal column. Neurosurg Clin N Am 2008;19:5–15.
5. Walcott BP, Nahed BV, Mohyeldin A, et al. Chordoma: Current concepts, management, and future directions. Lancet Oncol 2012;13:e69–76.

Chapter 19

Cornelia Wenokor

History

▶ A 9-year-old girl presents with worsening back pain and radiculopathy (**Figures 19.1 and 19.2**).

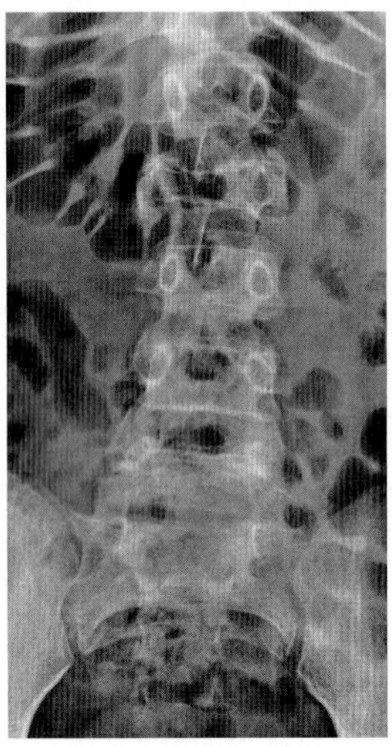

Figure 19.1

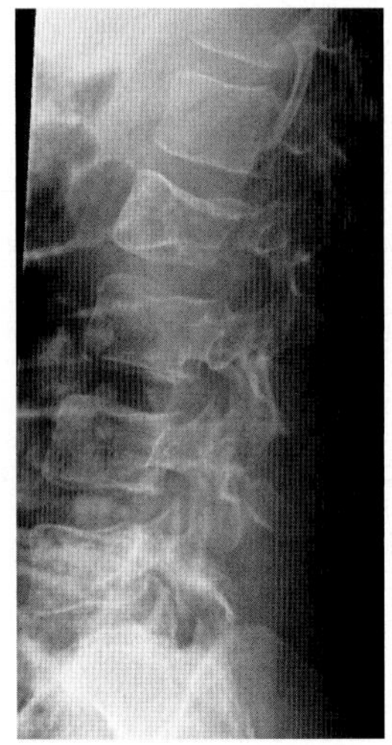

Figure 19.2

Findings

Aneurysmal bone cyst. On the radiographs (Figures 19.1 and 19.2) there is a bubbly, lytic lesion involving the L2 vertebra. There is moderate loss of height, consistent with a pathologic fracture. The vertebra is slightly expanded in a transverse direction. The endplates are intact and there is no apparent periosteal new bone formation or soft tissue mass.

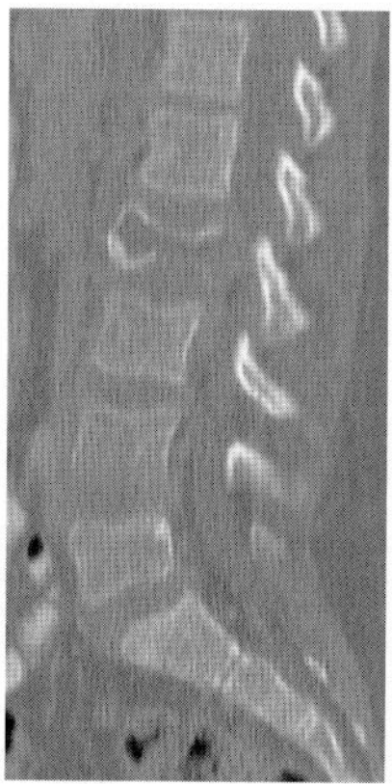

Figure 19.3

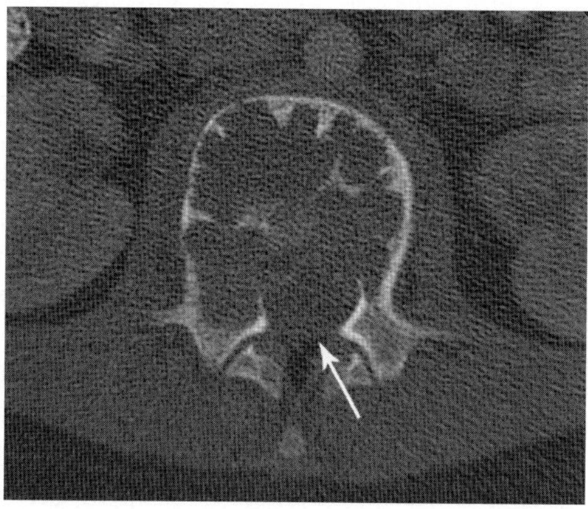

Figure 19.4

Findings on the CT scan (**Figures 19.3 and 19.4**) are similar to the radiographic findings, but demonstrate destruction of the posterior vertebral cortex with lesion extension into the spinal canal (arrow) and resultant severe spinal stenosis. There is no matrix; the lesion is purely lytic.

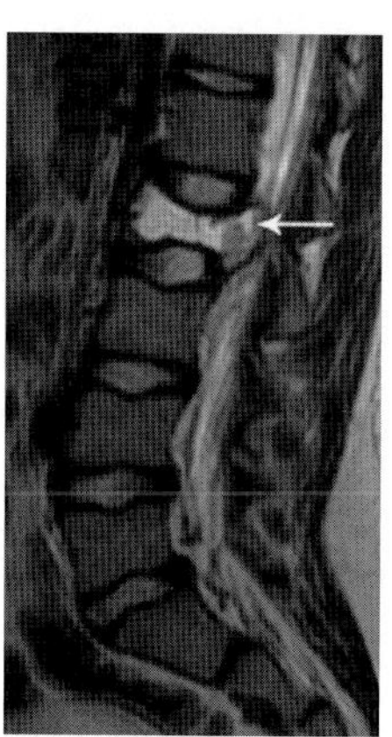

Figure 19.5

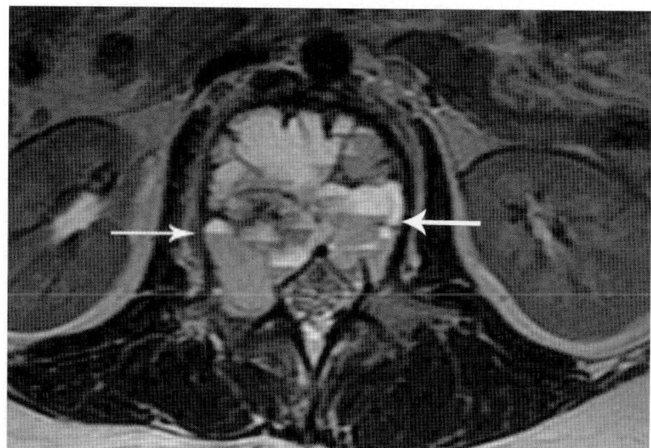

Figure 19.6

The MR images (**Figure 19.5: sagittal T2–weighted image; Figure 19.6: axial T2-weighted image**) demonstrate that the lesion is cystic in nature with numerous fluid–fluid levels (white arrows), which is typical for an aneurysmal bone cyst (ABC).

Differential Diagnosis

► Eosinophilic granuloma (Langerhans cell histiocytosis)
► Osteoblastoma
► Infection

Discussion

An ABC is a benign bone lesion. The spine is involved in up to 20–30% of cases. The origin of these lesions is unknown. One hypothesis is that the lesion is formed from hemorrhage into a preexisting lesion, the most common of which is a giant cell tumor but also includes other lesions such as an osteoblastoma or chondroblastoma. These lesions are termed secondary ABCs. ABCs are primarily seen in children and adolescents, with 80% occurring in patients under age 20 years. When seen in the spine, they typically involve the posterior elements but can extend into the vertebral body. If found in the long bones, ABCs are mostly metaphyseal in location (50–60%).

Radiological Evaluation

Patient age is of utmost importance in the evaluation of bone tumors, as is lesion location. Lytic lesions in the spinal column include an eosinophilic granuloma and aneurysmal bone cyst for children. Osteoblastoma is also found in this age group, but is generally found in the posterior elements, rather than in the vertebral body. For older patients, a hemangioma could be considered, in which the vertebra has a striated appearance, due to prominent vertical trabeculation. Metastasis and multiple myeloma are more likely to represent a lytic lesion in a patient older than 40 years of age. Sarcomas can occur in the spinal column, but typically are rare. Infection can mimic tumors, but usually manifests as discitis/osteomyelitis with resultant endplate destruction, which is not present in this case.

Radiographs will often demonstrate a lytic, expansile lesion. CT will have similar findings, although a fluid–fluid level may be evident. On MRI, fluid–fluid levels are typically more apparent; in addition, a solid component is sometimes visualized, which would suggest the presence of a secondary ABC. The cystic portion of the lesion has variable signal characteristics due to the varying ages of internal blood products. Fluid–fluid levels are not diagnostic of an ABC and can be seen in several other benign and malignant entities such as a giant cell tumor and telangiectatic osteosarcoma.

Management

Complete excision of ABCs used to offer the best chance of cure and spinal decompression if neurological deficits are present, but recent literature indicates excellent outcomes using percutaneous ablation techniques.

Teaching Points

▶ Aneurysmal bone cysts are primarily seen in children and adolescents, with 80% occurring in patients under the age of 20 years. Up to a third of ABCs are secondary to an underlying lesion such as chondroblastoma, fibrous dysplasia, giant cell tumor, or osteosarcoma.

▶ If found in the long bones ABCs are mostly metaphyseal in location (50–60%): 40% are found in the lower extremities, 20% in the upper extremities and 20–30% in the spine.

▶ Fluid–fluid levels are characteristic for ABCs, but nonspecific, as they can be seen in both benign and malignant lesions (e.g., giant cell tumor, chondroblastoma, simple bone cysts, and telangiectatic osteosarcoma).

Further Reading

1. Ameli NO, Abbassioun K, Saleh H, et al. Aneurysmal bone cyst of the spine. Report of 17 cases. J Neurosurg 1985;63:685–690.
2. Bush CH, Adler Z, Drane WE, et al. Percutaneous ablation of axial aneurysmal bone cysts. AJR Am J Roentgenol 2010;194:W84–W90.
3. Kransdorf MJ and Sweet DE. Aneurysmal bone cyst: Concept, controversy, clinical presentation, and imaging. AJR Am J Roentgenol 1995;164 (3):573–580.

Nima Jadidi and Sylvie Destian

History

▶ A 62-year-old female presents with back pain (**Figures 20.1, 20.2, 20.3, and 20.4**).

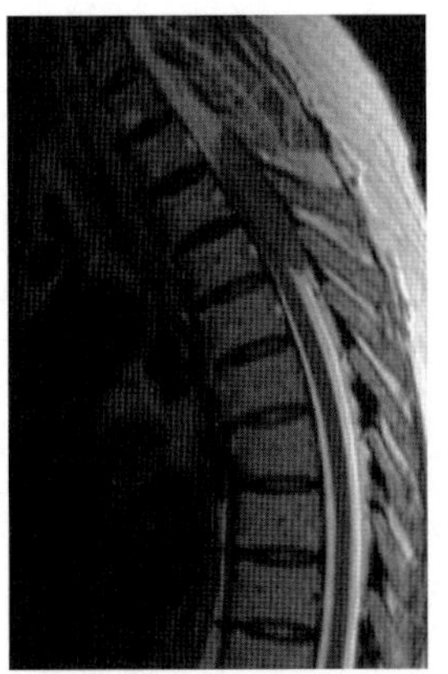

Figure 20.1

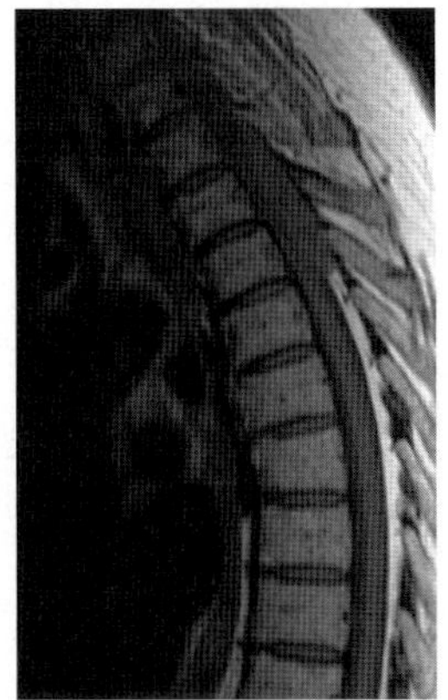

Figure 20.2

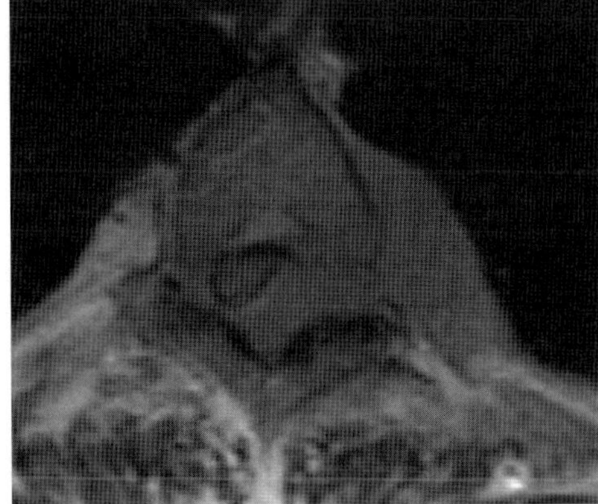

Figure 20.3

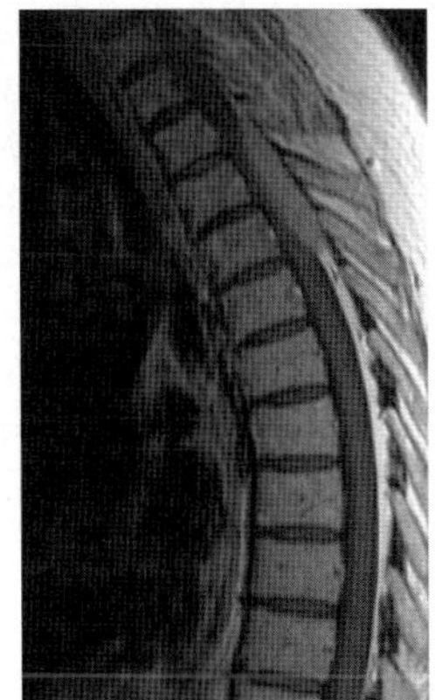

Figure 20.4

Chapter 20 **Lymphoma**

Findings

Spinal lymphoma. Sagittal T2WI and T1WI (Figures 20.1 and 20.2) depict a posterior soft tissue mass in the upper thoracic spine that is minimally hyperintense to the cord. The mass compresses the cord. Note the lack of bone involvement. Axial T1WI (Figure 20.3) depicts compression of the thecal sac and cord by an epidural soft tissue mass that extends into the left paraspinal space. A postcontrast T1-weighted image (Figure 20.4) shows homogeneous enhancement of the epidural soft tissue mass.

Differential Diagnosis

▶ Metastasis

▶ Epidural abscess

▶ Meningioma

▶ Peripheral nerve sheath tumor

Discussion

Epidural lymphoma comprises less than 10% of all lymphomas. A subset of these is considered a primary spinal epidural lymphoma if the diagnostic workup elsewhere in the body is negative. Non-Hodgkin's lymphoma accounts for the majority of the reported cases. Patients may initially present with localized back pain. If the lesion progresses to cause significant spinal cord compression, rapid neurological deterioration may then be observed.

Radiological Evaluation

The most common location for epidural lymphoma is the thoracic spine followed by the lumbar and cervical spine. The lesions typically extend across a few vertebral levels. Radiography is a poor demonstrator of this lesion. Myelography can demonstrate the extent of compression well; however, MRI offers several additional advantages including visualization of multiple lesions, evaluation for paraspinal involvement, and extent of disease. Epidural lymphoma typically occurs dorsal to the spinal cord. Imaging findings are somewhat nonspecific. MRI characteristics are iso to low intensity on T1WI and iso to hyperintense on T2WI. There is usually marked homogeneous enhancement of the lesion (Figures 20.2, 20.3, and 20.4). Metastatic disease typically is more hyperintense on T2WI. An epidural abscess shows peripheral enhancing or low intensity within epidural fat. Meningiomas may have similar signal characteristics; however, they are more often intradural lesions.

Management

Lymphomas are typically amenable to combined chemotherapy and radiation treatment. If there is compression of the spinal cord by the tumor, then surgery is usually considered. Surgery usually involves laminectomy for decompression with partial or total resection of the tumor.

Teaching Points

▶ Spinal epidural lymphoma most commonly occurs in the extradural space along the thoracic spine.

▶ Patients present with neurological symptoms from cord and nerve root compression due to mass effect.

Further Reading

1. Grossman RI and Yousem DM. *Neuroradiology, the Requisites.* St. Louis, MO: Mosby, 2003, p. 819.
2. Cugati G, Singh M, Pande A, et al. Primary spinal epidural lymphomas. J Craniovertebr Junction Spine 2011;2:3–11.

Justin Morris Honce

History

▶ A 22-year-old male presents with a 6 year history of slowly progressive low back pain, with some radiation into his legs and buttocks, and lower extremity weakness (**Figures 21.1, 21.2, 21.3, and 21.4**).

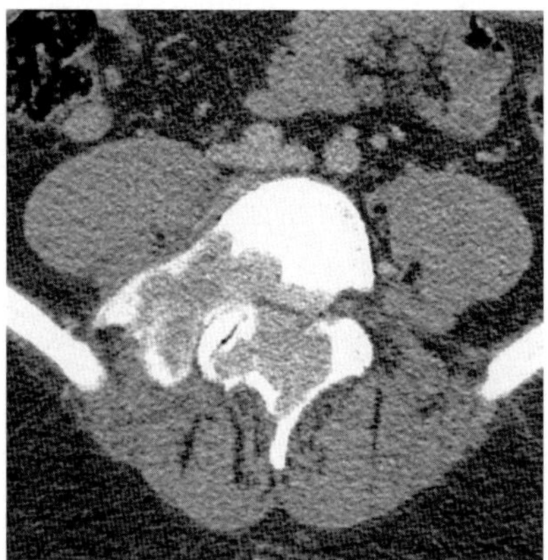

Figure 21.1

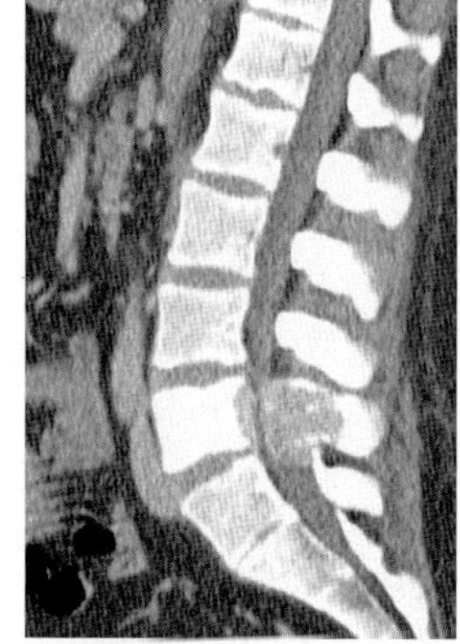

Figure 21.2

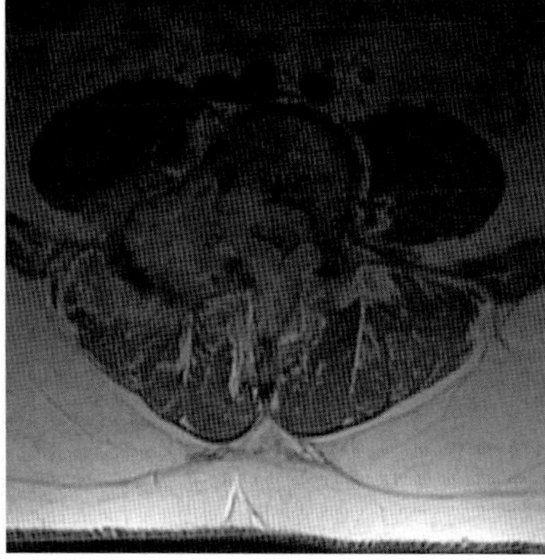

Figure 21.3

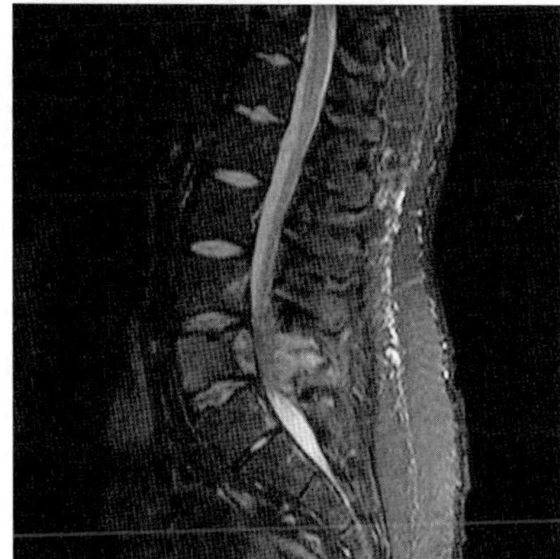

Figure 21.4

Chapter 21 Osteoblastoma

Findings

Spinal osteoblastoma (Figures 21.1, 21.2, 21.3, and 21.4). Axial (Figure 21.1) and sagittal (Figure 21.2) CT images through the lumbar spine show an expansile, soft tissue mass replacing much of the right side of the L4 vertebral body, expanding the right transverse process and posterior elements. The soft tissue extends into the spinal canal, causing severe spinal canal stenosis. The remainder of the L4 vertebral body is diffusely sclerotic. Axial postcontrast T1-weighted images (Figure 21.3) demonstrate an enhancing soft tissue mass that has replaced the right side of the L4 vertebral body, and expands/replaces the right transverse process, facet, lamina, and base of the spinous process. On sagittal STIR (Figure 21.4) the mass is hyperintense. There is resultant severe spinal canal stenosis and compression of the cauda equina nerve roots.

Differential Diagnosis

▶ Osteoblastoma
▶ Lymphoma
▶ Metastatic disease
▶ Plasmacytoma

Discussion

Osteoblastomas are benign neoplasms of the bone, representing approximately 1% of primary bone tumors. While osteoblastomas can occur in virtually any bone, between 25% and 50% of osteoblastomas occur within the spine. The lumbar spine is most frequently affected. Osteoblastomas appear to have a predilection for the posterior elements, rather than the vertebral bodies themselves. Most commonly the transverse process or pedicle is affected. These lesions are larger variants of the more common osteoid osteoma, and are distinguished from the latter by a vascular nidus measuring >1.5 cm.

The diagnosis of osteoblastoma occurs in the majority of cases before 30 years of age, and patients most commonly present with symptoms in their second or third decade. Males are more frequently affected than females. The most common presenting symptom is pain and focal tenderness. This pain can be quite severe resulting in alterations in spinal curvature (scoliosis) or muscular contractions/shortening (torticollis).

Radiological Evaluation

The initial workup of patients typically will include plain radiographs and computed tomography. MRI can provide additional information in those patients in whom the symptomatology is not typical, or if there is associated neurological deficits (as in this case). Typical features on plain films include reactive sclerosis. On CT, especially in larger lesions, regions of lucency and osseous destruction can be seen. Overall then, the appearance can be that of a densely calcified mass, or an expansile, soft tissue mass. There may be multifocal areas of mineralization within the tumor matrix. The T1 and T2 signal is heterogeneous and will vary greatly depending on the degree of mineralization. All of these tumors enhance with gadolinium. A rare but classic imaging feature is that of diffuse sclerosis of the vertebral body, producing a radiographic "ivory vertebra" (as in this case). Of note, this sclerosis may extend over multiple levels. On bone scintigraphy osteoblastomas will have marked uptake of radiotracer.

Management

The primary goal of all treatment is for symptomatic relief of the pain and focal tenderness classic for these lesions. If there is no osseous destruction or neurological deficits as a result of compression, nonoperative management is usually the first therapeutic approach. Patients may respond to nonsteroidal antiinflammatory drugs (NSAIDs). If medical therapy fails, the lesions are typically ablated, either via radiofrequency or laser approaches. If these more conservative options fail, or there are substantial neurological deficits due to compression, or there is spinal instability, surgical curettage or resection is indicated. Complete resection of the lesion is preferred and spinal stabilization with instrumentation may be necessary.

Teaching Points

▶ Osteoblastomas most commonly occur within the spine, frequently the lumbar spine, and have a predilection for the transverse process or pedicle.

▶ Osteoblastomas are distinguished from osteoid osteomas by the size of the vascular nidus, which measures >1.5 cm in osteoblastomas.

▶ Lesions can be sclerotic, lytic, or mixed, with varying signal on T1/T2 but all lesions enhance. A rare but classic feature of osteoblastoma is associated sclerosis of the vertebral body creating a so-called "ivory vertebrae" appearance.

Further Reading

1. Burn SC, Ansorge O, Zeller R, and Drake JM. Management of osteoblastoma and osteoid osteoma of the spine in childhood. J Neurosurg: Pediatr 2009;4(5):434–438.
2. Kroon HM and Schurmans J. Osteoblastoma: Clinical and radiologic findings in 98 new cases. Radiology 1990;175(3):783–790.
3. Murphey MD, Andrews CL, Flemming DJ, et al. From the archives of the AFIP—Primary tumors of the spine: Radiologic pathologic correlation. Radiographics 1996;16:1131–1158.
4. Shaikh MI, Saifuddin A, Pringle J, et al. Spinal osteoblastoma: CT and MR imaging with pathological correlation. Skeletal Radiol 1999;28(1):33–40.
5. Sherazi Z, Saifuddin A, Shaikh MI, et al. Unusual imaging findings in association with spinal osteoblastoma. Clin Radiol 1996;51:644–648.
6. Zileli M, Çagli S, Basdemir G, and Ersahin Y. Osteoid osteomas and osteoblastomas of the spine. Neurosurg Focus 2003;15(5):1–7.

Chapter 22

Joseph Boonsiri, Cynthia A. Britton, and Vikas Agarwal

History

► A 61-year-old female presents with progressive back pain and paresthesias (**Figures 22.1, 22.2, and 22.3**).

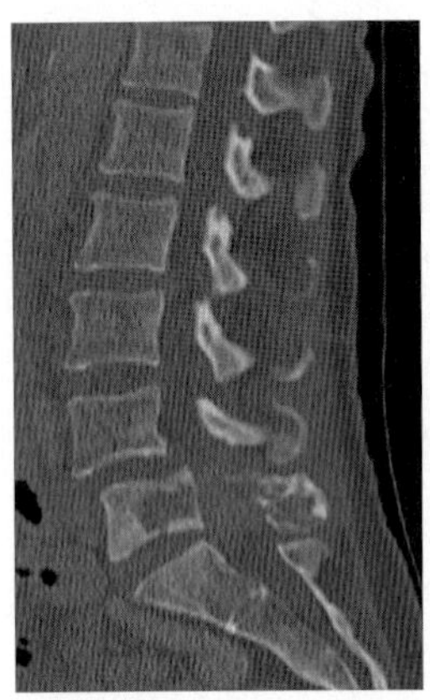

Figure 22.1

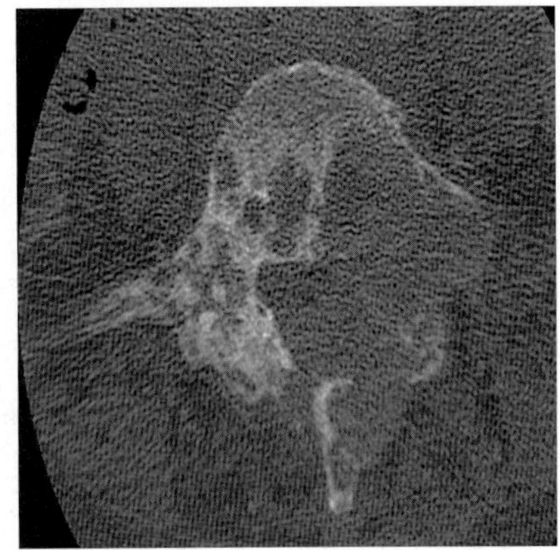

Figure 22.2

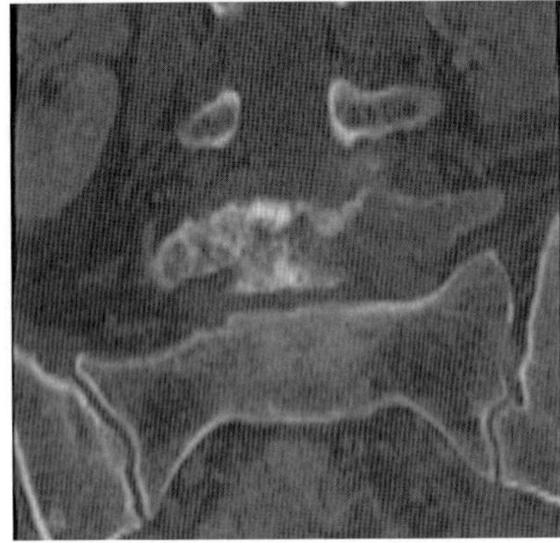

Figure 22.3

Findings

Spinal osteosarcoma (Figures 22.1, 22.2, and 22.3). Sagittal, axial and coronal CT images demonstrate an expansive, destructive mixed sclerotic-lytic mass involving the posterior L5 vertebral body and posterior elements (Figures 22.1, 22.2, and 22.3). There is invasion of the spinal canal.

Differential Diagnosis

- ▶ Osteoblastoma
- ▶ Ewing sarcoma/primitive neuroectodermal tumor
- ▶ Chordoma
- ▶ Chondrosarcoma
- ▶ Hemangioma
- ▶ Telangiectatic osteosarcoma
- ▶ Hematogenous metastasis
- ▶ Osteomyelitis

Discussion

Only 0.6–3.2% of osteosarcomas occur in the spine and represent 3–5% of all spinal malignancies. Osteosarcomas may be associated with Paget's disease (approximately 1% of patients with Paget's disease develop osteosarcoma) or with mutations in tumor suppressor genes: hereditary retinoblastoma, Li–Fraumeni Syndrome, Rothmund–Thomson Syndrome, Werner Syndrome, Diamond Blackfan Anemia, and Bloom Syndrome.

Patients may present with progressive pain and elevated alkaline phosphatase. Osteosarcoma is more common in the sacrum than the thoracolumbar spine. The radiological appearance and clinical behavior depend on the subtype: conventional osteosarcoma (with osteoblastic, chondroblastic, and fibroblastic subsubtypes), surface, telangiectatic, and fibroblastic.

Radiographic Evaluation

On plain films, an ivory vertebral body can be seen. CT is useful in the assessment of mineralization and bone destruction. Up to 80% of conventional osteosarcomas demonstrate osteoid matrix mineralization. Mixed sclerotic lytic lesions with bony destruction, a wide zone of transition, or permeative patterns may be seen.

MRI is useful for the evaluation of soft tissue extension (**Figures 22.4, 22.5, 22.6, 22.7, 22.8, and 22.9**). Lesions can have a variable appearance, including aggressive permeative lesions with - variable signal on T1- and T2-weighted images depending on the degree of mineralization (more mineralized portions are low on T1- and T2-weighted sequences, nonmineralized portions are T2 hyperintense). Contrast enhancement is heterogeneous.

Spinal osteosarcomas involve the posterior elements in up to 79% of cases. Cortical destruction is common. Spinal canal or dural invasion is also common, seen in up to 84% of cases. The Enneking staging system is based on histopathology and degree of spread, and is as follows:

- ▶ Stage I: Low-grade, localized tumors
- ▶ Stage II: High-grade, localized tumors
- ▶ Stage III: Distant metastases
- ▶ Stage IA or IIA if the tumor remains within the bone, Stage IB or IIB if it extends outside the bone locally

The imaging appearance of an osteosarcoma in the spine is often nonspecific, and may require further work-up with a biopsy.

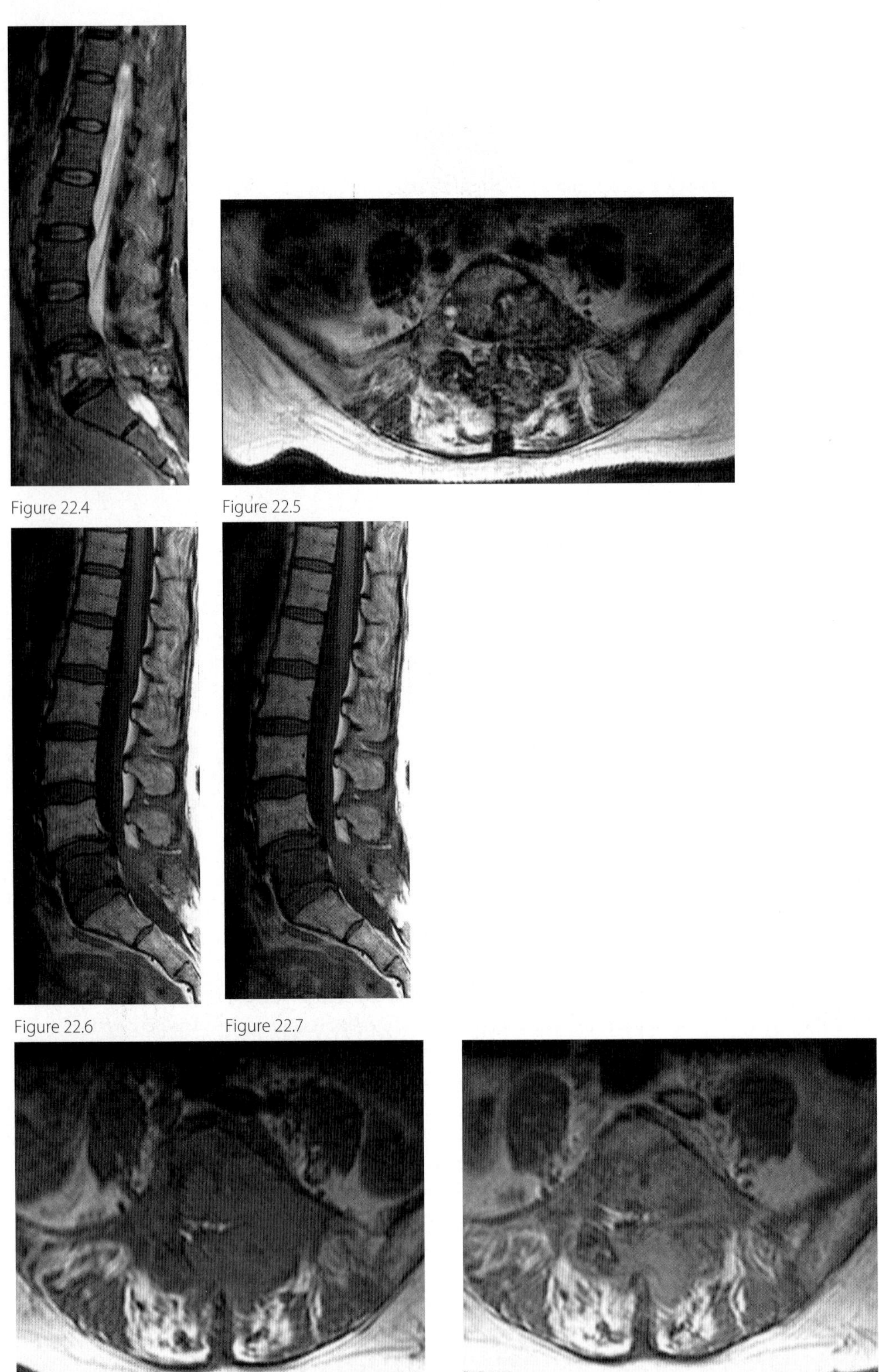

Figure 22.4

Figure 22.5

Figure 22.6

Figure 22.7

Figure 22.8

Figure 22.9

MRI evaluation of an osteosarcoma (Figures 22.4, 22.5, 22.6, 22.7, 22.8, and 22.9). A bubbly appearance of The osseous portion of the tumor is noted on T2-weighted sequences (Figures 22.4 and 22.5) whereas the soft tissue component is hypointense to marrow on T1 and enhances following the administration of gadolinium (Figures 22.6, 22.7, 22.8, and 22.9). Pathological examination revealed a high-grade osteosarcoma with giant cell features—the latter may account for the bubbly appearance of the lytic component on T2-weighted sequences.

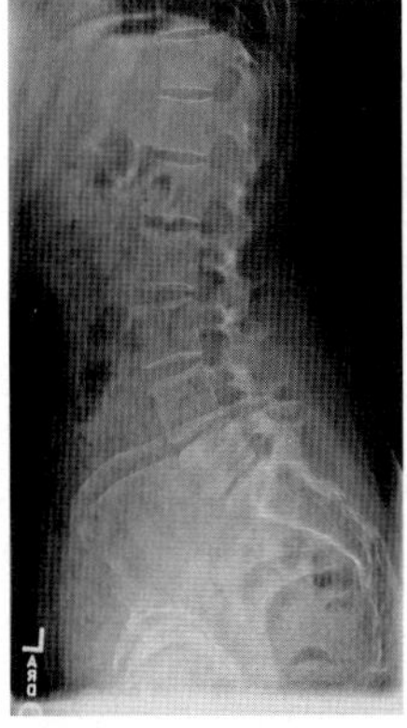

Figure 22.10

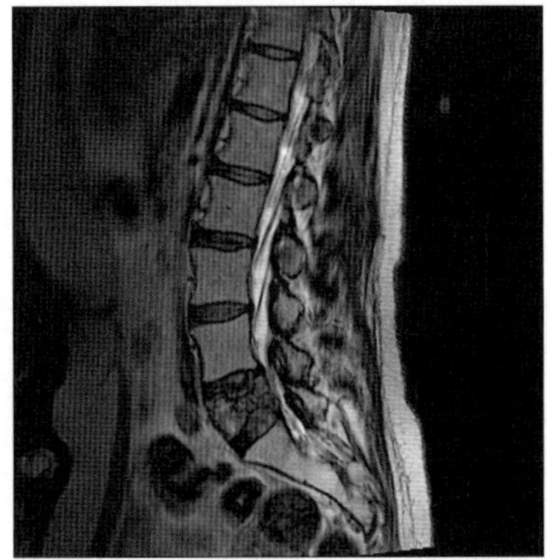

Figure 22.11

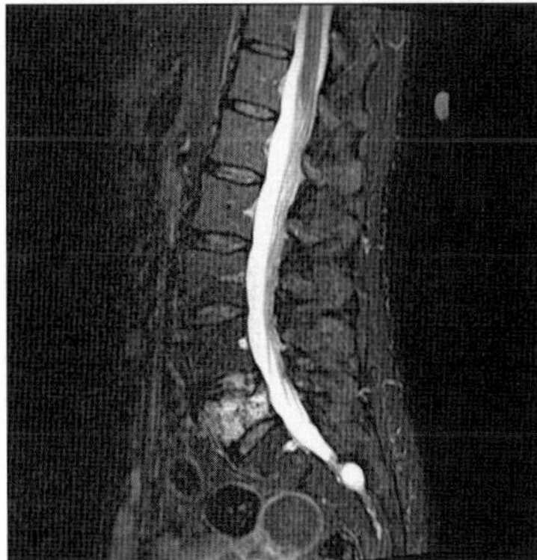

Figure 22.12

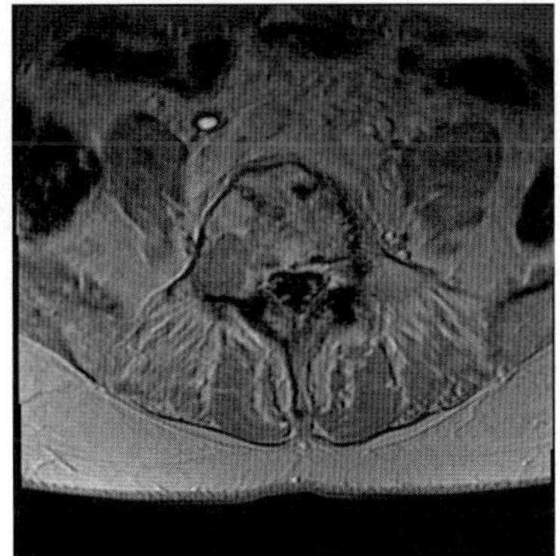

Figure 22.13

Lumbar spine osteosarcoma in a 53-year-old patient (**Figures 22.10, 22.11, 22.12, and 22.13**). A lateral view of the lumbar spine (Figure 22.10) demonstrates subtle increased density of L5. Sagittal T2 (Figure 22.11) and STIR (Figure 22.12) MR images better depict the abnormal marrow signal at L5. Heterogeneous enhancement is seen on an axial T1 postcontrast image (Figure 22.13). This was a pathologically proven osteosarcoma. The overall imaging appearance is nonspecific, and easily could have been secondary to metastatic disease, among other possible entities.

Management

The prognosis is poor despite surgical resection, adjuvant chemotherapy, and radiation (mean survival is reported to be between 30 and 38 months). En-bloc resection of the tumor is difficult due to the proximity of the spinal cord and other sensitive structures. Local recurrence after resection ranges from 20% to 60%. Pulmonary, bone, and liver metastases are more common than local recurrence.

Teaching Points

▶ Spinal osteosarcoma may have a variable appearance depending on the subtype.
▶ Dural or intraspinal involvement is common.
▶ Clinical suspicion for osteosarcoma should be higher in the setting of Paget's disease, prior radiation therapy, or various tumor suppressor gene mutations.

Further Reading

1. Katonis P, Datsis G, Karantanas A, et al. Spinal osteosarcoma. Clin Med Insights: Oncol 2013;7:199–208.
2. Orguc S and Remide A. Primary tumors of the spine. Semin Musculoskel Radiol 2014;18:280–299.

Chapter 23

Nima Jadidi and Sylvie Destian

History

► A 47-year-old woman presents with lower extremity weakness (**Figures 23.1, 23.2, and 23.3**).

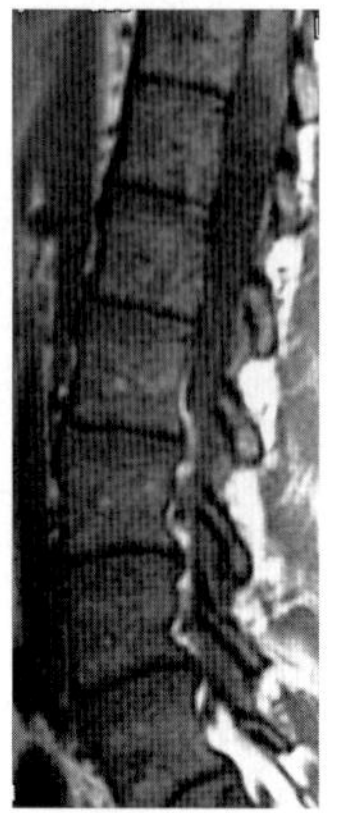

Figure 23.1

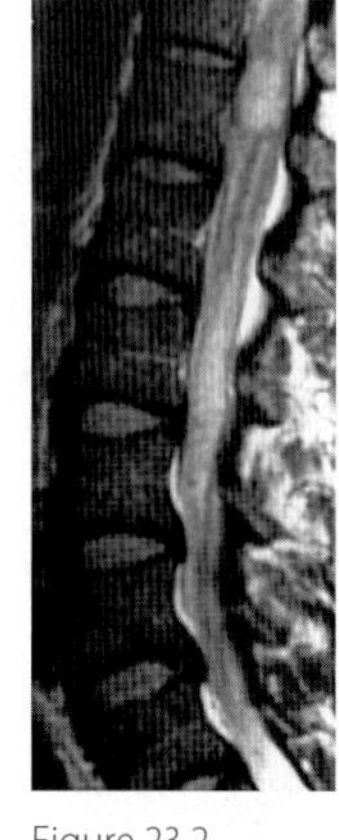

Figure 23.2

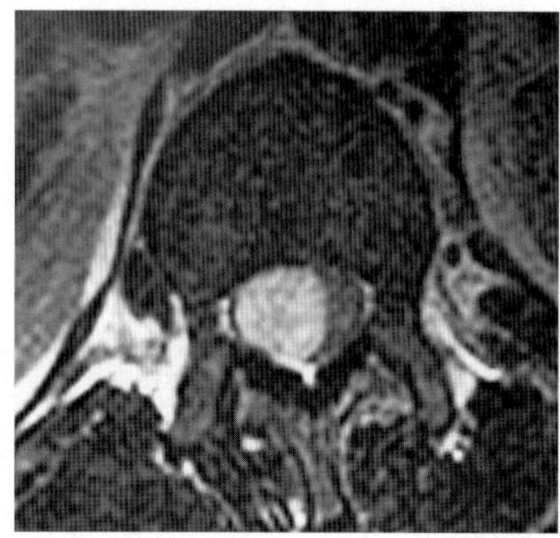

Figure 23.3

Findings

Filum terminale ependymoma (Figures 23.1, 23.2, and 23.3). Sagittal T1- and T2-weighted images (Figures 23.1 and 23.2) and a postcontrast T1-weighted image (Figure 23.3) demonstrate an ovoid lesion at the T12 level that is iso- to slightly hyperintense to the cauda equina on T1WI, hyperintense on the T2WI, and enhances homogeneously with contrast. This lesion is intradural and intramedullary.

Differential Diagnosis

▶ Spinal schwannoma
▶ Spinal metastases

Discussion

Filum terminale ependymomas specifically arise from ependymal cells around the filum terminale and conus medullaris. Histologically, the more common myxopapillary variant is classified as WHO grade 1. They make up approximately 10% of spinal ependymomas, have a slight male predominance, and tend to occur around the fourth decade of life. Patients may have myelopathic or radicular pain and can present with symptoms mimicking cauda equina syndrome.

Radiological Findings

Although most ependymomas elsewhere in the spine tend to be intramedullary, ependymomas of the filum terminale are intradural and extramedullary. They often have a lobulated appearance. If the tumor becomes large, they can remodel the spinal canal making it difficult to distinguish from a bone lesion such as an aneurysmal bone cyst. On MRI, they are usually isointense on T1W and hyperintense on T2WI unless there is hemorrhage or calcification present. Proteinaceous material within the tumor can cause a hyperintense signal on T1WI. The tumor enhances on postcontrast images.

Management

Although these tumors tend to be WHO grade I, there is a belief that the tumor location is a better prognostic indicator than the grade, as there is literature to support the claim that lower spinal tumors tend to have a higher rate of recurrence. Nevertheless, treatment of this tumor usually requires total surgical resection. The extent of the tumor's insinuation among the nerve roots may complicate total resection. If the tumor is large, debulking of the tumor may be required. The benefits of adjunct therapy after resection, such as with radiotherapy, are somewhat uncertain.

Teaching Points

▶ The myxopapillary variant is most common and has the best prognosis.
▶ They occur later in life compared to the more classic pediatric ependymomas occurring elsewhere in the spine and brain.
▶ They can have calcifications and undergo hemorrhage.

Further Reading

1. Grossman RI and Yousem DM. *Neuroradiology, the Requisites.* St. Louis, MO: Mosby, 2003, p. 815.
2. Mechael C, et al. Prognosis by tumor location in adults with spinal ependymomas. J Neurosurg: Spine 2013;18(3):226–235.

Chapter 24

Justin Morris Honce

History

▶ A 40-year-old male presents with a 1 month history of interscapular pain and numbness and tingling in his hands (**Figures 24.1, 24.2, 24.3, and 24.4**).

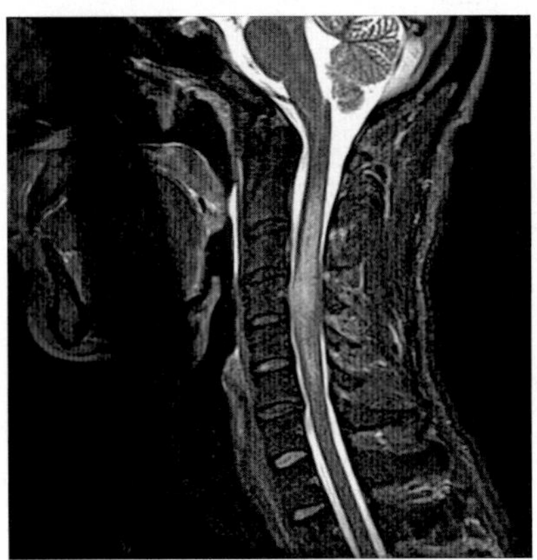

Figure 24.1

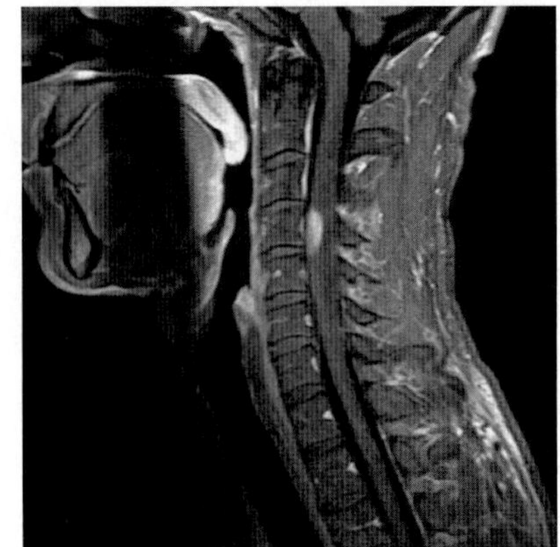

Figure 24.2

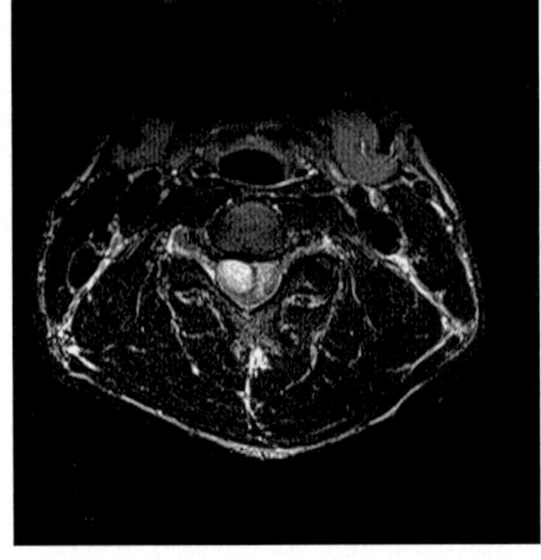

Figure 24.3

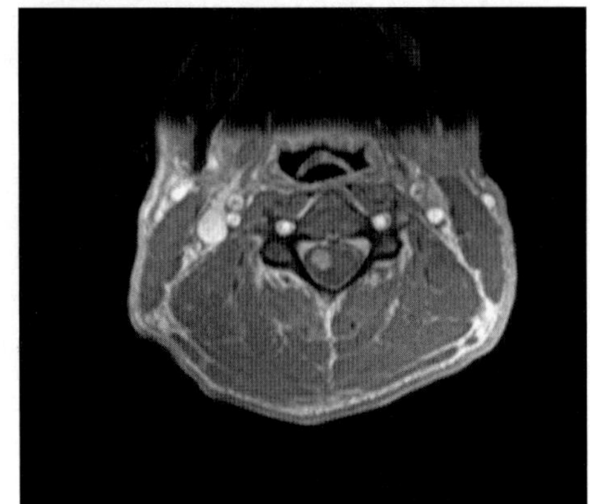

Figure 24.4

Findings

Spinal oligoastrocytoma (Figures 24.1, 24.2, 24.3, and 24.4). Sagittal STIR image (Figure 24.1) demonstrates diffuse T2 hyperintensity within the cervical cord extending from about the C1–C2 level inferiorly to C6–C7. The signal abnormality is centered at the C4 level, where there is associated cord expansion, with signal abnormality extending from about C1–C2 through C6–C7. A sagittal postcontrast T1-weighted fat-saturated image (Figure 24.2) demonstrates that within the ventral cord at the level of C4, there is a focal intramedullary enhancement. Axial T2-weighted imaging (Figure 24.3) demonstrates that the T2 hyperintense mass is located in the mid and right side of the cord. Postcontrast axial T1-weighted imaging (Figure 24.4) shows the corresponding contrast enhancement.

Differential Diagnosis

► Astrocytoma
► Ependymoma
► Ganglioglioma
► Metastases
► Lymphoma
► Hemangioblastoma

Discussion

Spinal cord gliomas comprise approximately 20% of all spinal tumors and two-thirds to one-half of these gliomas are astrocytomas, which are neoplastic proliferations of astrocytic cells. Mixed type glial neoplasms also occur, most commonly oligoastrocytomas (as is the diagnosis in this case). Oligoastrocytomas are exceedingly rare in the spinal cord and require the identification of two separate neoplastic glial components to make the diagnosis (typically oligodendroglial and astrocytic). They are indistinguishable from conventional astrocytoma on imaging.

The peak incidence of spinal astrocytomas is 20–40 years of age, but they are quite frequent in children, comprising up to 50% of all pediatric spinal cord tumors. These lesions are slightly more common in males than in females. They are frequently located within the thoracic cord, with the cervical cord being the second most commonly involved region. Astrocytomas are uncommon in the lower thoracic cord or conus. In the pediatric population nearly all spinal cord astrocytomas are WHO grade I, but can be WHO grade I–IV, though only 2–5% are high grade (IV).

The differential diagnosis of intramedullary spinal cord astrocytoma (or oligoastrocytoma) is that of an intramedullary spinal cord tumor and includes diagnoses such as ependymoma, ganglioglioma, hemangioblastoma, and lymphoma. Most of the time these lesions are indistinguishable from the other lesions, but a few features can at times help order the differential. Astrocytomas are slightly more frequently off midline in the cord compared with the centrally located ependymoma. Hemorrhage and calcification are more frequent in ependymoma, as are tumor cysts. Gangliogliomas typically have longer spinal cord involvement (>8 vertebral body segments). Hemangioblastomas are typically smaller, more focal, and many have associated T2 flow voids due to associated vessels.

Radiological Evaluation

MR imaging is the modality of choice for the evaluation of spinal cord astrocytomas. Lesions typically appear as large expansile T2 hyperintense lesions centered within the cord. They are more often asymmetric in the cord than ependyomomas, which are typically central. Most lesions enhance on postcontrast imaging and this enhancement may be diffuse, patchy, or focal. While signal characteristics are typically fairly homogeneous, marked heterogeneity in lesions can be seen due to rare intratumoral hemorrhage or calcification. Reactive and neoplastic cysts can be seen within or adjacent to these masses and these can sometimes be differentiated: tumor cysts typically will have some degree of peripheral enhancement, while reactive cysts will not. Both reactive and tumor cysts may contain varying levels of protein and/or blood and as such their appearance of MRI is otherwise quite variable.

Management

Surgical excision followed by radiation therapy is the recommended treatment of choice. Complete resection of the tumor is rarely achieved given the infiltrative nature of the lesion. The most important predictor of prognosis is the histological grade. Low-grade lesions tend to have an indolent course, whereas high-grade lesions usually result in rapid progression and deterioration of clinical status.

Teaching Points

▶ Astrocytomas most frequently occur in the thoracic cord, followed by the cervical cord. They are very rare in the lower cord and conus.
▶ The classic appearance is that of an infiltrative, expansile T2 hyperintense mass within the spinal cord. Enhancement may be diffuse, patchy, or focal.
▶ Astrocytomas are frequently indistinguishable from ependymomas, but are more commonly eccentrically located within the cord, and less frequently have internal hemorrhage/calcification or peritumoral cysts.

Further Reading

1. Constantini S, Houten J, Miller DC, et al. Intramedullary spinal cord tumors in children under the age of 3 years. J Neurosurg 1996;85:1036–1043.
2. Miller DC. Surgical pathology of intramedullary spinal cord neoplasms. J Neurooncol 2000;47:189–194.
3. Shaw EG, Scheithauer BW, O'Fallon JR, and Davis DH. Mixed oligoastrocytomas: A survival and prognostic factor analysis. Neurosurgery 1994;34:577–578.
4. Shimizu T, Saito N, Aihara M, et al. Primary spinal oligoastrocytoma: A case report. Surg Neurol 2004;61(1):77–81.
5. Traul DE, Shaffrey ME, and Schiff D. Part I: Spinal-cord neoplasms—intradural neoplasms. Lancet Oncol 2007;8(1):35–45.
6. Waldron JS and Cha S. Radiographic features of intramedullary spinal cord tumors. Neurosurg Clin N Am 2006;17(1):13–19.

Freddie R. Swain

History

▶ A 42-year-old patient presents with chronic lower back pain (**Figures 25.1, 25.2, and 25.3**).

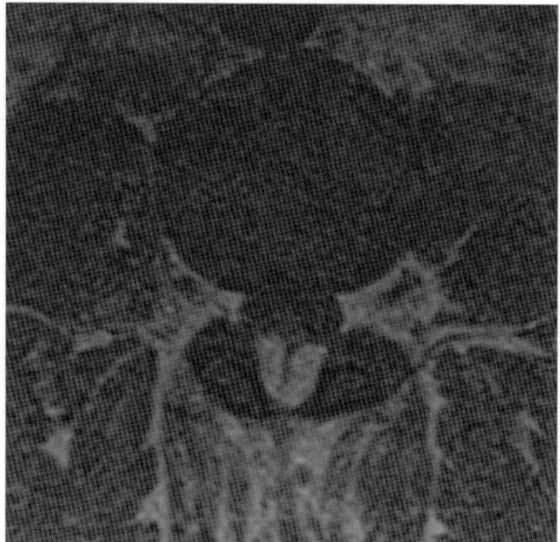

Figure 25.1

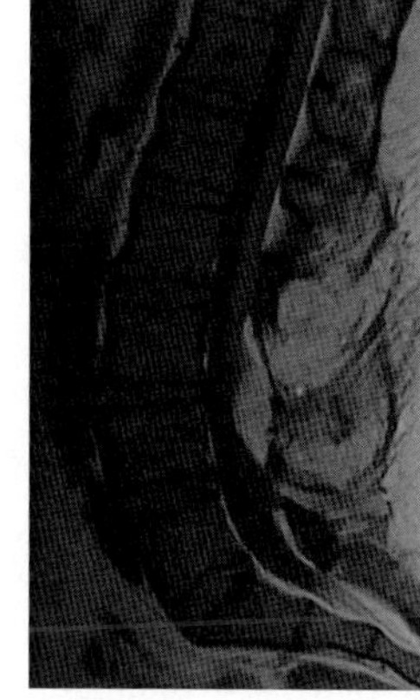

Figure 25.2

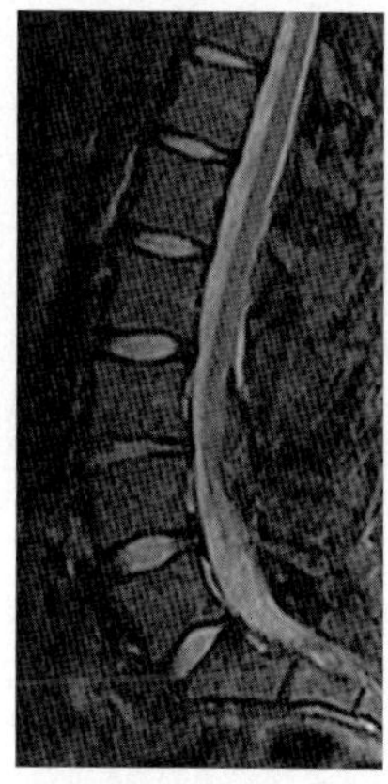

Figure 25.3

Chapter 25 **Lipoma**

Findings

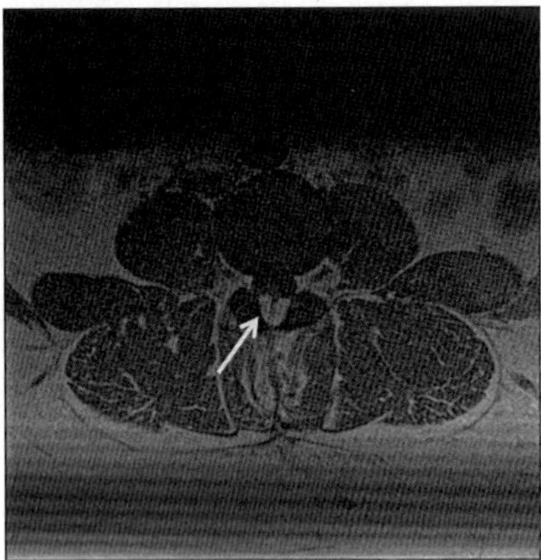

Figure 25.4

Intradural lipoma. An axial T1-weighted MR image (**Figure 25.4**) demonstrates an intrathecal/intradural mass, which shows bright signal identical to fat (arrow).

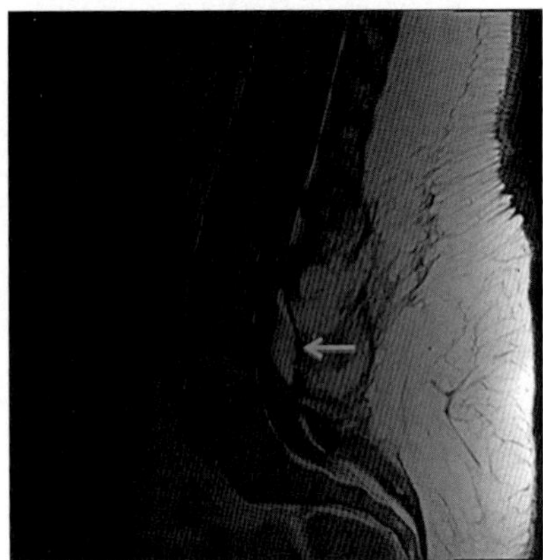

Figure 25.5

A sagittal T1-weighted MR image (**Figure 25.5**) also exhibits fat signal within the lesion (arrow).

A T2-weighted sagittal image with fat saturation (**Figure 25.3**) demonstrates signal drop out of the previously seen mass. This is consistent with a fat-containing lesion.

Differential Diagnosis

► Lipomyelomeningocele
► Lipoma of the terminal filum
► Dermoid

Discussion

Intradural lipomas can be intradural, subpial, or juxtamedullary in location. They are usually seen in the second or third decade of life and are not associated with vertebral and dermal abnormalities. Back pain is a common presenting symptom, as well as neurological signs secondary to mass effect. Radicular pain is not typically seen. In adults, the most common location is the thoracic spine, whereas in children, the most common location is the cervical spine. They tend to be located along the dorsal aspect of the spinal canal.

Radiological Evaluation

CT imaging depicts a lesion with increased fat attenuation within the spinal canal. However, MR imaging is the best diagnostic tool to evaluate spinal lipomas. Intradural lipomas will follow fat signal characteristics on all sequences and will not enhance. Fat-suppressed images are useful. Chemical shift artifact may be seen.

Management

The treatment of choice for an intradural lipoma is surgical resection. These lesions are often difficult to completely excise, but a subtotal resection can produce satisfactory results with adequate surgical decompression.

Teaching Points

▶ Intradural lipomas follow signal characteristics of fat on all sequences.
▶ MR imaging is the best diagnostic tool to evaluate spinal lipomas.

Further Reading

1. Rufener SL, Ibrahim M, Raybaud CA, et al. Congenital spine and spinal cord malformations—pictorial review. AJR Am J Roentgenol 2010;194 (3):S26–37.
2. Osborn AG. *Diagnostic Neuroradiology*. St. Louis, MO: Mosby, 1994.
3. Fujiwara F, Tamaki N, Nagashima T, et al. Intradural spinal lipomas not associated with spinal dysraphism: A report of four cases. Neurosurgery 1995;37(6):1212–1215.

Chapter 26

Anant Krishnan and Richard Silbergleit

History

▶ A 50-year-old woman presents with increasing back pain (**Figures 26.1, 26.2, and 26.3**).

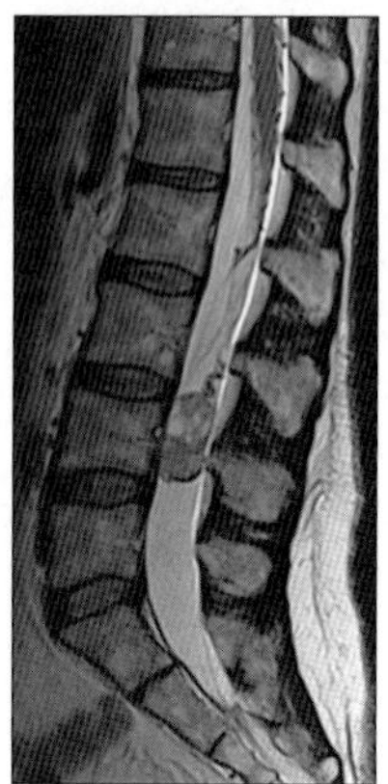

Figure 26.1

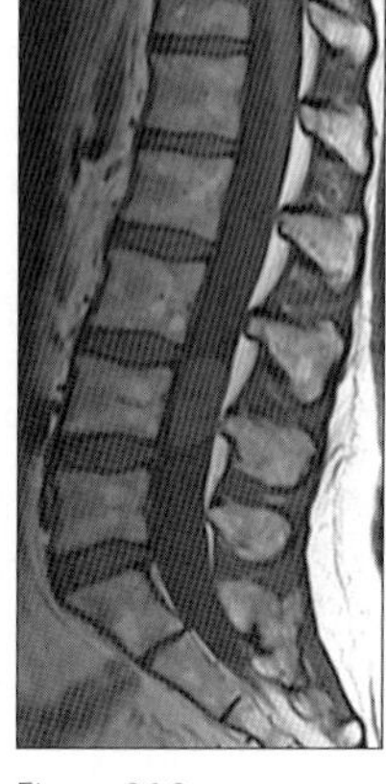

Figure 26.2

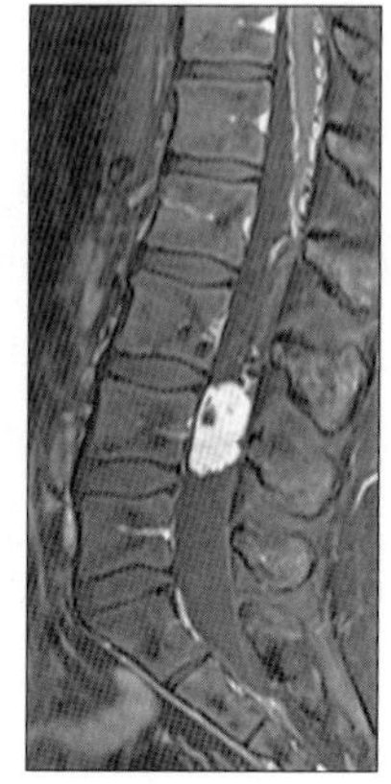

Figure 26.3

Findings

Paraglioma. Sagittal T2-weighted (**Figure 26.4**) and sagittal T1-weighted (**Figure 26.5**) images demonstrate an intradural extramedullary mass in the lower lumbar spine with a slightly heterogeneous T2 signal and isointense (to spinal cord) T1 signal. On closer review, there is a hypointense curved rim along the inferior margin of the mass on the T2WI (short black arrow in Figure 26.4) potentially representing blood. Most strikingly, serpiginous structures are seen extending superior to the mass and surrounding the conus (long white arrows).

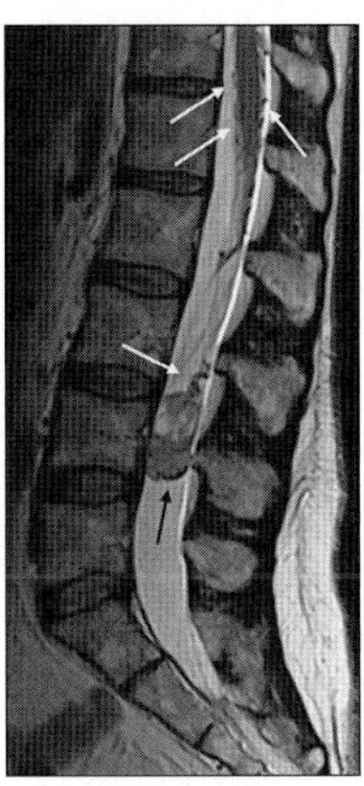

Figure 26.4

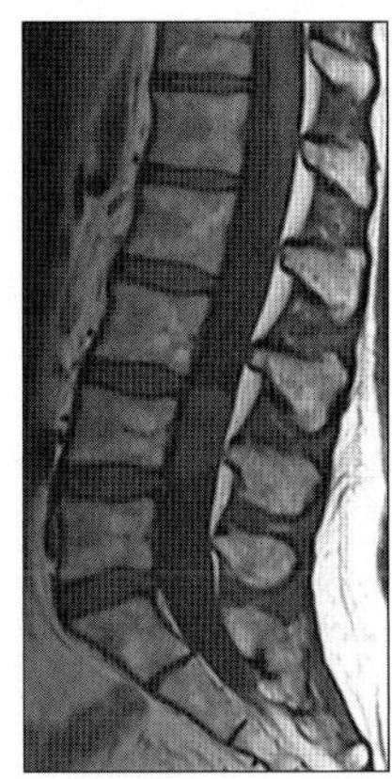

Figure 26.5

A fat-saturated postcontrast T1-weighted image (**Figure 26.6**) demonstrates intense enhancement of the mass with further demonstration of the serpiginous structures, suspicious for prominent vessels (arrows). This combination of findings raises concern for a hypervascular mass or lesion.

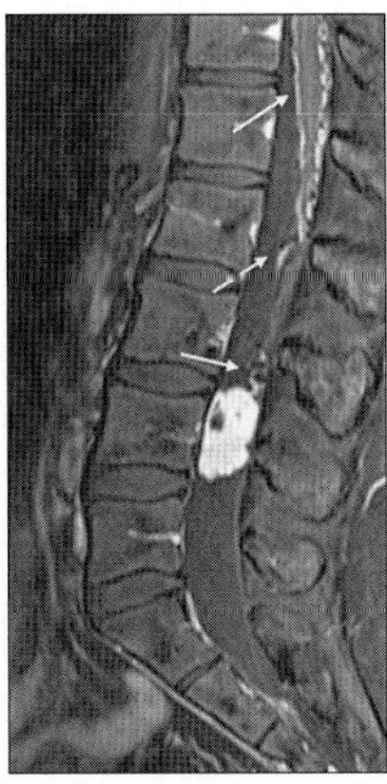

Figure 26.6

Additional Imaging

A sagittal STIR (Short Tau Inversion Recovery) image through the thoracic cord (**Figure 26.7**) and a fat-suppressed postcontrast T1-weighted image (**Figure 26.8**) demonstrate prominent flow voids (long arrows) along the lower aspect of the thoracic spinal cord and corresponding serpiginous enhancement (short arrows) without intracord edema.

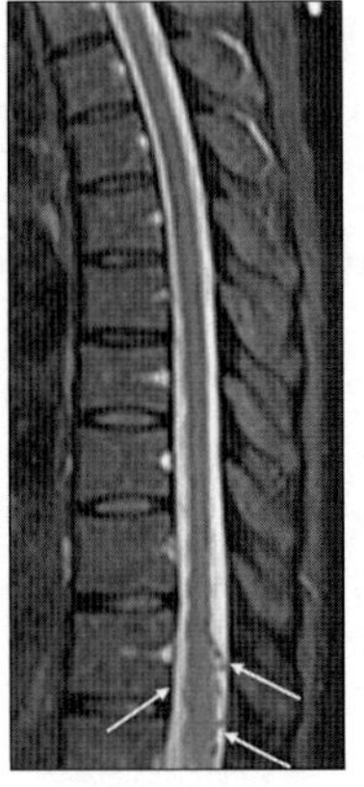 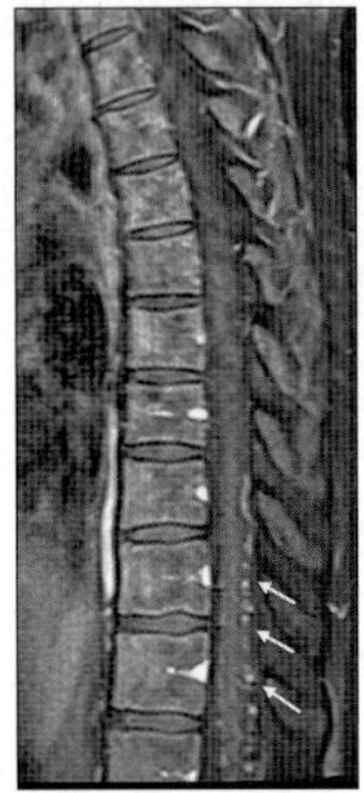

Figure 26.7   Figure 26.8

Differential Diagnoses

Intradural extramedullary mass in the lumbar spine:
- ► Ependymoma (specifically myxopapillary ependymoma), which is sometimes indistinguishable from a paraganglioma
- ► Nerve sheath tumors (most commonly a schwannoma)
- ► Drop lesions including those from intracranial masses, leptomeningeal, and other metastases
- ► Meningiomas (much less common in the lumbar spine compared to the thoracic spine)

Prominent flow voids in the thoracolumbar region:
- ► Dural arteriovenous fistula (AVF) (and other malformations)
- ► Paraganglioma
- ► Myxopapillary ependymoma
- ► Hemangioblastomas (Can be multiple and part of Von Hippel Lindau Syndrome and can present similar to paragangliomas as masses with flow voids. However, they are usually multiple with extensive intramedullary edema.)
- ► Rare: Hemangiopericytoma, solitary fibrous tumor, hypervascular metastases

Discussion

Spinal paragangliomas (which are a subset of extraadrenal paragangliomas) are uncommon tumors, occur most commonly within the filum terminale, and are rarely reported in the cervical or thoracic spine. They can also occur in the vertebrae, epidural soft tissues, and paraspinal regions. Interestingly, while most extraadrenal paragangliomas are of the parasympathetic type, those in the spinal canal are reported to be of the sympathetic type.

Both radiologically and pathologically, the primary differential is the myxopapillary ependymoma. This is a much more common tumor of this region. Microscopic features of paragangliomas include a nesting pattern called "Zellballen," but additional methods such as immunohistochemical staining and electron microscopy may be required in the atypical variants of paragangliomas to distinguish them from ependymomas. Some authors suspect that this histological difficulty in differentiation may have resulted in paragangliomas being underestimated in earlier studies.

Paragangliomas in the lumbar spine primarily present with symptoms of mass effect on neighboring structures including sensory and motor loss, bowel and bladder dysfunction, and lower lumbar pain. The mean duration of symptoms is 48 months. Very rarely do these tumors have secretory effects. Cervical paragangliomas can present with neck and arm pain while spastic gait may be a manifestation of thoracic lesions.

Radiological Evaluation

While some authors believe that the above described imaging features are non specific, certain features are fairly suggestive of a paraganglioma. The mass is often encapsulated and heterogeneous on T2, partly from hemorrhage. This hemorrhage may be detected as a hypointense rim. As in other parts of the body, these tumors are hypervascular, enhance intensely, and can demonstrate flow voids adjacent to them. The classic salt and pepper appearance is, however, not typically seen in these locations. The combination of enhancing intradural mass and adjacent flow voids/prominent vessels should raise the possibility of a paraganglioma. However, ependymomas are much more common lesions, and share some of the imaging features including hemorrhage and occasionally can be hypervascular.

Management

Typically, slow growing tumors are managed with surgical excision. The prognosis is dependent on successful total resection. Up to 10% of these tumors can recur between 4 and 22 years after gross total resection. Patients can present with distant metastases and long-term clinical–radiological follow-up is warranted. A small number may be malignant; among all extraadrenal paragangliomas, malignancy is seen in 6.5%.

Teaching Points

- ▶ An enhancing intradural extramedullary mass in the lumbar spine along the cauda equina with prominent flow voids should raise the possibility of a paraganglioma, though myxopapillary ependymoma (which is overall a more common tumor) should still be the leading differential.
- ▶ In the presence of flow voids in the lumbar spine, evaluation of the thoracic spine should be considered to exclude other common causes such as dural AVF (often associated with intramedullary edema) and multiple hypervascular masses such as hemangioblastomas.

Further Reading

1. Sundgren P, Annertz M, Englund E, et al. Paragangliomas of the spinal canal. Neuroradiology 1999;41(10):788–794.
2. Makhdoomi R, Nayil K, and Santosh V. Primary spinal paragangliomas: A review. Neurosurg Quart 2009;19(3):196–199.
3. Hayes E, Lippa C, and Davidson R. Paragangliomas of the cauda equina. AJNR Am J Neuroradiol 1989;10(Suppl):S45–S47.
4. Aggarwal S, Deck JH, and Kucharczyk W. Neuroendocrine tumor (paraganglioma) of the cauda equina: MR and pathologic findings. AJNR Am J Neuroradiol 1993;14(4):1003–1007.
5. Toyota B, Barr HW, and Ramsay D. Hemodynamic activity associated with a paraganglioma of the cauda equina. Case report. J Neurosurg 1993;79(3):451–455.
6. Shin JY, Lee SM, Hwang MY, et al. MR findings of the spinal paraganglioma: Report of three cases. J Korean Med Sci 2001;16(4):522–526.

Chapter 27

Keith A. Cauley and Christopher G. Filippi

History

► A 41-year-old male presents with Von Hippel–Lindau Syndrome (**Figure 27.1**).

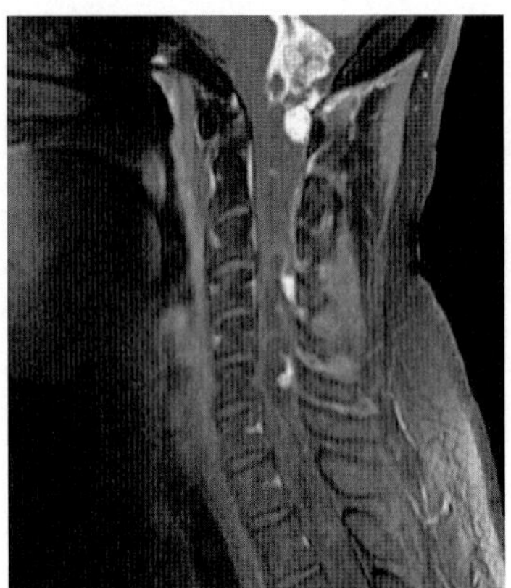

Figure 27.1

Findings

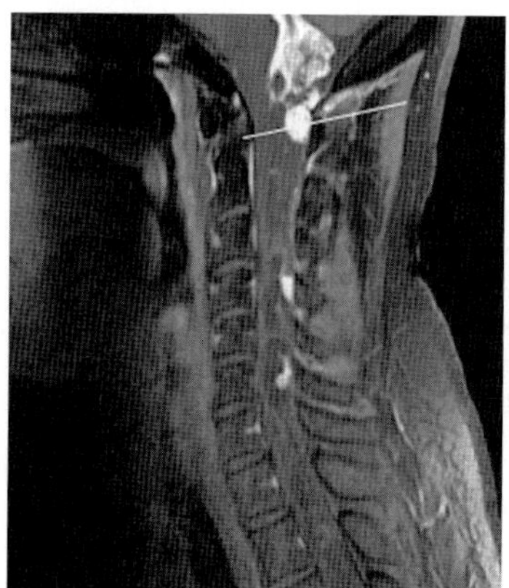

Figure 27.2

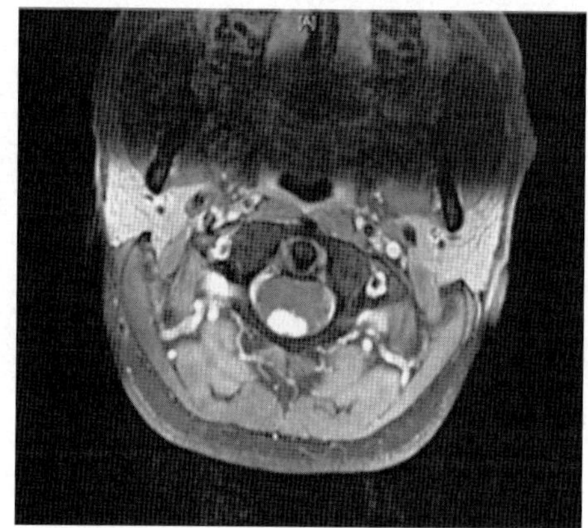

Figure 27.3

Spinal hemangioblastoma (**Figures 27.2 and 27.3**). A sagittal postcontrast T1-weighted MR (Figure 27.2) image shows an enhancing mass in the posterior fossa and brainstem. Additional lesions are seen at C4 and C6 levels. An axial T1-weighted postcontrast image (Figure 27.3) shows a rounded, brightly enhancing intramedullary lesion at the upper C2 level, centered posteriorly with the upper cervical cord.

Differential Diagnosis

Metastasis is the most common posterior fossa mass in a middle-aged or older patient. In children, pilocytic astrocytoma is a leading consideration; glioblastoma multiforme is seen in adults. Ependymoma, medulloblastoma, arteriovenous malformation (AVM), cavernoma, and subacute infarction might all present as enhancing intramedullary lesions.

Discussion

Hemangioblastomas are benign (WHO Grade 1) tumors of vascular origin that can occur in the cerebellum, brainstem and spinal cord. The majority of lesions are confined to the posterior fossa; only 3–13% of lesions are seen in the spinal cord. Symptoms are varied and arise from the mass effect of the tumor on adjacent structures.

Most hemangioblastomas occur as a single lesion; however, multiple lesions are seen in the setting of Von Hippel–Lindau (VHL) disease, a rare autosomal dominant genetic condition. Reports state that 45% of VHL patients develop a hemangioblastoma, and 20% of people with a hemangioblastoma have VHL.

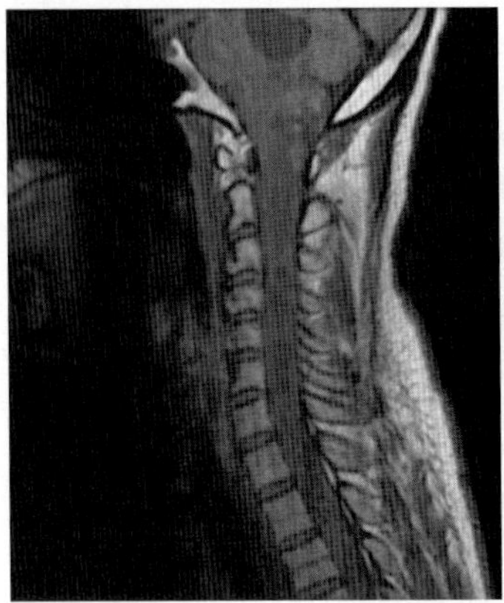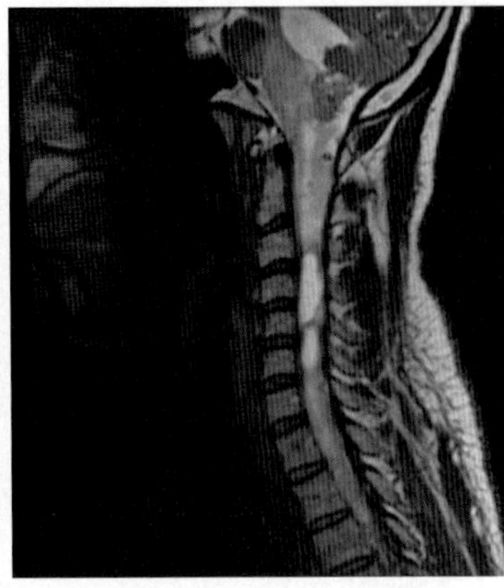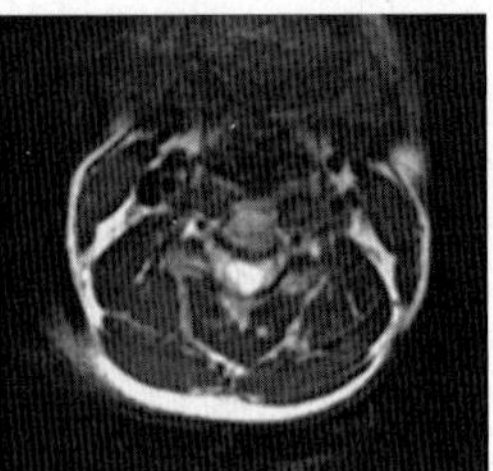

Figure 27.4

Hemangioblastoma causing hydrocephalus and syrinx formation (**Figure 27.4**). Sagittal T1- and T2-weighted images of the cervical spine demonstrate hydrocephalus seen on the sagittal T2 image (middle) and a syrinx seen on sagittal and axial T2 images (middle and right).

Hemangioblastomas typically appear as sharply demarcated masses composed of a cyst with enhancing mural nodule (60% of cases). The remaining 40% of cases are a solid tumor with no cystic cavity.

MRI is most sensitive for the evaluation of a spinal hemangioblastoma. The solid portion of the tumor is hypointense to isointense on T1-weighted images, and enhances brightly with contrast. The mural nodule is typically hyperintense on T2-weighted images. The cyst has signal characteristics similar to cerebrospinal fluid (CSF). Tumors can cause hydrocephalus (Figure 27.4); spinal tumors can also cause syrinx formation. Brain imaging is often performed to look for additional lesions. (**Figures 27.5, 27.6, and 27.7**).

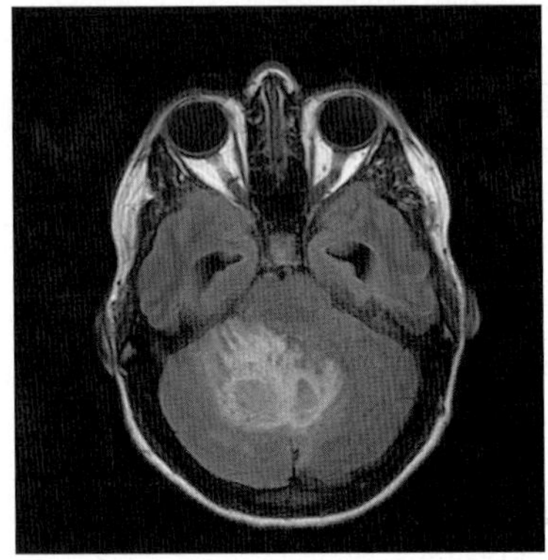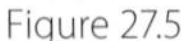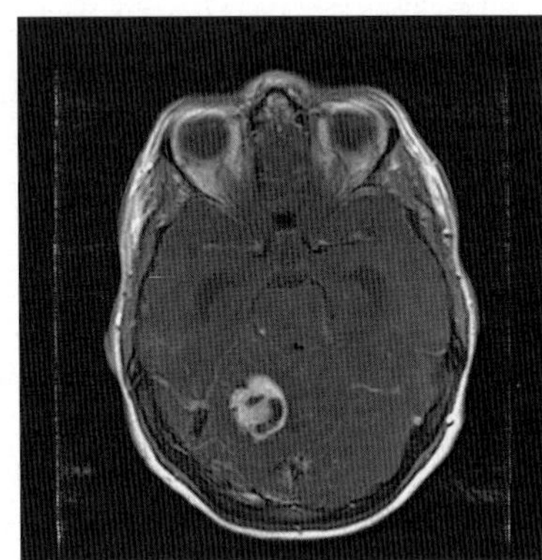

Figure 27.5

Figure 27.6

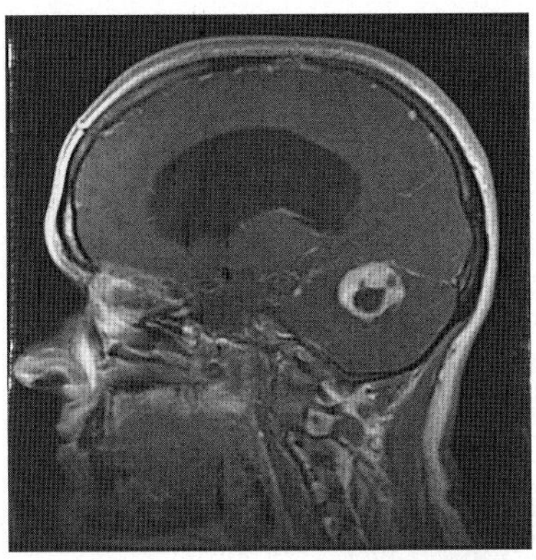

Figure 27.7

Cerebellar hemangioblastoma is seen in a 43-year-old patient with VHL (**Figures 27.5, 27.6, and 27.7**). Axial T2/FLAIR (Figure 27.5) and postcontrast axial (Figure 27.6) and sagittal (Figure 27.7) T1-weighted images demonstrate an enhancing lesion in the right cerebellar fossa with surrounding vasogenic edema. This lesion was a pathologically proven to be a hemangioblastoma.

Management

Hemangioblastomas are typically treated by surgical excision. Tumors recur in 20% of patients. Stereotactic radiosurgery has been used to treat recurrences and control tumor growth. Hydrocephalus or syrinx formation may require decompression. Patients with VHL disease are screened routinely for CNS hemangioblastomas, retinal angiomas, clear-cell renal carcinomas, and pheochromocytomas.

Teaching Points

► Hemangioblastomas are benign tumors of vascular origin typically seen in the posterior fossa and less frequently seen in the spinal cord.
► Hemangioblastomas are seen in association with von Hippel–Lindau disease but are also seen in patients without a genetic condition.
► Tumors are treated surgically; in von Hippel–Lindau disease, the likelihood for recurrence necessitates follow-up imaging.

Further Reading

1. Ho VB, Smirniotopoulos JG, Murphy FM, et al. Radiologic-pathologic correlation: Hemangioblastoma. AJNR Am J Neuroradiol 1992;13(5):1343–1352.
2. Farrukh HM. Cerebellar hemangioblastoma presenting as secondary erythrocytosis and aspiration pneumonia. West J Med 1996;164 (2):169–171.

Chapter 28

Justin Morris Honce

History

► A 49-year-old female with neurofibromatosis type 1 presents with a 1 year history of severe neck pain and bilateral upper extremity and thoracic paresthesias (**Figures 28.1, 28.2, 28.3, and 28.4**).

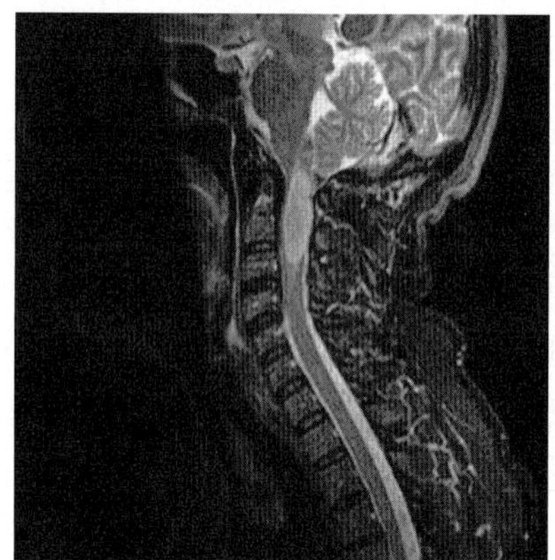

Figure 28.1

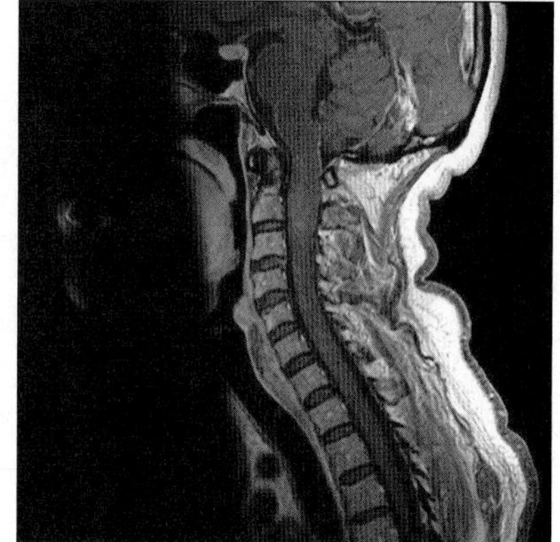

Figure 28.2

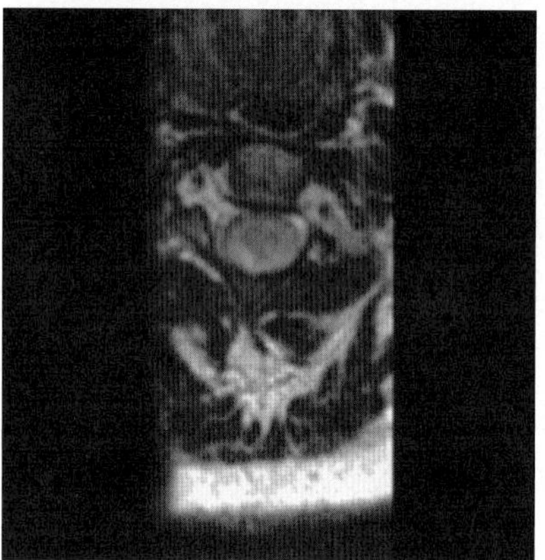

Figure 28.3

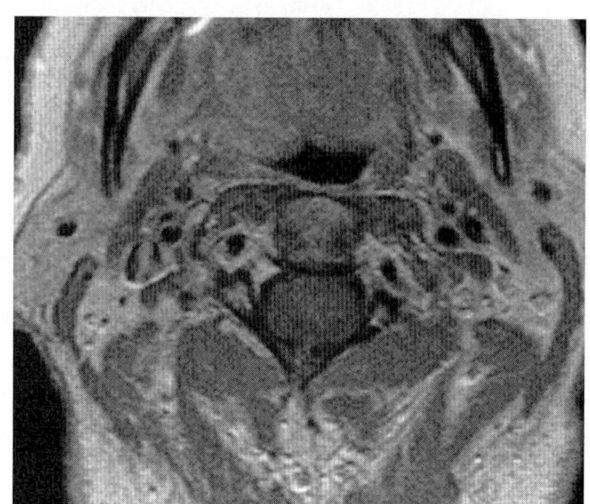

Figure 28.4

Findings

Ganglioglioma. A sagittal STIR image (Figure 28.1) demonstrates an ovoid T2 hyperintense expansile intramedullary mass within the upper cervical cord, spanning from the obex at the cervicomedullary junction to about the C3 level. A postcontrast T1-weighted image (Figure 28.2) shows faint patchy enhancement.

An axial T2-weighted image (Figure 28.3) demonstrates an expansile T2 hyperintense mass within the cord. An axial postcontrast T1-weighted image (Figure 28.4) demonstrates subtle associated enhancement.

Differential Diagnosis

- ▶ Astrocytoma
- ▶ Ependymoma
- ▶ Ganglioglioma
- ▶ Hemangioblastoma
- ▶ Lymphoma

Discussion

Gangliogliomas are WHO grade II rare intramedullary tumors of the spinal cord, accounting for approximately 1% of all spinal cord neoplasms. These tumors contain both neoplastic astrocytes and neurons and are generally slow growing, benign neoplasms with little risk of malignant degeneration. As the name implies, on histopathology these lesions are composed of both differentiated neurons and glial cells.

Gangliogliomas most commonly occur in children and young adults but have been reported in up to the fifth decade of life. In younger patients ganglioglioma is the second most common intramedullary spinal cord tumor (astrocytoma is the most common). The most common presenting symptom is back pain and weakness of the extremities. Paresthesias are also reported. Patients will typically have upper motor neuron signs on neurological examination.

These lesions occur more commonly in the cervical cord, but on occasion are present within the thoracic cord or conus. Long segment involvement of the cord has been reported, commonly involving more than eight vertebral body segments and in some cases involving the entire length of the spinal cord.

Radiological Evaluation

On MR imaging the ganglioglioma is variable. On T1-weighted imaging lesions may appear hypointense, isointense, or hyperintense, but are usually hyperintense on T2-weighted imaging. Enhancement is heterogeneous when present but up to 15% of cases may not enhance at all. Intratumoral hemorrhage is quite uncommon but calcifications are noted (more commonly in children than older patients).

The differential diagnosis of intramedullary spinal cord ganglioglioma is that of an intramedullary spinal cord tumor and includes diagnoses such as astrocytoma, ependymoma, hemangioblastoma, and lymphoma. Ependymomas more commonly have intralesional hemorrhage and calcifications are more frequent in adults than in children. Vascular flow voids in and around a lesion can help distinguish hemangioblastoma from ganglioglioma. Associated scoliosis and osseous remodeling are seen more commonly with ganglioglioma than with these other considerations.

Management

The standard treatment for gangliogliomas of the spinal cord is total surgical resection if possible. The extent of resection is the main factor determining final patient outcome. Progression free survival has been reported to be 67% at 5 years and 48–48% at 10 years with aggressive surgical approaches.

Teaching Points

- ▶ Gangliogliomas are rare intramedullary spinal cord tumors that most commonly occur in the cervical cord, but can involve the thoracic cord or conus.

▶ The extent of the lesion is much larger than for other intramedullary tumors (greater than eight segments) and can on occasion involve the entire spinal cord.

▶ Gangliogliomas are often mistaken for astrocytomas, and at times are diagnosed only after surgery.

▶ Gangliogliomas rarely hemorrhage, but can contain calcium. Up to 15% of lesions will not enhance.

Further Reading

1. Albright L and Byrd RP. Ganglioglioma of the entire spinal cord. Pediatr Neurosurg 1980;6:274–280.
2. Constantini S, Miller DC, Allen JC, et al. Radical excision of intramedullary spinal cord tumors: Surgical morbidity and long-term follow-up evaluation in 164 children and young adults. J Neurosurg: Spine 2000;93(2):183–193.
3. Jallo GI, Freed D, and Epstein FJ. Spinal cord gangliogliomas: A review of 56 patients. J Neuro-Oncol 2004;68(1):71–77.
4. Koeller KK, Rosenblum RS, and MorrisonAL. Neoplasms of the spinal cord and filum terminale: Radiologic-pathologic correlation 1. Radiographics 2000;20(6):1721–1749.
5. Patel U, Pinto RS, Miller DC, et al. MR of spinal cord ganglioglioma. AJNR Am J Neuroradiol 1998;19(5):879–887.
6. Park C-K, Chung C-K, Choe G-Y, et al. Intramedullary spinal cord ganglioglioma: A report of five cases. Acta Neurochirurg 2000;142(5):547–552.
7. Koeller KK, Rosenblum RS, and Morrison AL. Neoplasms of the spinal cord and filum terminale: Radiologic-pathologic correlation 1. Radiographics 2000;20(6):1721–1749.

History

▶ A 51-year-old male presents with mid to lower back pain (**Figures 29.1, 29.2, 29.3, and 29.4**).

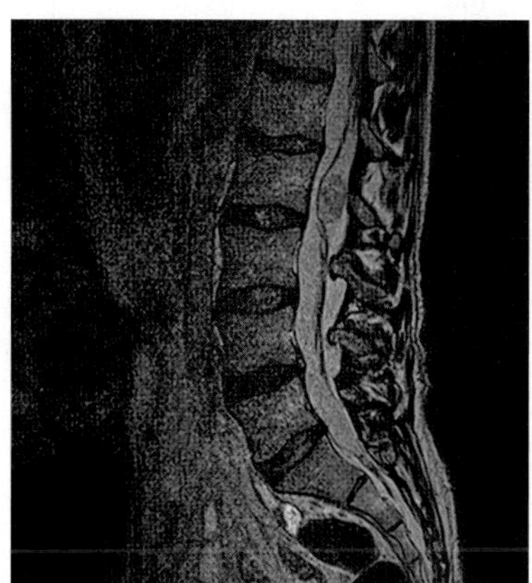

Figure 29.1

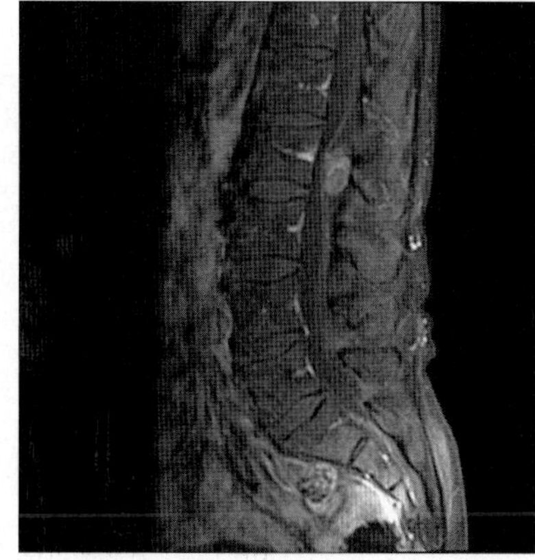

Figure 29.2

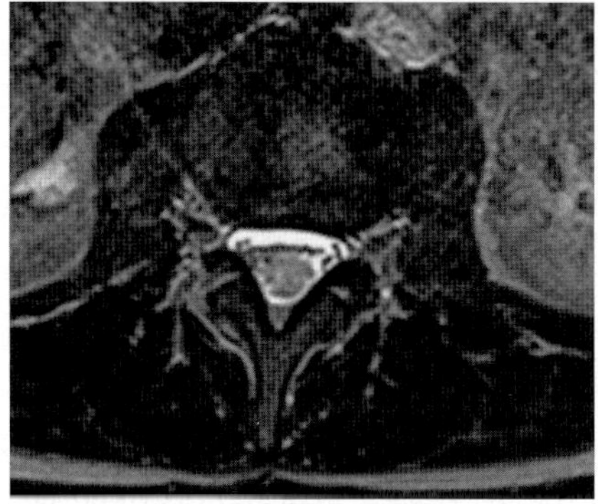

Figure 29.3

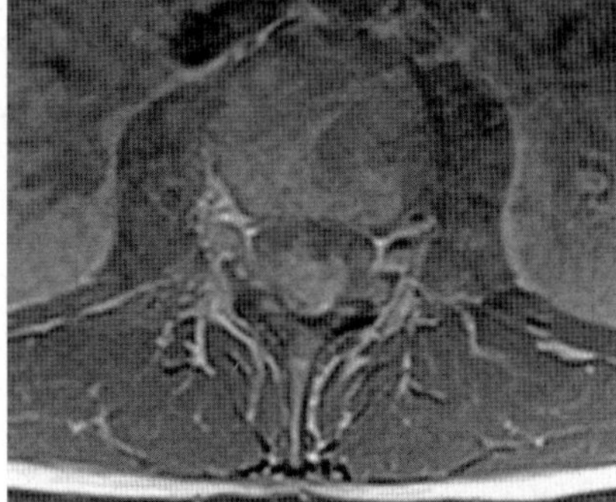

Figure 29.4

Chapter 29 **Myxopapillary Ependymoma**

Findings

Myxopapillary ependymoma (**Figure 29.1, Figure 29.2, Figure 29.3, and Figure 29.4**). A sagittal T2-weighted image (Figure 29.1) demonstrates an ovoid, heterogeneous, apparently intradural extramedullary mass within the spinal canal at the level of L2. The mass is seen displacing several nerve roots of the cauda equina anteriorly. A postcontrast T1-weigthed fat-saturated image (Figure 29.2) shows that the mass is avidly but heterogeneously enhancing.

An axial T2-weighted image (Figure 29.3) demonstrates an intradural, extramedullary mass within the thecal sac, predominantly displacing the nerve roots of the cauda equina anteriorly and laterally. A postcontrast T1-weighted image (Figure 29.4) demonstrates that the mass is enhancing and it does not involve the neural foramina.

Differential Diagnosis

- ▶ Myxopapillary ependymoma
- ▶ Schwannoma
- ▶ Metastases
- ▶ Paraganglioma
- ▶ Meningioma
- ▶ Hemangioblastoma

Discussion

Myxopapillary ependymomas are World Health Organization (WHO) grade 1 neoplasms, typically occurring in the young adult population, most commonly in the fourth decade. Males are affected more frequently that females. They comprise ~13% of all spinal ependymomas. These neoplasms most frequently occur within the lumbosacral region, typically involving the filum terminale and are usually limited to the cauda equina. Infrequently they may extend into the sacrum/coccyx and surrounding tissues extending along nerve roots and rarely they can be found in the brain or other areas of the spinal cord. It is theorized that these tumors arise from neoplastic proliferation of ependymal cell rests within the filum terminale. On microscopic examination they are characterized by an accumulation of mucin in the extracellular spaces around vessels. Despite being ependymal in origin, these tumors are a distinct clinical entity given that they are quite amenable to complete surgical resection, much more so than other intramedullary ependymoma variants.

Patients with myxopapillary ependymoma may present with low back pain, with or without radicular pain along lumbosacral nerve root distributions. A classic symptom is pain that is worse at night or in a recumbent position. As the mass enlarges there is progressive lower extremity weakness and urinary incontinence may develop. Given the slow indolent course of clinical presentation with myxopapillary ependymomas, the average symptom duration approaches 21 months.

Radiological Evaluation

MR imaging is the optimal imaging modality for an evaluation of these patients as it allows direct visualization of the mass and its effect on the conus and cauda equina nerve roots. Evaluation of the relationship of the mass to adjacent structures is of paramount importance as this dictates the degree of resection that can be performed. Myxopapillary ependymomas are typically lobulated, well-circumscribed and typically encapsulated, sausage-shaped tumors. These tumors are usually isointense on T1-weighted imaging, hyperintense on T2-weigthed imaging, and enhance diffusely but heterogeneously. As noted above, internal hemorrhage and calcification can result in substantial heterogeneity of the signal. Rostral or caudal cystic degeneration can also occur. As the mass enlarges there is increasing displacement and eventually compression of adjacent nerve roots of the cauda equine. Eventually the mass may extend into the sacrum or along the lumbosacral nerve roots, mimicking nerve sheath tumors. Given the slow clinical course of the disease, myxopapillary ependymomas can be fairly large at the time of diagnosis, frequently spanning several vertebral body levels.

The differential diagnosis of myxopapillary ependymoma is that of a soft tissue mass within the conus medullaris. Common diagnoses that can mimic myxopapillary ependymoma include schwannoma, metastases, paraganglioma, meningioma, and hemangioblastoma. While it is often quite difficult to differentiate between these various masses, there are some features that can be of use. Schwannomas, as opposed to myxopapillary ependymomas, are typically smaller lesions, enhance more homogeneously, and importantly arise directly from a nerve root rather than from the filum terminale. Intradural metastases are frequently multiple and can present with caking/sugar coating of the nerve roots. Paragangliomas may have a characteristic "salt-and-pepper" appearance on T2 imaging and tortuous flow voids are sometimes seen. Flow voids can also be seen in patients with hemangioblastoma.

Management

Myxopapillary ependymomas are slow growing, encapsulated masses that are amenable to complete surgical excision in most cases. However, it should be noted that local recurrence is not uncommon, especially in those patients in whom complete resection could not be performed. Rarely, metastases within the central nervous system can occur. In general, outcomes are best in patients who have undergone aggressive initial resections to remove as much of the tumor as possible, and in a recently reported patient cohort, the 11.5 year survival rate was 94%. Treatment in patients in whom complete resection cannot be performed may include directed radiotherapy to the operative site. Given the slow growing nature of the mass, there is no convincing evidence that chemotherapeutic regimens are effective.

Teaching Points

► Myxopapillary ependymomas are a prototypically sausage-shaped mass centered within the cauda equina, typically along the filum terminale.
► Given their well-defined appearance, slow growth, and encapsulation they are amenable to aggressive surgical resection, typically complete. Local recurrence can occur, especially in those in whom complete resections cannot be performed.
► Internal hemorrhage and calcification can lead to a heterogeneous signal.

Further Reading

1. Akyurek S, et al. Spinal myxopapillary ependymoma outcomes in patients treated with surgery and radiotherapy at MD Anderson Cancer Center. J Neuro-Oncol 2006;80(2):177–183.
2. Chan HSL, Becker LE, Hoffman HJ, et al. Myxopapillary ependymoma of the filum terminale and cauda equina in childhood: Report of seven cases and review of the literature. Neurosurgery 1984;14(2):204–210.
3. Sato H, Ohmura K, Mizushima M, et al. Myxopapillary ependymoma of the lateral ventricle. Pathol Int 1983;33(5):1017–1025.
4. Sonneland PR, Scheithauer BW, and Onofrio BM. Myxopapillary ependymoma, a clinicopathologic and immunocytochemical study of 77 cases. Cancer 1985;56:883–893.
5. Wippold FJ II, Smirniotopoulos JG, and Moran CJ. MR imaging of myxopapillary ependymoma: Findings and value to determine extent of tumor and its relation to intraspinal structures. AJR Am J Roentgenol 1995;165:1263–1267.
6. Wippold FJ II, Smirniotopoulos JG, and Pilgram TK. Lesions of the cauda equina: A clinical and pathology review from the Armed Forces Institute of Pathology. Clin Neurol Neurosurg 1997;99(4):229–234.

Chapter 30

David Rodriguez, Camilo G. Borrero, and Vikas Agarwal

History

▶ A 66-year-old female presents with mid-thoracic pain, burning, and pressure (**Figures 30.1, 30.2, 30.3, and 30.4**).

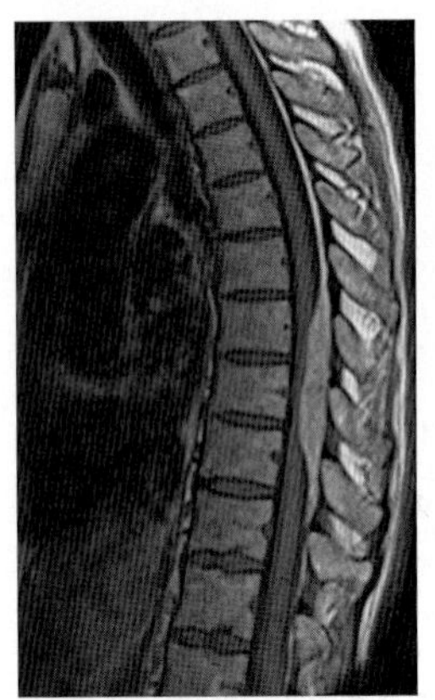

Figure 30.1

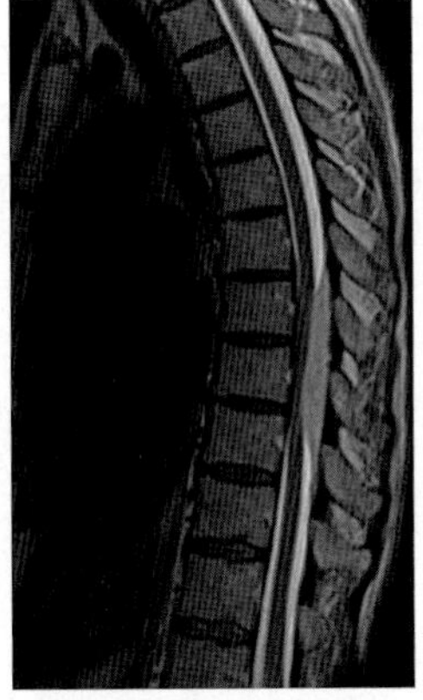

Figure 30.2

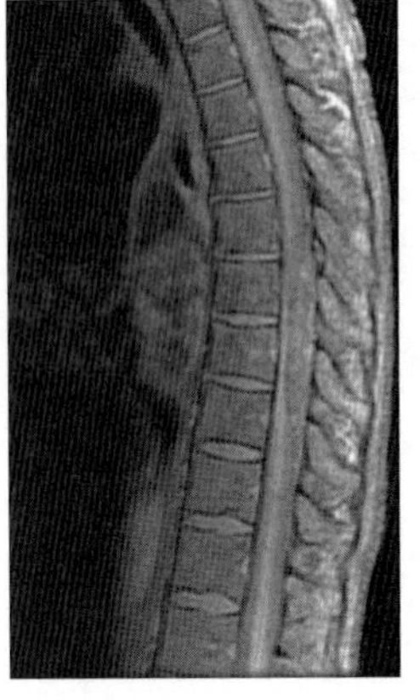

Figure 30.3

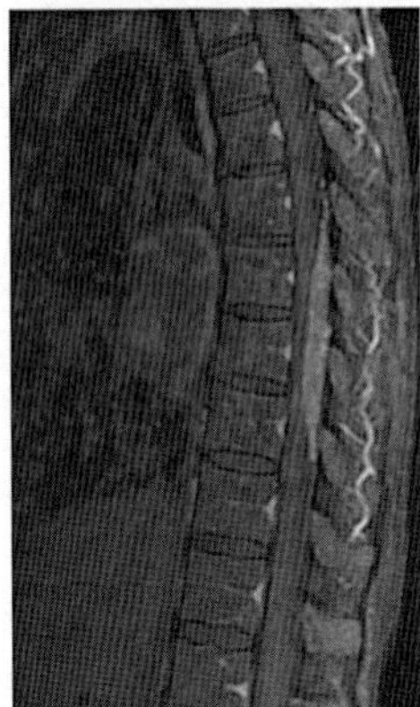

Figure 30.4

Findings

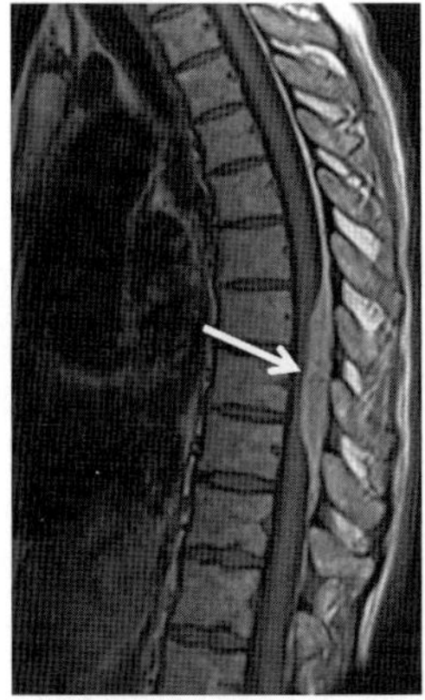

Figure 30.5

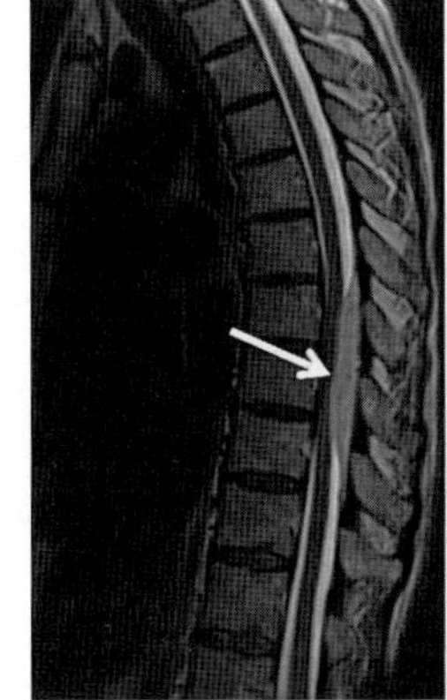

Figure 30.6

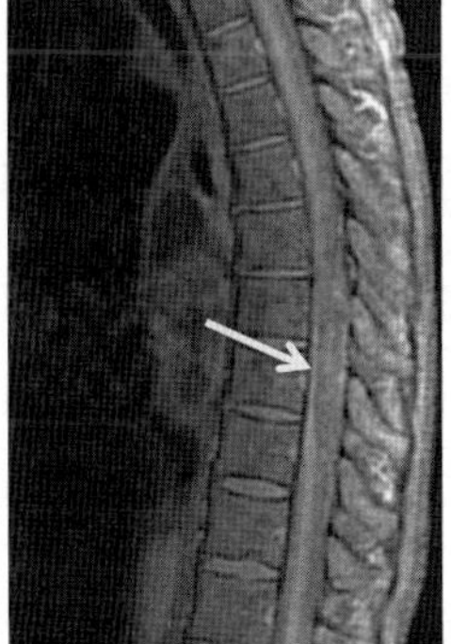

Figure 30.7

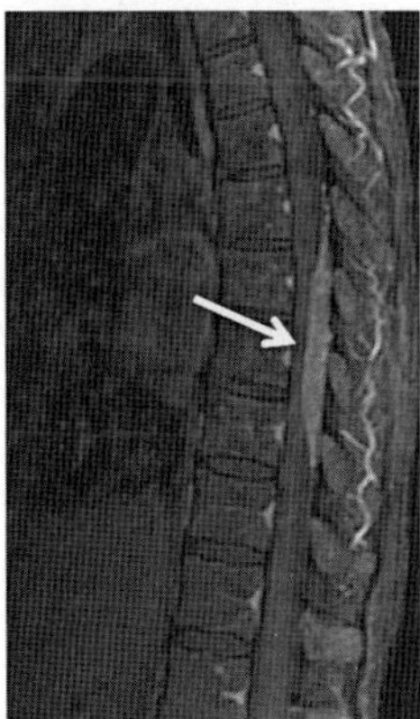

Figure 30.8

Angiolipoma of the thoracic spine. T1- and T2-weighted MR images of the thoracic spine demonstrate a T1 hyperintense (**Figure 30.5**) and mildly T2 hyperintense (**Figure 30.6**) intradural, extramedullary mass. The lipomatous composition of the lesion is evident by loss of signal on T1-weighted images with fat saturation (**Figure 30.7**). The avid enhancement (**Figure 30.8**) and location of the mass allow a specific diagnosis of angiolipoma to be made.

Differential Diagnosis

- ▶ Lipoma
- ▶ Epidural lipomatosis
- ▶ Liposarcoma
- ▶ Hematoma
- ▶ Spinal epidural metastases
- ▶ Neurogenic tumor
- ▶ Meningioma
- ▶ Lymphoma

Discussion

Angiolipoma is an uncommon spinal tumor, but it can be suggested when a predominately fat-containing mass demonstrates avid homogeneous enhancement.

Radiological Evaluation

The approach to a spinal tumor begins with identifying its location within the spine, either epidural, intradural extramedullary, or intramedullary. The tumor's location helps narrow the differential diagnosis, as certain tumors have a predilection for specific locations.

▶ Intramedullary tumors expand the spinal cord.

▶ Intradural extramedullary tumors expand the intradural cerebrospinal fluid (CSF).

▶ Extradural tumors compress the intradural CSF.

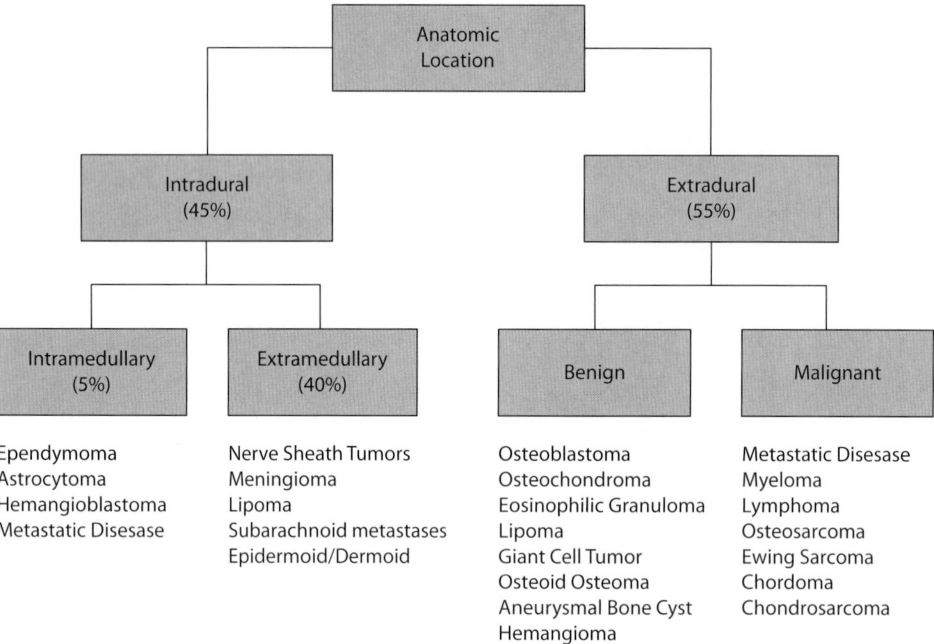

Figure 30.9

The tumor is this case can be identified as arising from the epidural space, as most easily depicted on the T2-weighted sequence (**Figure 30.6**), where the mass effect by the tumor on the CSF can be clearly demonstrated. Once the location of the tumor is identified, a differential diagnosis of the most common tumors in these locations can be given (**Figure 30.9**).

In our case, this extradural spinal tumor does not appear to arise from the spinal vertebrae, and there is no known primary malignancy to suggest metastasis. Thus, less common extradural spinal tumors must be considered in this case. Given the high fat content of the tumor, as evidenced by its bright signal on T1 that suppresses on T1 with fat saturation, a primarily fatty tumor rises to the top of our differential. The most common fatty extradural spinal tumor is a benign lipoma, but such a tumor would not homogeneously enhance as this tumor does. The most likely diagnosis then becomes an angiolipoma, which is a predominantly fatty tumor that homogeneously enhances, and is usually found in the posterior mid-thoracic spine, such as in this case. This patient was taken to surgery for removal of the tumor, with pathological analysis confirming the diagnosis of angiolipoma.

Management

Angiolipomas are benign lesions, but can enlarge and compress neurological structures. When compression results in progressive neurological symptoms, surgical excision is the primary approach to these symptomatic tumors.

Teaching Points

- ▶ The spinal tumor location helps narrow the differential diagnosis.
- ▶ Predominantly fatty tumors have a short differential, with homogeneous enhancement a distinguishing characteristic of angiolipoma.

Further Reading

1. http://www.jefferson.edu/university/jmc/departments/neurosurgery/divisions_programs/spinal_tumors/spine.html
2. Provenzale JM and McLendon RE. Spinal angiolipomas: MR features. Am J Neuroradiol 1996;17:713–719.
3. Gelabert-Gonzalez M and Garcia-Allut A. Spinal extradural angiolipoma: Report of two cases and review of the literature. Eur Spine J 2009;18:324–335.

Chapter 31

Ismail Tawakol Ali, Shamir Rai, Savvas Nicolaou, Shivani Gupta, and Daniel M. Sciubba

History

▶ A 27-year-old female complains of worsening bladder symptoms and numbness in the left leg (**Figures 31.1, 31.2, and 31.3**).

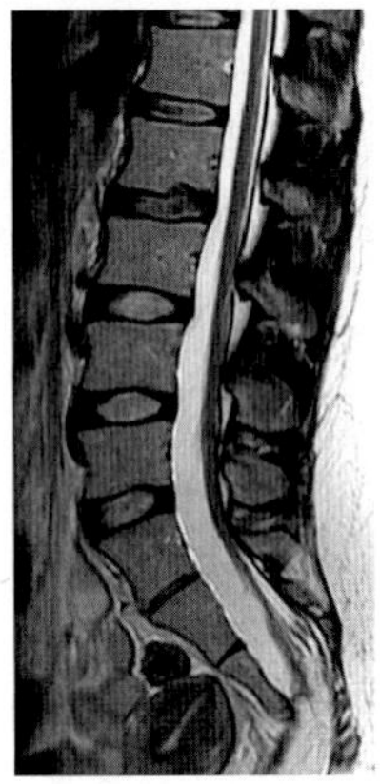

Figure 31.1

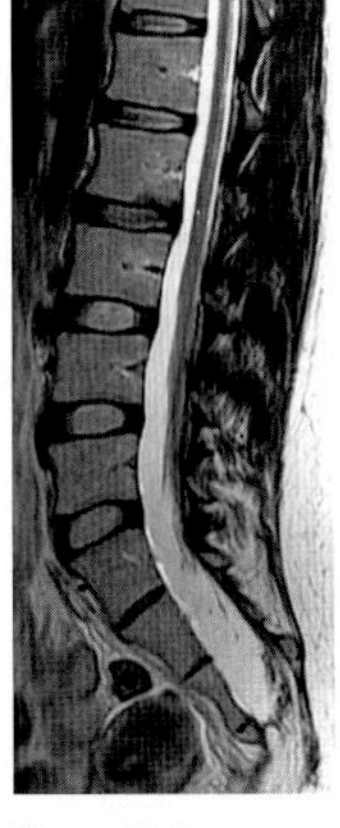

Figure 31.2

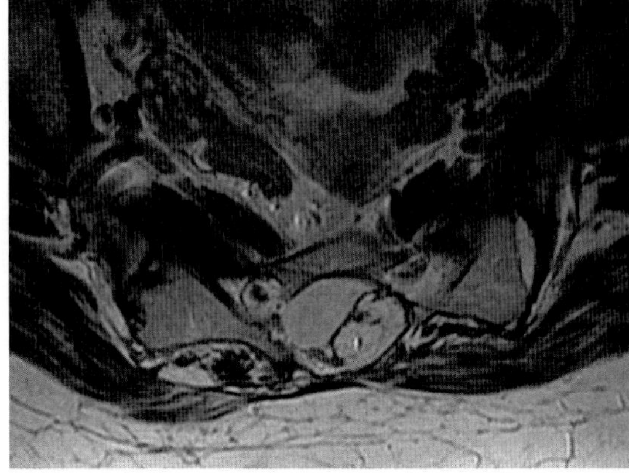

Figure 31.3

Findings

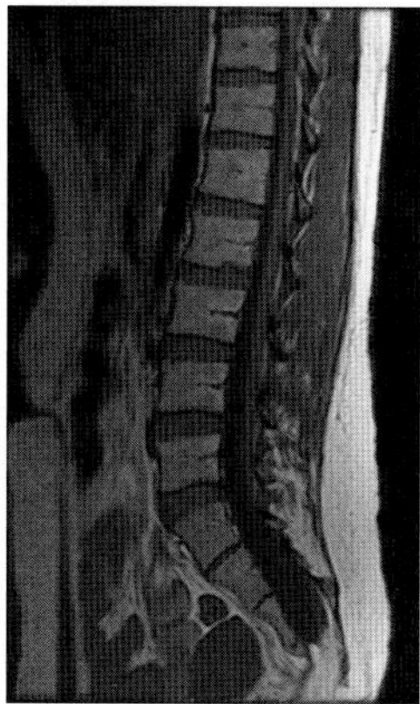
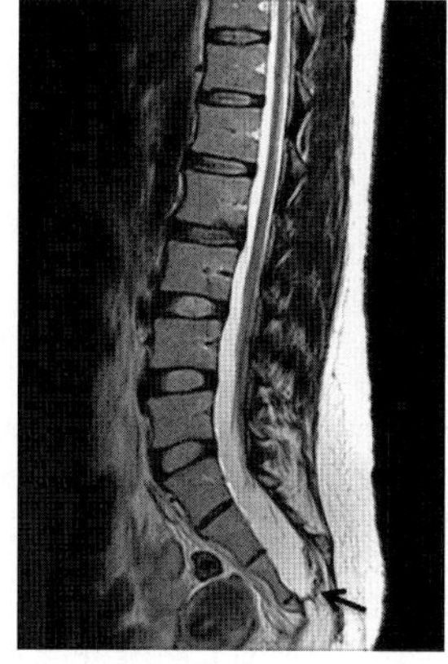
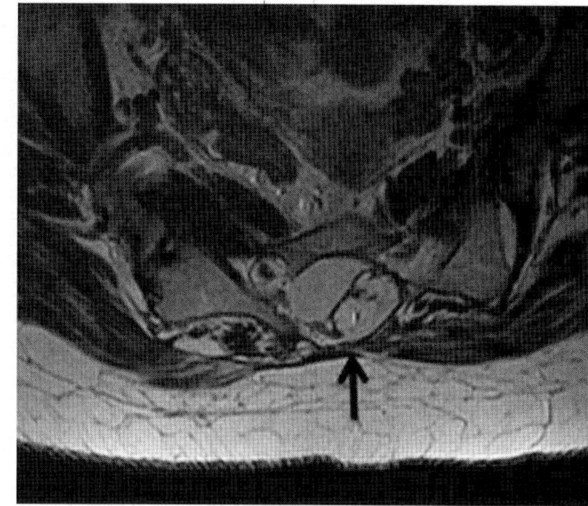

Figure 31.4

Figure 31.5

Figure 31.6

Lipomyelomeningocele (Figures 31.4, 31.5, and 31.6). Sagittal T1 (Figure 31.4) and T2-weighted (Figure 31.5) MR images demonstrate a tethered cord with the conus noted at L5 and the thecal sac noted at the S2–S3 level (black arrow in Figure 31.5). An axial T2 MRI (Figure 31.6) demonstrates distortion of the sacrum to the right side. The left-sided sacral bony elements are poorly formed. A sacral lipomyelomeningocele is present (black arrow).

Differential Diagnosis

▶ Lipomyelocele (the placode–lipoma interface is within the spinal canal as opposed to outside it)
▶ Spinal intradural lipoma (this lesion, discussed elsewhere in the book, is within the spinal canal and is not related to spinal dysraphism)

Discussion

A lipomyelomeningocele is a closed spinal dysraphism. It is made up of a subcutaneous mass (covered by skin) that contains fat, neural tissue, cerebrospinal fluid (CSF), and meninges. Patients typically present with a soft tissue mass just superior to the intergluteal cleft. Other patients present with neurological deterioration secondary to an underlying tethered spinal cord. This entity is a result of premature separation of the neural ectoderm prior to the adequate formation of the neural tube.

Radiological Evaluation

The imaging modality of choice in the evaluation of a lipomyelomeningocele is MRI. A spinal defect is best seen on T2-weighted sagittal images. Through this defect, tissue matching that of fat signal is seen (T1 and T2 hyperintense). The overlying defect is covered by skin. The placode–lipoma interface is outside the spinal canal (whereas it is within the spinal canal in a lipomyelocele). This entity is usually associated with a low-lying spinal cord, often tethered. The size of the canal can be increased, and is often ballooned (whereas in a lipomyelocele, the size of the subarachnoid space ventral to the cord is normal). CT imaging can occasionally play a role, particularly to evaluate the surrounding osseous structures.

Management

Although the lipomatous tissue in a lipomyelomeningocele is abnormal, it is not neoplastic, and thus it cannot be treated with radiation or chemotherapy. Treatment of a lipomyelomeningocele is focused around surgical untethering of neural elements and debulking the lipomatous mass in an effort to ameliorate or stabilize neurological symptoms, which is generally safe and effective. Of note, although surgery may be deemed technically successful, a follow-up MRI often still reveals a low-lying conus and persistence of some lipomatous tissue. Therefore, clinical correlation should always be used as a guide in concert with repeat imaging when considering further surgical debulking.

Teaching Points

- ▶ A lipomyelomeningocele is a closed spinal dysraphism.
- ▶ It is made up of a subcutaneous mass (covered by skin) that contains fat, neural tissue, CSF, and meninges.
- ▶ Look for other associated findings such as a tethered cord and hydromyelia.

Further Reading

1. Sarris CE, Tomei KL, Carmel PW, et al. Lipomyelomeningocele: Pathology, treatment, and outcomes. Neurosurg Focus 2012;33(4):E3.
2. Brophy JD, Sutton LN, Zimmerman RA, et al. Magnetic resonance imaging of lipomyelomeningocele and tethered cord. Neurosurgery 1989;25(3):336–340.
3. Lee SH, Je BK, Kim SB, et al. Adult with sacral lipomyelomeningocele covered by an anomalous bone articulated with iliac bone: Computed tomography and magnetic resonance images. Congenit Anom (Kyoto). 2012;52(2):115–118.
4. Sutton LN. Lipomyelomeningocele. Neurosurg Clin N Am 1995;6(2):325–338.

Rakesh Mannava, Joseph M. Mettenburg, Vikas Agarwal, and Daniel M. Sciubba

History

▶ A 45-year-old female presents with 3 years of slowly progressive numbness in the left hand and both feet (**Figures 32.1, 32.2, and 32.3**).

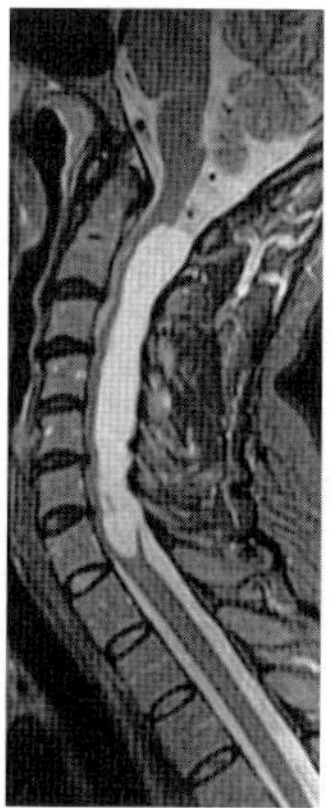

Figure 32.1

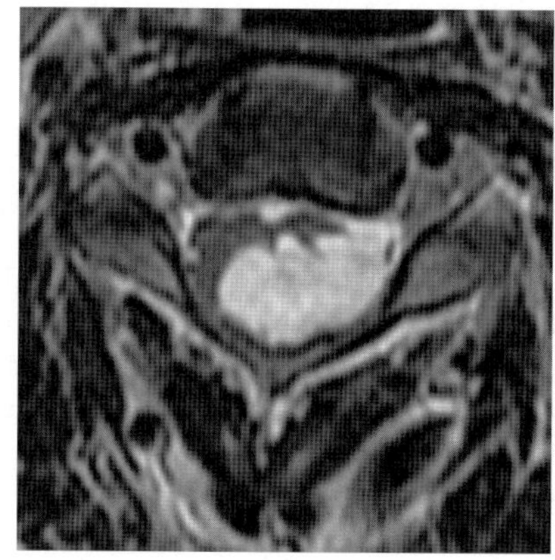

Figure 32.2

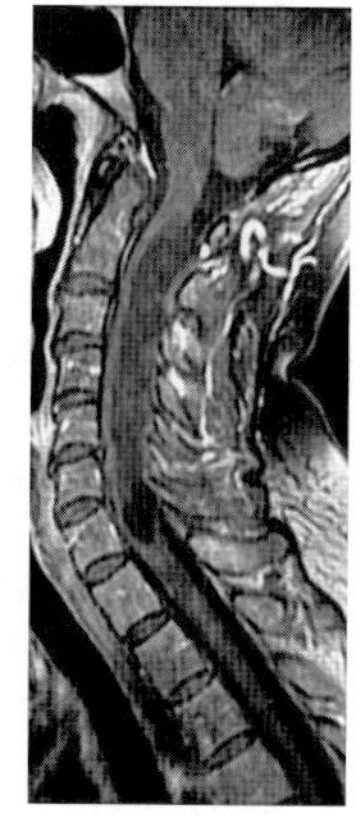

Figure 32.3

Chapter 32 **Spinal Subependymoma**

Findings

Spinal subependymoma (Figures 32.1, 32.2, and 32.3). Sagittal and axial long TR, long TE images (Figures 32.1 and 32.2) show a circumscribed, homogeneous intensity intramedullary mass with prolonged T2 signal eccentrically expanding the cervical cord. A "claw" of normal cord is present along the margins of the mass. Figure 32.3 shows no enhancement of the mass following contrast administration. The signal characteristics of the mass do not follow those of cerebrospinal fluid (CSF).

Differential Diagnosis

► Arachnoid cyst
► Epidermoid cyst
► Spinal ependymoma
► Syrinx

Discussion

Subependymomas are rare tumors more commonly found in an intraventricular location, with a predilection for the inferior fourth ventricle (Figures 32.4 and 32.5). They are slow-growing, WHO grade I tumors that infrequently recur following resection. Spinal subependymomas are exceedingly rare, with less than 50 cases reported in the English literature since their first description in 1954. Most spinal subependymomas are in the cervical spine and are intramedullary, thought to arise from the subependymal lining of the central canal. Spinal subependymomas typically have characteristics similar to their intracranial counterparts.

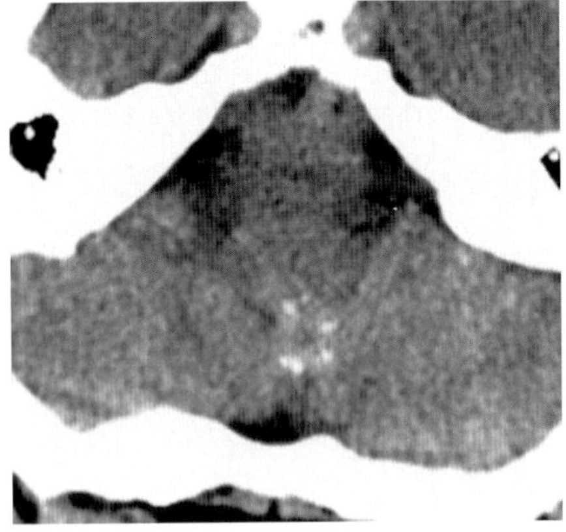

Figure 32.4

Fourth ventricular subependymoma (**Figures 32.4, 32.5, and 32.6**). Partially calcified fourth ventricular subependymoma is seen on axial unenhanced CT (Figure 32.4). Sagittal T1 precontrast and postcontrast (Figures 32.5 and 32.6) images show lack of enhancement of this fourth ventricular subependymoma.

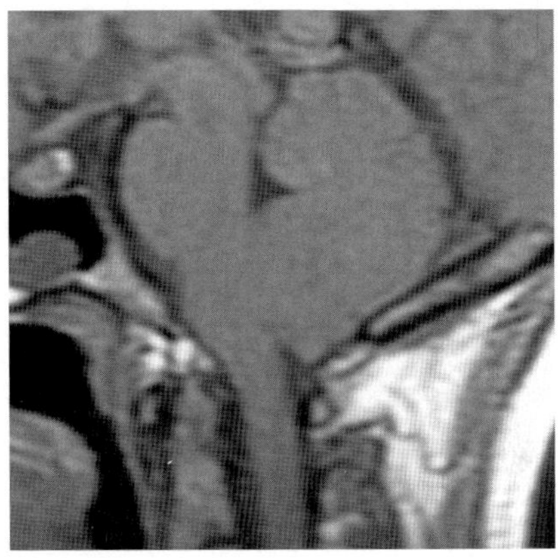
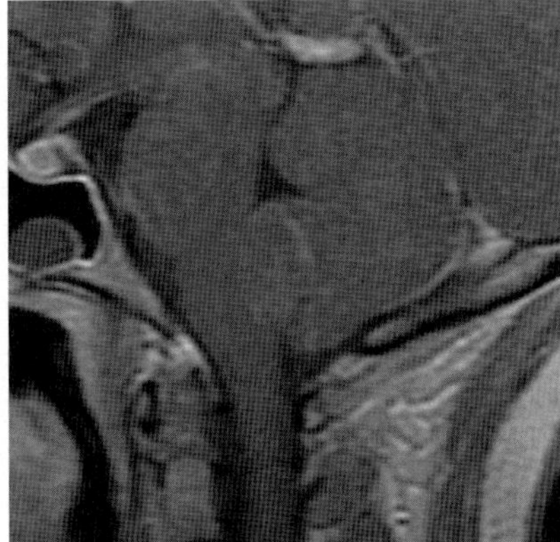

Figure 32.5   Figure 32.6

Radiological Evaluation

Contrast-enhanced MRI is the study of choice for the evaluation of a spinal subependymoma. On T1-weighted imaging, they are most commonly hypointense or isointense to white matter. On T2 imaging they are hyperintense to white matter. They demonstrate no to minimal enhancement. They do not suppress like CSF on FLAIR sequences. The lack of enhancement differentiates subependymoma from other spinal neoplasms such as an ependymoma. The case above (Figure 32.2) shows a "claw" of normal spinal cord surrounding the mass, compatible with an intramedullary location, subsequently proven at surgery.

Management

Spinal subependymomas are slow growing masses that can be considered for surgical resection when symptomatic. Although these lesions may be amenable to gross total resection like other benign intramedullary spinal cord neoplasms (e.g., ependymomas, astrocytomas, hemangioblastomas), these tumors may often have a less discrete border between tumor and normal spinal cord tracts. Therefore, a conservative approach to total resection of these lesions is appropriate given that small residual lesions may be extremely slow growing. Wu et al.[3] found that gross total resection was possible in 9 of 13 patients. In those patients undergoing total resection, there was no recurrence during a mean follow-up of 62 months, and in those with subtotal resection, no increase in residual was found during follow-up. All patients either improved or had no worsening of preoperative clinical presentation. Given the slow growing nature of the mass, there is no convincing evidence that radiation or chemotherapeutic regimens are effective.

Teaching Points

▶ Spinal subependymomas are exceedingly rare, low-grade nonenhancing tumors most frequently found as an intramedullary mass in the cervical spine.

▶ They have low rates of recurrence following resection.

Further Reading

1. Hoeffel C, Boukobza M, Polivka M, et al. MR manifestations of subependymomas. AJNR Am J Neuroradiol 1995;16(10):2121–2129.
2. Krishnan SS, Panigrahi M, Pendyala S, et al. Cervical subependymoma: A rare case report with possible histogenesis. J Neurosci Rural Pract 2012;3(3):366–369.
3. Wu L, Yang T, Deng X, et al. Surgical outcomes in spinal cord subependymomas: An institutional experience. J Neurooncol 2014;116(1):99–106.

Section 3   Degenerative Conditions and Arthropathies

Malisa S. Lester, Michelle Naidich, Ismail Tawakol Ali, and Savvas Nicolaou

History

► A 33-year-old man presents with chronic back pain (**Figures 33.1, 33.2, and 33.3**).

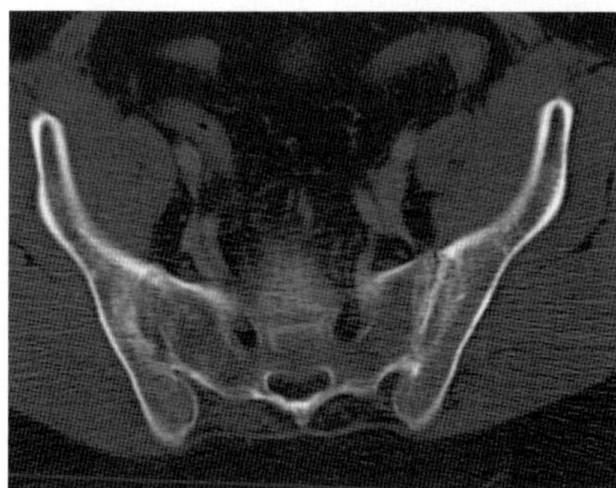

Figure 33.1

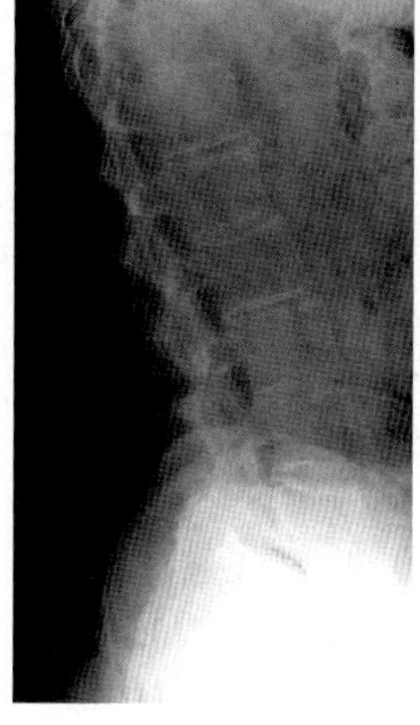

Figure 33.2

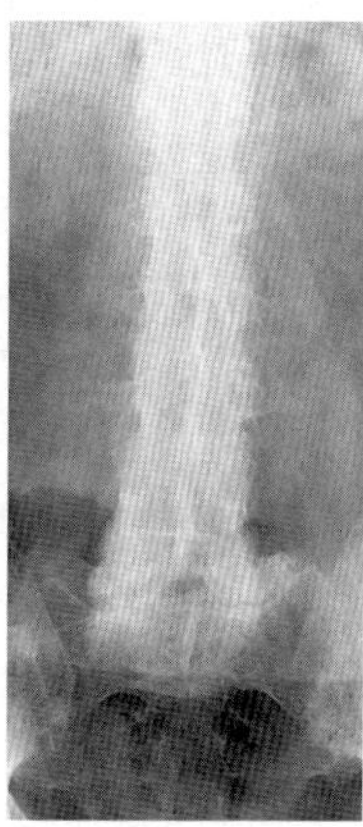

Figure 33.3

Chapter 33 Ankylosing Spondylitis

Findings

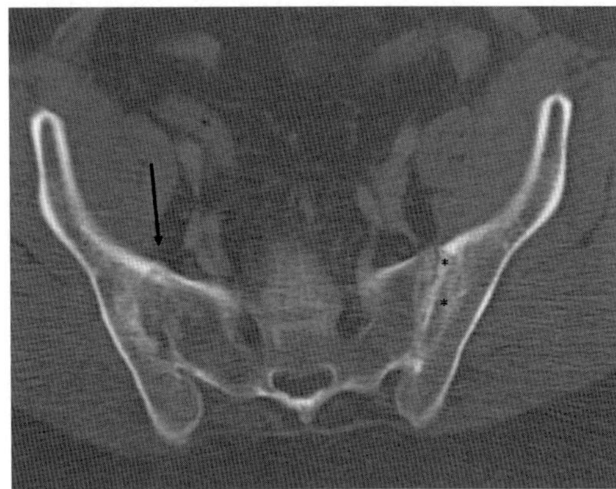

Figure 33.4

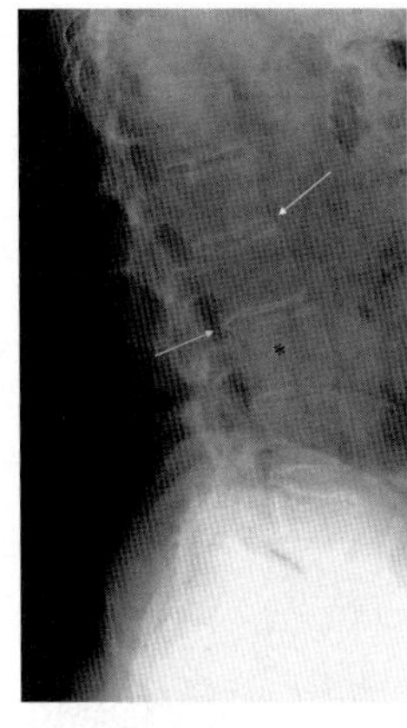

Figure 33.5

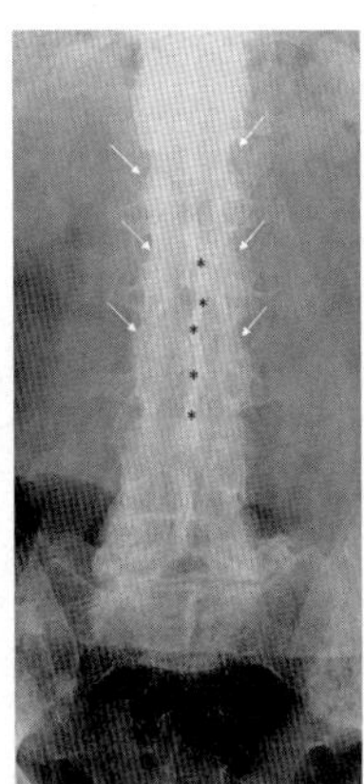

Figure 33.6

Ankylosing spondylitis (**Figures 33.4, 33.5, and 33.6**). An axial CT image through the pelvis (Figure 33.4) demonstrates subchondral sclerosis (asterisks) and the beginning of ankylosis with bony bridges (arrow). A lateral view of a lumbar spine radiograph (Figure 33.5) shows syndesmophyte formation along the anterior (top right arrow) and posterior (bottom left arrow) annulus of the intervertebral disc bridging the vertebral bodies, and squaring of the vertebral margins (asterisk). An anteroposterior (AP) view of a lumbar spine radiograph (Figure 33.6) demonstrates multiple bridging syndesmophytes, ankylosis of the facet joints, and ossification of the interspinous ligaments in combination creating a trolley track (arrows) and a central dagger sign (asterisks).

Differential Diagnosis

▶ Diffuse idiopathic skeletal hypertrophy (DISH)

Discussion

Ankylosing spondylitis is a seronegative spondyloarthropathy associated with HLA-B27. The histological process reflected in imaging is a combination of inflammation, bony repair, and ossification. Sacroiliitis is a hallmark with subsequent involvement of the thoracolumbar spine and lumbosacral spine. Classically, these changes ascend up the axial skeleton to involve the entire spine.

Radiological Evaluation

The radiographic appearance varies with the chronicity of the disease. Ill-defined articular contours, erosions, and pseudodilatation of the joint are early findings of sacroiliitis. Involvement of both sides of the joint is expected. Subsequently, there is reactive bony proliferation with bridging and narrowing of the joint space eventually resulting in complete bony ankylosis. Early spondylitis is reflected by small erosions at the corners of the vertebral bodies with reactive sclerosis, resulting in the "shiny corner sign" or "Romanus lesion." Squaring of the vertebral bodies results from a combination of corner erosions and new periosteal bone formation along the anterior vertebral bodies. Further inflammation leads to syndesmophyte formation, which results from ossification of the outer fibers of the annulus fibrosis that form bony bridges between the inflamed corners of adjacent vertebrae.

Ossification within fibers of the adjacent paravertebral connective tissues, i.e., the posterior interspinous ligaments, links sequential spinous processes into a solid vertebral midline "bone," which appears as a dense line, or "dagger sign". Involvement of the facet joints and costovertebral junctions results in erosions followed by ossification and eventually fusion, and can be seen as the "trolley" or "tram-track sign." Complete fusion of the vertebral bodies by syndesmophytes and related paraspinal ossification results in a "bamboo spine" appearance. Calcification of the intervertebral discs may or may not be present.

These findings are all reflected on conventional radiography. CT may be able to identify the early findings sooner and MR is often useful in established disease to assess for complications related to the disease and to evaluate neurological symptoms.

One differential consideration based on imaging is DISH, in which there is ossification along the anterolateral aspect of at least four consecutive vertebral bodies with intervertebral height loss. However, DISH does not involve the sacroiliac joints and lacks the erosive and sclerotic changes typically seen in AS.

Patients with AS are predisposed to fractures at the thoracolumbar and cervicothoracic junctions, which may be seen as horizontally oriented fractures through an unossified intervertebral disc (**33.7, 33.8, 33.9**). These fractures often represent highly instable patterns and can result in serious neurological injury. Patients may then have subsequent complications due to pseudoarthrosis at the fracture site, with resultant discovertebral destruction and adjacent sclerosis, also known as an "Anderson lesion." This may mimic an infective spondylodiscitis.

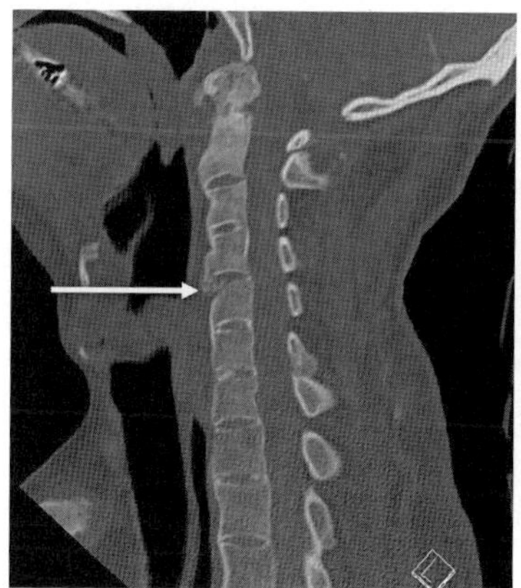

Figure 33.7

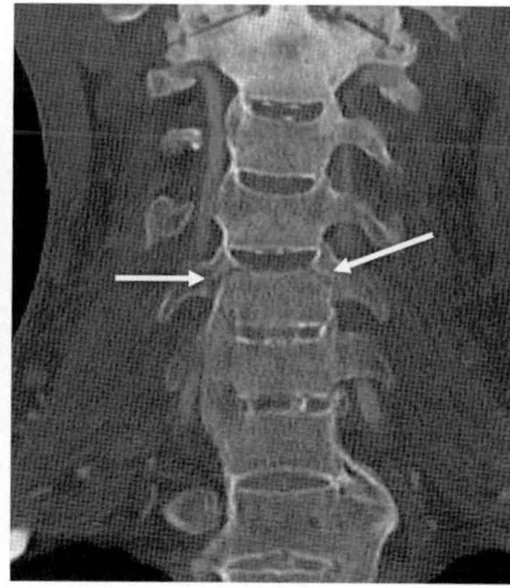

Figure 33.8

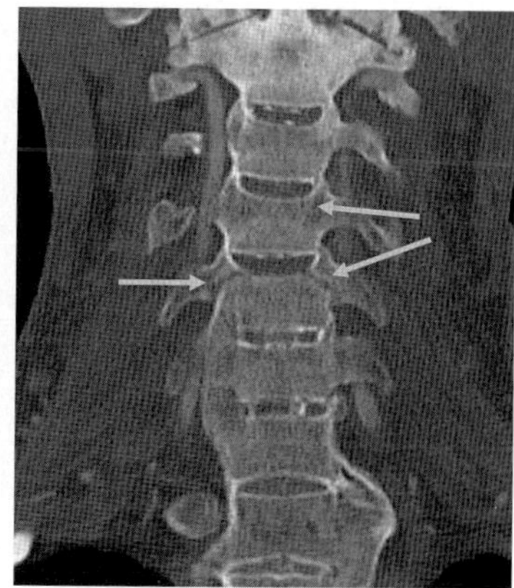

Figure 33.9

Acute trauma in AS (**Figures 33.7, 33.8, 33.9**). Sagittal reformatted CT images of the cervical spine (Figures 33.7 and 33.8), demonstrate the ankylosis with bridging syndesmophytes between the cervical vertebral bodies in this 51-year-old male involved in a motor vehicle accident. A fracture is noted at the anteroinferior aspect of the C4 vertebra and the anterosuperior aspect of the C5 vertebra. This fracture also extends across the C4/C5 disc space with disruption of the disc space as evidenced by the widening of the disc space (arrow, Figure 33.8). Coronal reformatted CT image of the cervical spine for the same patient, (Figure 33.11), demonstrates the ankylosis with bony bridges between the cervical vertebral bodies and the facet joints. A fracture is noted in the posterior elements of the C5 vertebrae (arrows).

Management

Ankylosing spondylitis predisposes patients to unstable, three-column fractures, even from low-energy injuries such as a ground level fall. As the spine becomes progressively ossified, seemingly innocuous fractures will commonly involve all three vertebral columns; furthermore, such fractures are highly unstable because of the large moment arms that act across them. Fractures commonly occur in anatomic areas that are difficult to fully evaluate with plain radiographs, for example, at the cervicothoracic junction and within the thoracic spine. Providers should have a high index of suspicion for three-column injuries in any patient with known ankylosing spondylitis, and a CT scan, in addition to plain films, is the imaging modality of choice. Fractures in patients with ankylosing spondylitis are treated with surgical stabilization using long pedicle screw constructs spanning at least three vertebral segments above and below the fracture. These patients commonly have severe osteoporosis.

Cervicothoracic junctional kyphosis with resultant "chin-on-chest" deformity is relatively unique to patients with ankylosing spondylitis. Sagittal decompensation and an inability to achieve horizontal gaze are the primary indications for surgery. Surgical treatment of these complex deformities frequently includes a posterior-based vertebral column resection and long pedicle screw construct, most commonly at the cervicothoracic junction.

Teaching Points

- ► AS is associated with HLA-B27.
- ► Look for bilateral disease involving the sacroiliac joints.
- ► Patients are at risk for fractures, even in the setting of minimal trauma.

Further Reading

1. Lacout A, Rousselin B, and Pelage JP. CT and MRI of spine and sacroiliac involvement in spondyloarthropathy. AJR 2008;191:1016–1023.
2. Van Goethem J, van de Hauwe L, and Parizel PM. *Spinal Imaging: Diagnostic Imaging of the Spine and Spinal Cord.* Berlin, Germany: Springer, 2007.
3. Naidich TB. *Imaging of the Spine.* Philadelphia, PA: Elsevier, 2011.

Malisa S. Lester, Michelle Naidich, and Gary Shapiro

History

▶ A 52-year-old man presents with a history of low back pain intermittently over 10 years. He is able to work full time as a mechanic without restrictions. He has had physical therapy and epidural steroid injections on several occasions over the years with excellent results.

Over the past 3 months, he has had radiating right leg pain in an S1 nerve root distribution. Physical therapy has been ineffective. He has tried oral steroids, pain medications, nonsteroidal antiinflammatory drugs (NSAIDs), and three epidural steroid injections. He is having difficulty working secondary to the right leg pain. The ratio of leg pain to low back pain is 90:10 (**Figures 34.1 and 34.2**).

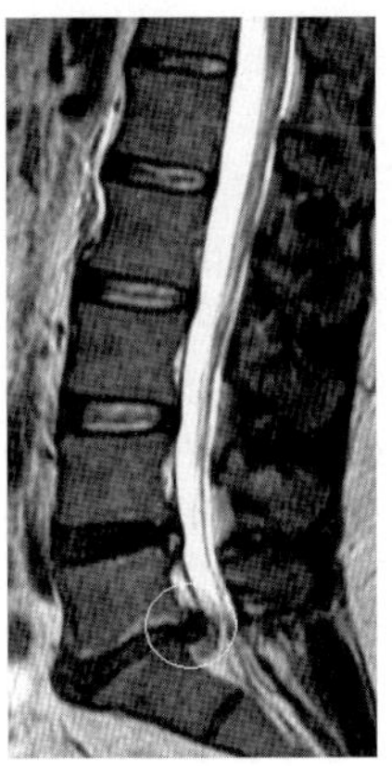

Figure 34.1

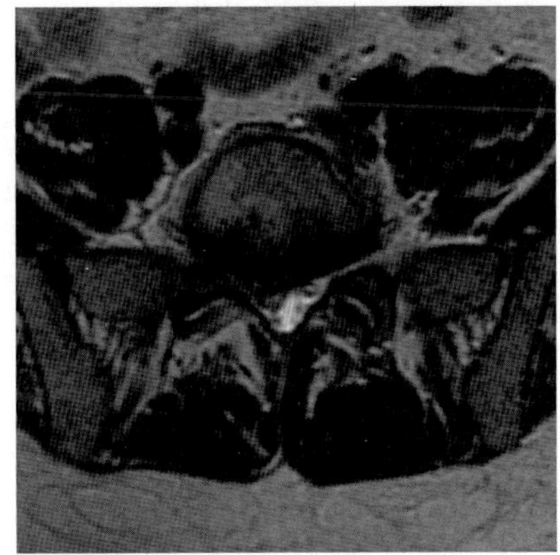

Figure 34.2

Chapter 34 **Disc Herniation, Degenerative Disc Disease, and Modic Changes**

Findings

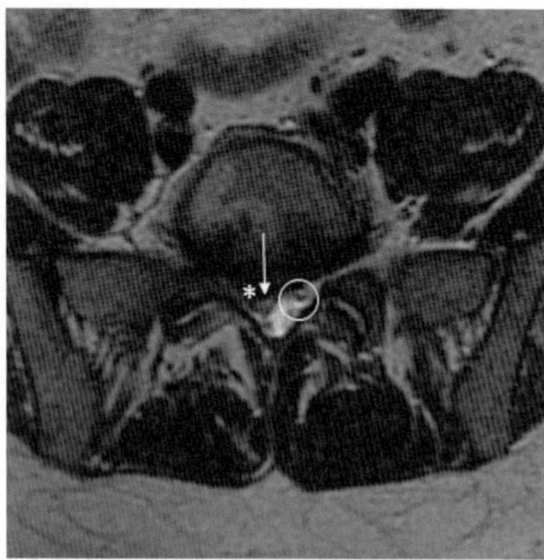

Figure 34.3

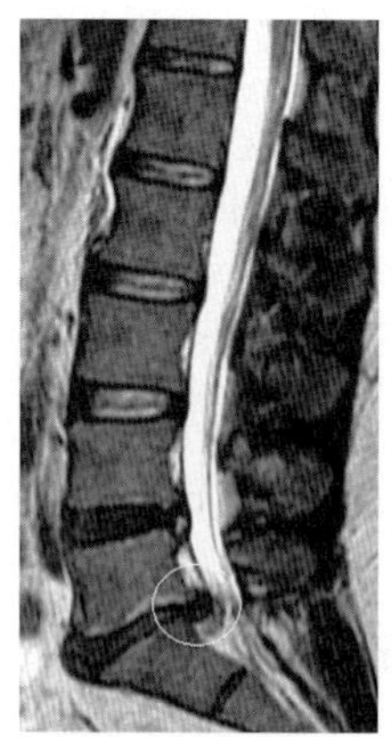

Figure 34.4

Disc degeneration with disc protrusion (Figures 34.3 and 34.4). A sagittal T2-weighted image (Figure 34.2 and Figure 34.3) demonstrates contour abnormality of the intervertebral disc at L5–S1, with posterior extension of the disc beyond the posterior margin of the adjacent vertebral bodies (circled). There is corresponding degenerative disc desiccation and loss of intervertebral disc height. Axial T2-weighted imaging (Figure 34.3 and 34.4) at the L5–S1 level demonstrates the hypointense disc material (arrow) in the right paracentral region protruding posteriorly into the spinal canal and contributing to spinal canal and right subarticular zone stenosis. The disc material compresses the adjacent traversing S1 nerve roots (asterisk). Note the noncompressed left S1 nerve roots (circled).

Differential Diagnosis

Disc degeneration can mimic discitis/osteomyelitis as well as pseudogout.

Discussion

To standardize the nomenclature used in describing degenerative disc disease, a combined task force of the North American Spine Society, American Society of Spine Radiology, and American Society of Neuroradiology created a classification system for describing the imaging findings, as further discussed in the Radiographic Evaluation section.

Radiological Evaluation

Disc Degeneration

On all imaging studies, loss of intervertebral disc height is an early signal of degenerative disc disease. Loss of T2 disc signal on MR imaging is compatible with degenerative disc desiccation. Occasionally, there may be areas of hyperintense T1 signal in the disc reflecting calcium deposition. Very low/absent signal within the disc on T1- and T2-weighted imaging is secondary to gas in the degenerating disc, known as "vacuum disc phenomenon".

Modic Changes

Modic first described the MR appearance of degenerative stages of the vertebral body endplates, which reflect the underlying histopathological changes (**Figures 34. 5, 34.6, 34.7, 34.8, 34.9, 34.10, and 34.11**). Modic

Type 1 represents marrow edema related to acute/subacute inflammation. Modic Type 2 reflects replacement of the normal bone marrow by fat. Modic Type 3 changes represent sclerosis of the adjacent endplates. Overall, Modic Type 2 is most commonly imaged, and Modic Type 3 changes are relatively rare. The clinical significance of these changes is uncertain.

The low signal on T1 and T2 hyperintense signal with the vertebral body endplates in Modic Type 1 changes reflects inflammation and bone marrow edema. Fatty marrow replacement of Modic Type 2 appears as a high signal intensity on both T1- and T2-weighted images. Sclerotic changes in Modic Type 3 result in a hypointense signal on T1- and T2-weighted images.

Osteomyelitis may have an appearance similar to the acute edematous changes seen with Modic Type 1. However, inflammatory changes within the adjacent intervertebral disk (discitis) and/or surrounding paraspinal soft tissues, as well as the appropriate clinical setting, will help make the clinical distinction.

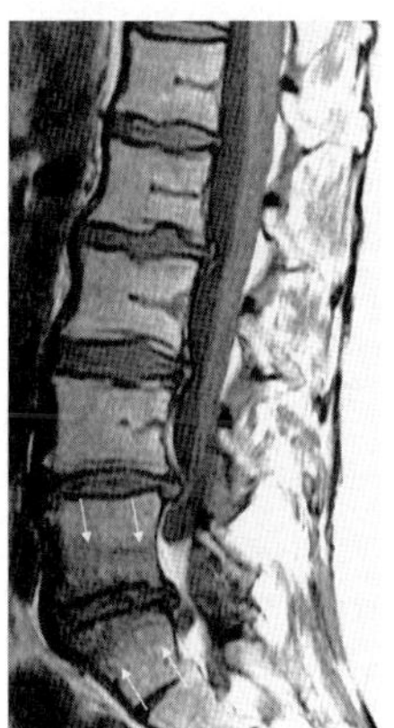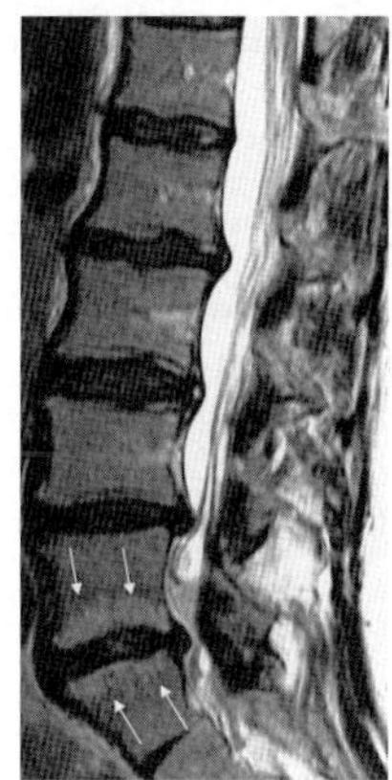

Figure 34.5   Figure 34.6

Modic Type 1 changes (**Figures 34.5 and 34.6**). Sagittal T1-weighted (Figure 34.5) and T2-weighted (Figure 34.6) images show low T1 and hyperintense T2 signal intensity along the adjacent vertebral body endplates at L5–S1 (arrows). The intervening disc demonstrates degenerative disc desiccation and loss of disc height.

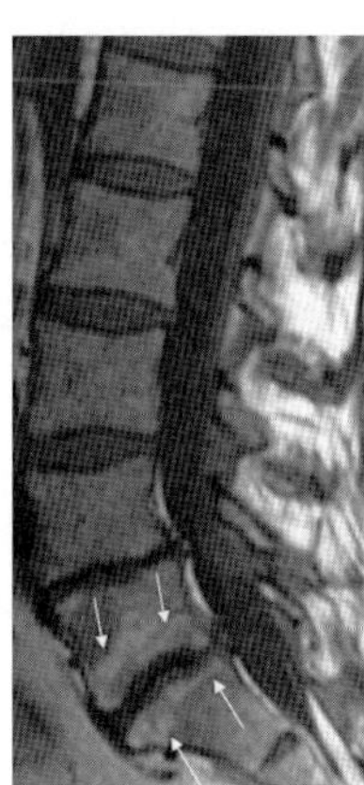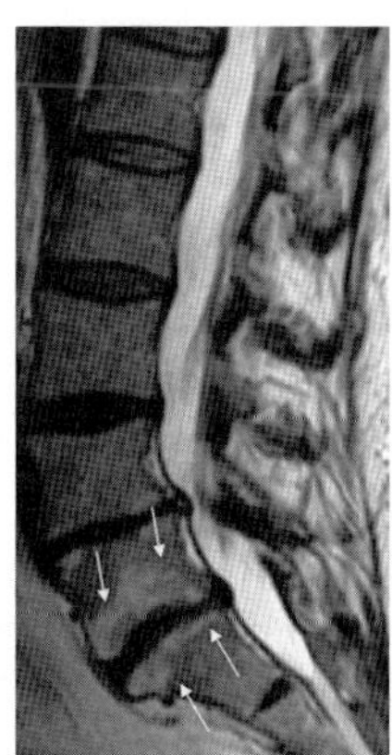

Figure 34.7   Figure 34.8

Modic Type 2 changes (**Figures 34.7 and 34.8**). Sagittal T1-weighted (Figure 34.7) and T2-weighted (Figure 34.8) images show hyperintense T1 and T2 signal (arrows) along the adjacent vertebral body endplates at L5–S1. The intervening disc demonstrates degenerative disc desiccation and loss of disc height.

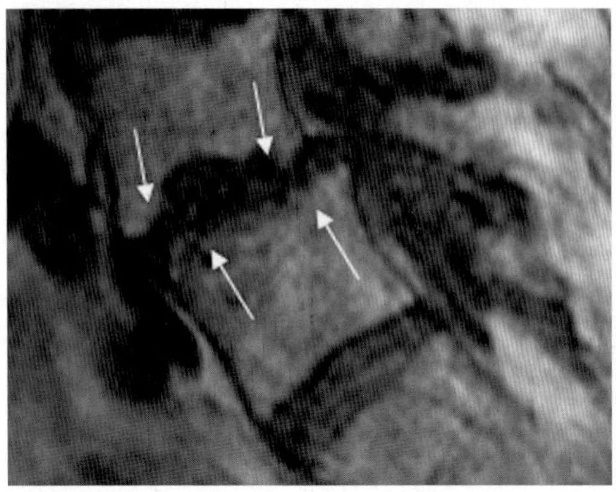

Figure 34.9

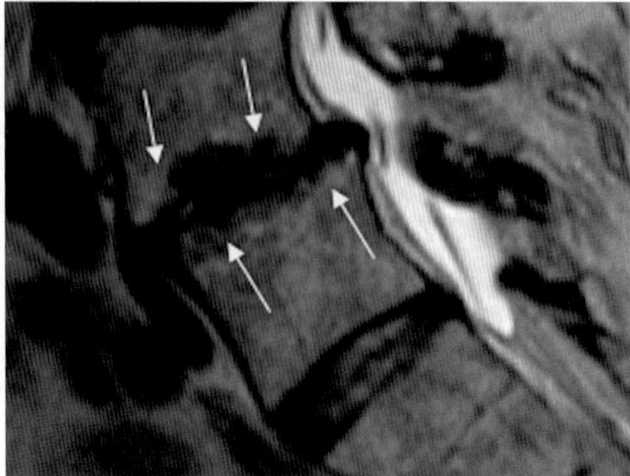

Figure 34.10

Modic Type 3 changes (**Figures 34.9 and 34.10**). Sagittal T1-weighted (Figure 34.9) and T2-weighted (Figure 34.10) images show hypointense T1 and T2 signal along the adjacent vertebral body endplates at L5–S1. The intervening disc demonstrates degenerative disc desiccation and loss of disc height.

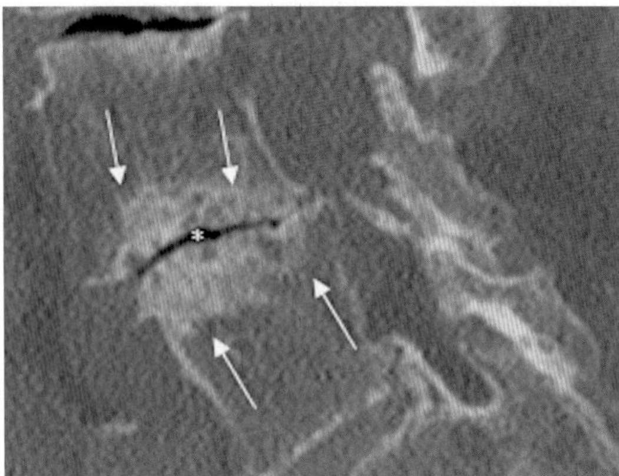

Figure 34.11

Modic Type 3 changes on CT (**Figure 34.11**). The sagittal CT image shows corresponding sclerosis along the adjacent vertebral body endplates at L5–S1. The intervening disc demonstrates advanced degenerative disc desiccation and vacuum disc phenomenon (asterisk).

Disc Herniation

A disc bulge is defined as circumferential disc displacement involving 50% or more of the disc circumference, extending beyond the posterior margins of the adjacent vertebral bodies. Bulging can be symmetrical or asymmetrical, particularly in the setting of superimposed scoliosis.

What is classically thought of as a herniated disc can more accurately be described as a disc protrusion or disc extrusion. A protruded disc is reported when the base of the displaced disc material is greater than the apex, i.e., there is a greater diameter at the base than at any other region (**Figures 34.3 and 33.4**). The location of the protrusion in the axial plane can be described as central, right/left paracentral, right/left foraminal, or right/left far lateral. In an extrusion, the base of the displaced disc material is narrower than the apex, i.e., the broadest diameter of the herniation lies away from the underlying disc rather than at the base of the herniation. Often the extruded disc material migrates in the craniocaudal direction. If the disc material is no longer contiguous with the parent disc, it is referred to as a "free" or "sequestered" fragment (**Figures 34.12, 34.13, 34.14, and 34.15**). The location of the disc protrusion/extrusion is important not only as a predicator of nerve root impingement, but also as a guide to the surgical approach when necessary.

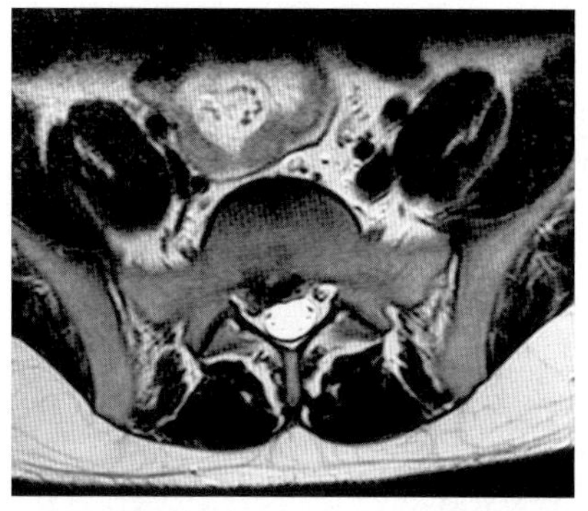

Figure 34.12

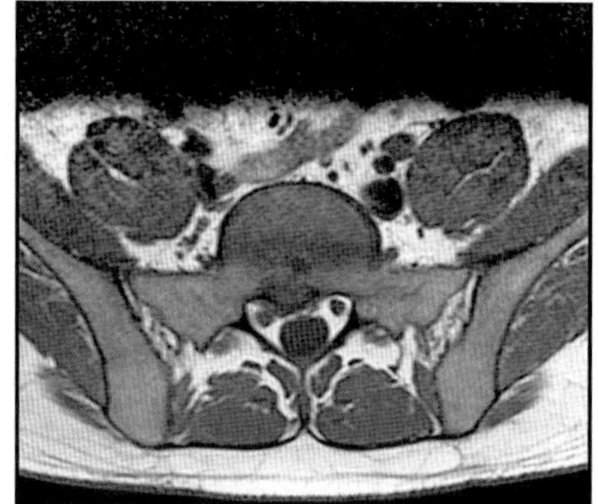

Figure 34.13

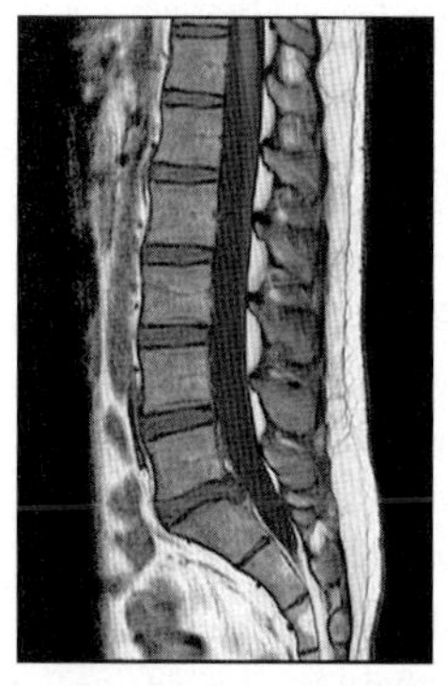

Figure 34.14

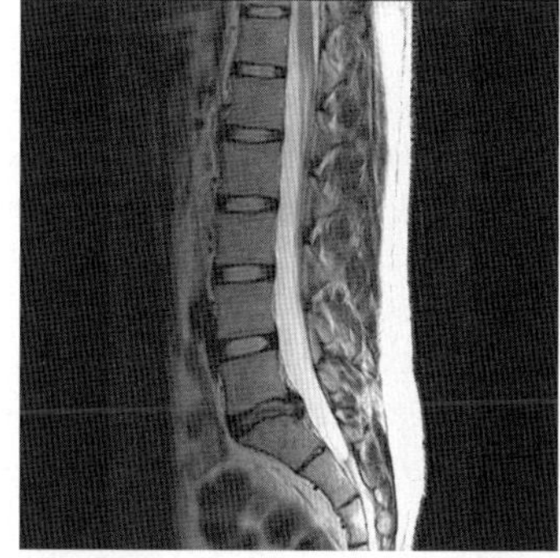

Figure 34.15

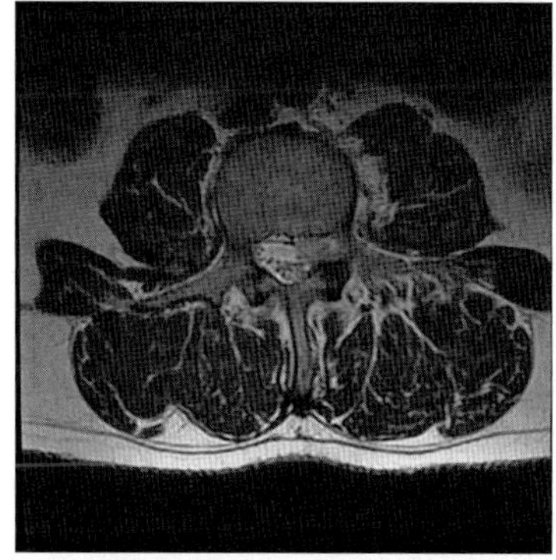

Figure 34.16

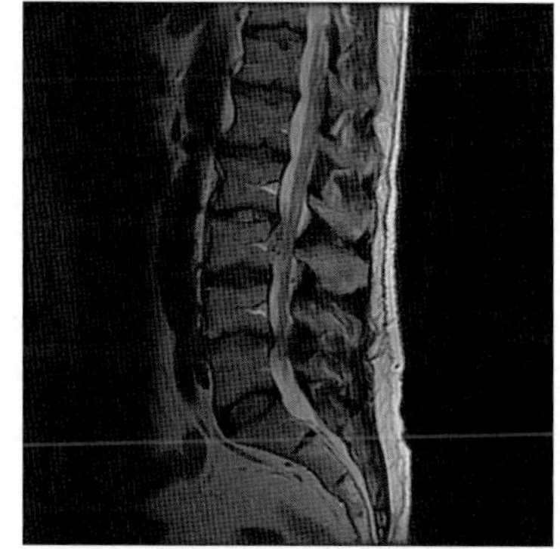

Figure 34.17

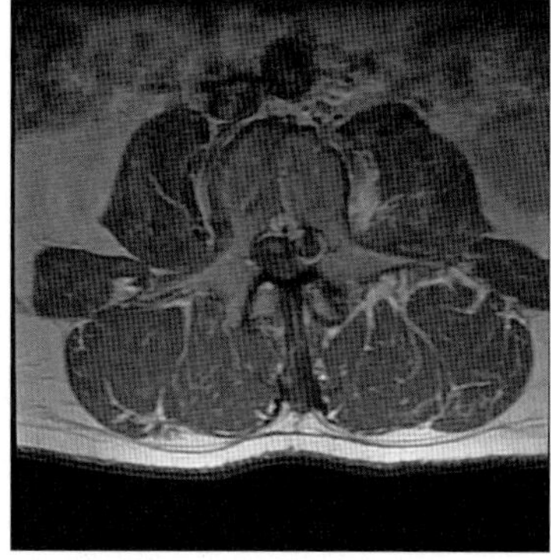

Figure 34.18

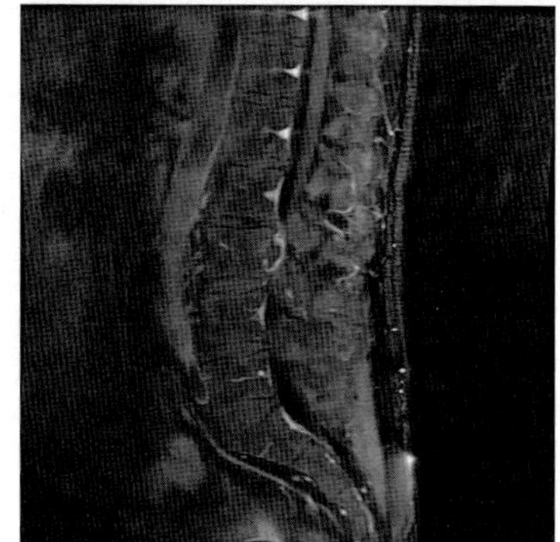

Figure 34.19

Sequestered disc fragment (**Figures 34.11, 34.12, 34.13, and 34.14**). Axial (Figure 34.11) and sagittal (Figure 34.12) T2-weighted images of the lumbar spine demonstrate a well-circumscribed extramedullary lesion in the spinal canal, posterior to the L3 vertebral body, in a left paracentral location (white arrows). Axial T1-weighted (Figure 34.13) and sagittal fat saturated T1-weighted (Figure 34.14) postcontrast images demonstrate enhancement surrounding the lesion, but not within it. Differential possibilities include a cystic schwannoma or sequestered disc. At surgery, this was consistent with a sequestered disc.

Management

Patients with radiculopathy secondary to a herniated disc are managed conservatively with physical therapy, medications, and epidural steroid injections for a period of 6 weeks to 3 months. Common medications prescribed by physicians include NSAIDs, pain medications, a brief course of oral steroids, and muscle relaxants. Pain management physicians may prescribe antidepressants, i.e., Cymbalta, and antiseizure medications, i.e., Lyrica and Neurontin.

Microsurgery is indicated in cases refractory to conservative management. It is also indicated with a progressive neurological deficit, intractable pain, and cauda equina syndrome. Surgery is performed under general anesthesia, with an excision of the herniated disc fragment. Most surgeries are ambulatory or a single night hospital stay. Clinical series have documented a 90% rate of good/excellent results.

Patients with degenerative disc disease are managed conservatively, similar to cases of radiculopathy. Pain management is a useful resource for patients trying to avoid surgery. Fusion surgery is indicated in cases of refractory pain that interferes with quality of life and activities of daily living. Patient selection is paramount with proper counseling including risks of nonunion, adjacent level disease, and overall expectations.

In the case example described above, a right L5–S1 microdiscectomy was performed with complete resolution of the right leg pain. The rationale for microsurgery, and not a fusion, is that his chronic back pain has been well tolerated. The current limitation is due to the right S1 nerve root impingement secondary to the herniated disc. Fusion surgery should be reserved for patients experiencing chronic back pain that is not well managed with conservative measures. As is the case demonstrated here, the MRI will often show degenerative changes. It is prudent to treat the patient, not the MRI.

Teaching Points
► Modic changes can occasionally be confused with osteomyelitis/discitis.
► The nomenclature to describe disc degenerative disease has been standardized to allow for better understanding of the findings among radiologists and clinicians.

Further Reading

1. Van Goethem J, van de Hauwe L, and Parizel PM. *Spinal Imaging: Diagnostic Imaging of the Spine and Spinal Cord.* Berlin, Germany: Springer, 2007.
2. Modic MT, Steinberg PM, Ross JS, et al. Degenerative disk disease: Assessment of changes in vertebral body marrow with MR imaging. Radiology 1988;166:193–199.
3. Fardon DF and Milette PC, for the Combined Task Forces of the North American Spine Society, American Society of Spine Radiology, and American Society of Neuroradiology. Nomenclature and classification of lumbar disc pathology: Recommendations of the combined task forces of the North American Spine Society, American Society of Spine Radiology, and American Society of Neuroradiology. Spine 2001;26:E93–113.
4. Matthews HH and Long, BH. Minimally invasive techniques for the treatment of intervertebral disk herniation. JAAOS 2002;10:80–85.
5. Phillips FM, Slosar PJ, Youssef JA, et al. Lumbar spine fusion for chronic low back pain due to degenerative disc disease: A systemic review. Spine 2013;38:409–422.

Malisa S. Lester, Michelle Naidich, and Mark M. Mikhael

History

▶ A 62-year-old man presents with back pain (**Figures 35.1 and 35.2**).

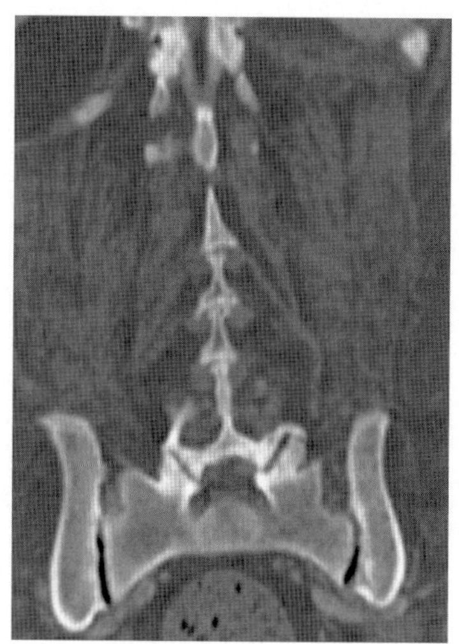

Figure 35.1

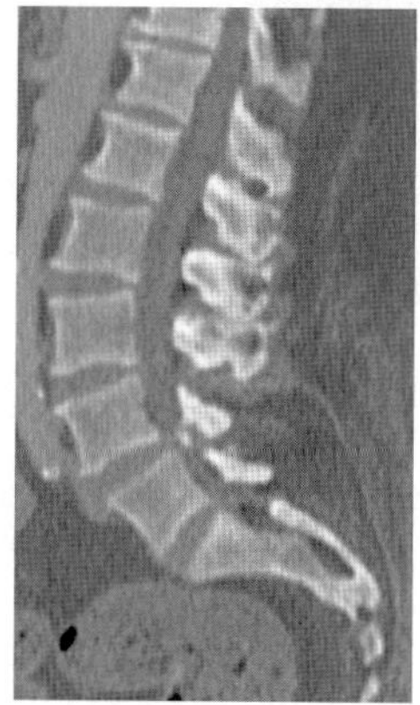

Figure 35.2

Chapter 35 Baastrup's Disease

Findings

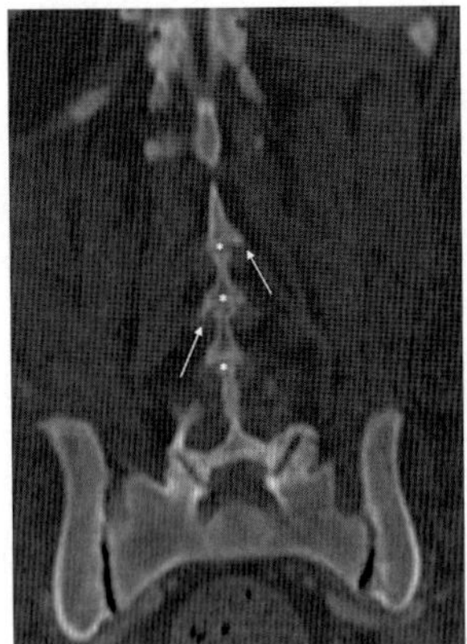

Figure 35.3

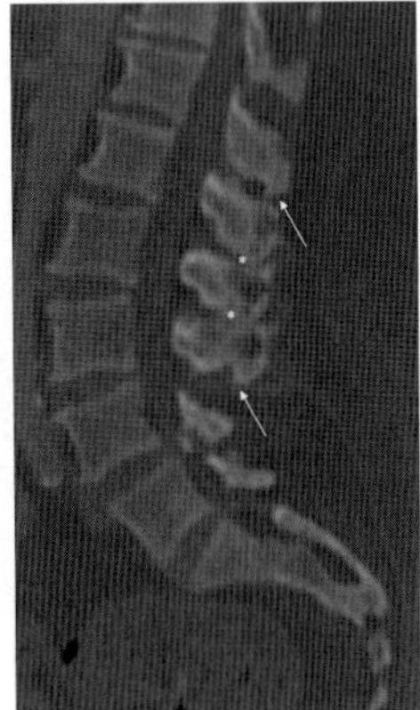

Figure 35.4

Baastrup's disease. A coronal image from a lumbar spine CT (**Figure 35.3**) demonstrates loss of interspinous joint space (asterisks) with apposition and hypertrophy (arrow) of the spinous processes. A sagittal image from a lumbar spine CT (**Figure 35.4**) demonstrates loss of interspinous joint space (asterisks) with apposition and hypertrophy (arrow) of the spinous processes.

Discussion

Baastrup's disease, or "kissing spine," is characterized by a close approximation of the adjacent spinous processes, resulting in inflammation and reactive changes. It is thought to be the result of repetitive strain upon the interspinous ligaments with degeneration and collapse of the ligaments. It is a cause of back pain and increases in frequency with age. It is most commonly reported at the L4–L5 level, but may be a multilevel process.

Radiographic Evaluation

With the collapse of the interspinous ligaments, the adjacent spinous processes come into contact. There is enlargement, flattening, and reactive sclerosis of the spinous processes. On MR, there may be hyperintense T2 signal between the spinous processes, consistent with fluid or inflammatory tissue. This process often occurs with other degenerative changes of the spine. Occasionally, a synovial cyst may form, which may extend into the epidural space and contribute to spinal canal stenosis.

Management

Management typically involves the associated symptomatic, degenerative conditions, such as stenosis, synovial cyst formation, or hypertrophy, causing radicular complaints. No treatment is required for the radiographic entity alone.

Teaching Points

▶ Baastrup's disease is most common at L4–L5.
▶ Look for enlargement, flattening, and reactive sclerosis of the spinous processes.

Further Reading

1. Kwong Y, Rao N, and Latief K. MDCT findings in Baastrup disease: Disease or normal feature of the aging spine? AJR 2011;196:1156–1159.

Cornelia Wenokor, Remi M. Ajiboye, and Arya N. Shamie

History

▶ A 26-year-old female athlete presents with back pain (**Figures 36.1 and 36.2**).

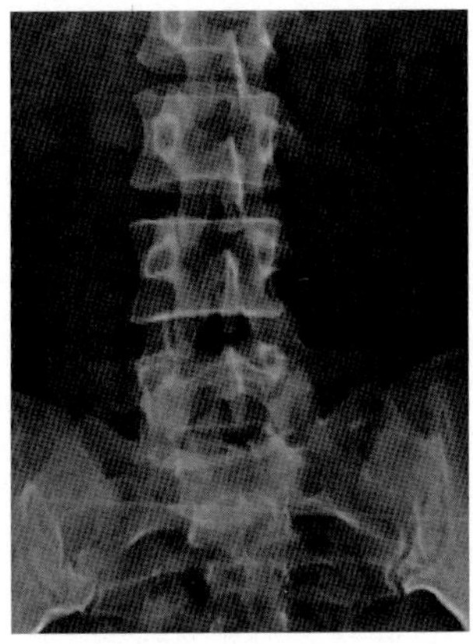

Figure 36.1

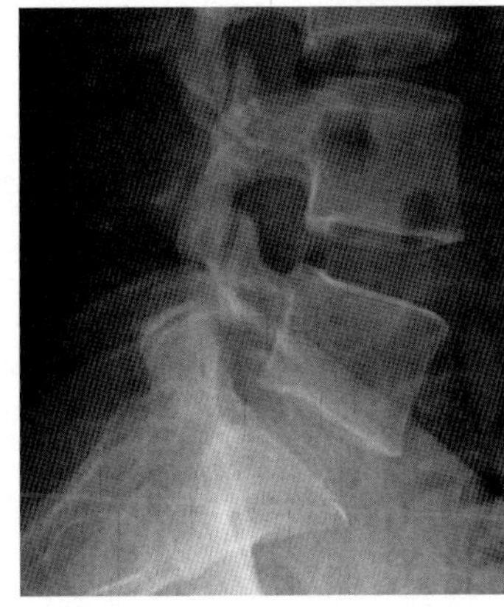

Figure 36.2

Chapter 36 **Pars Defects**

Findings

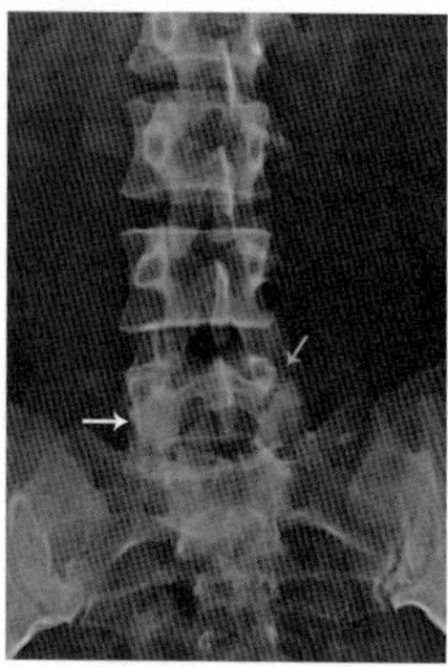
Figure 36.3

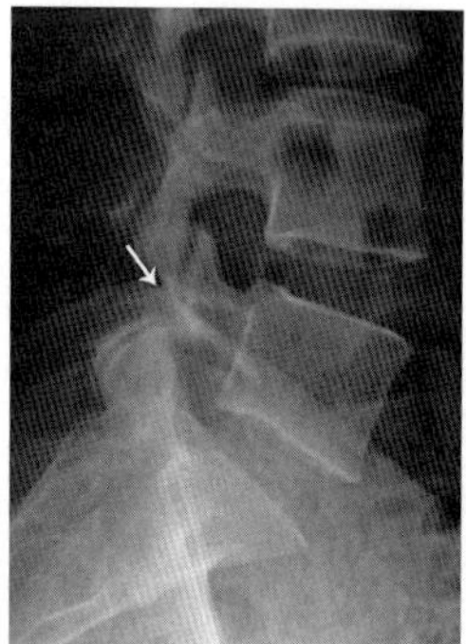
Figure 36.4

Unilateral spondylolysis defect (**Figures 36.3 and 36.4**). There is a unilateral spondylolysis defect on the left (Figure 36.3, grey arrow) at L5 with reactive sclerosis of the right-sided pedicle (Figure 36.3, white arrow). The white arrow on Figure 36.4 points to the spondylolysis defect.

Differential Diagnosis

► Osteoid osteoma (patients under 30 years of age, due to the focal sclerosis on the right)
► Metastatic disease (especially older patients)

Discussion

Spondylolysis defects can be unilateral or bilateral. If bilateral, then there may be an associated spondylolisthesis or slippage of the affected vertebra with respect to the vertebra below. A spondylolisthesis is graded by the degree of slippage of the vetrebrae with respect to each other (Figures 36.7 and 36.8):

1. Grade 1: <25% slippage
2. Grade 2: 25–50% slippage
3. Grade 3: 50–75% slippage
4. Grade 4: 75–100% slippage
5. Grade 5: >100% slippage

Radiographic Evaluation

The radiographic appearance in this case is quite typical of a unilateral spondylolysis defect. In Figure 36.3, there is a lucent defect just below the left pedicle, the pars defect (arrow). The right-sided pars is more sclerotic, just below the pedicle (white arrow). This represents a stress reaction. The lateral view also demonstrates the pars defect as a focal lucent line (arrow). Oblique radiographs are usually quite helpful (**Figures 36.5 and 36.6**).

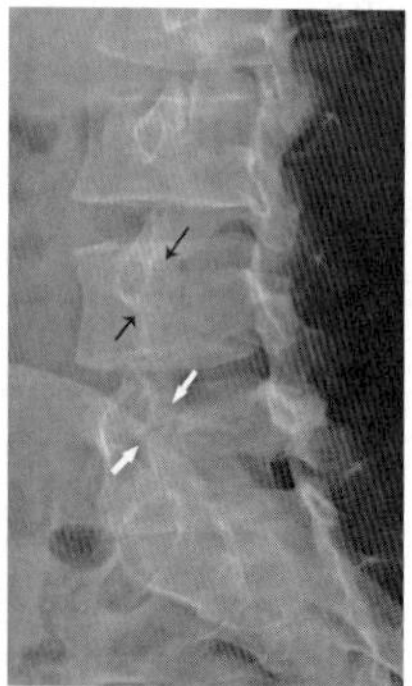
Figure 36.5

Figure 36.6

Oblique radiographs of the lumbar spine (**Figures 36.5 and 36.6**). Pars defects can also be evaluated with oblique views, seen in a different patient. The white arrows in Figure 36.5 are pointing to the pars defect. Compare this to the vertebra above, which demonstrates a normal pars (black arrows). Figure 36.6 shows increased sclerosis of the pars on the left (white arrow). This represents a stress reaction.

On CT a spondylolysis defect mimics a facet joint. However, the facet joint is seen at the neural foramina level, whereas the pars defect is seen at the pedicle level (**Figures 36.7 and 36.8**).

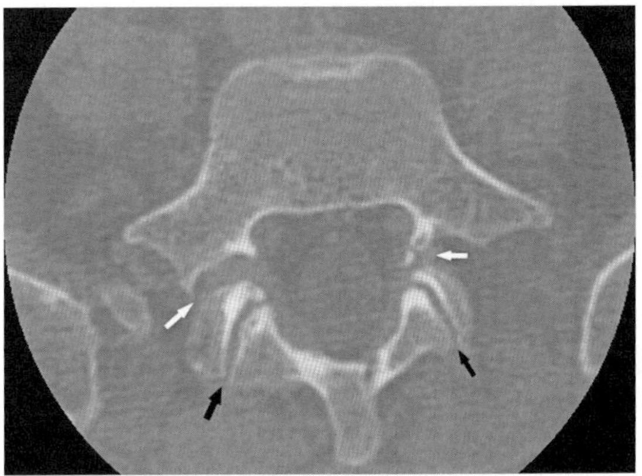

Figure 36.7

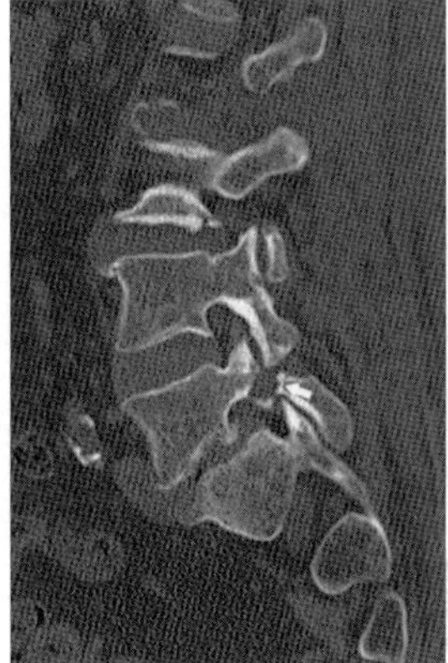

Figure 36.8

Bilateral spondylolysis defects seen on CT (Figure 36.7). Pars defects are seen bilaterally (white arrows) and the facets joints behind the pars defects (black arrows). Figure 36.8 (sagittal CT image) demonstrates a spondylolysis defect at L5 (white arrow).

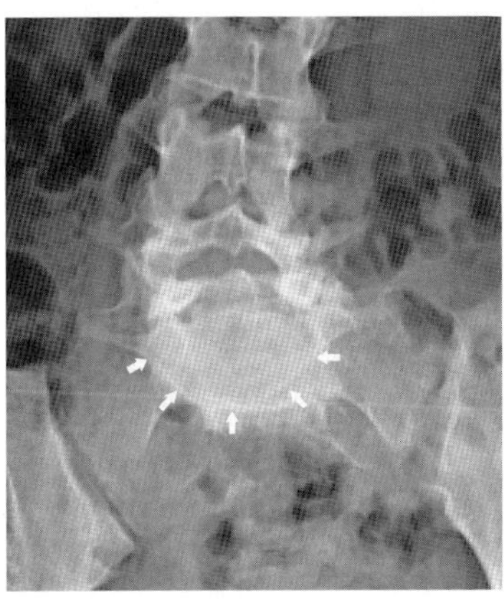

Figure 36.9

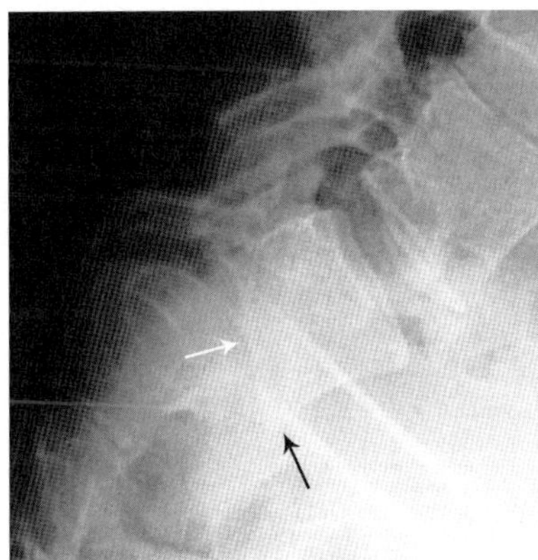

Figure 36.10

Spondylolisthesis (**Figures 36.9 and 36.10**). Radiographs demonstrate a high-grade spondylolisthesis with L5 (black arrow) having slipped anteriorly to S1 by about 40% of the vertebral body length. This can occur only with a bilateral spondylolysis defect, which is not seen on these radiographs, but must be present. Note the rounded anterior corner of S1 (white arrow) and the decreased height of the posterior vertebra of L5 due to longstanding abnormal alignment with resulting pressure erosion of the bone. Figure 36.9 demonstrates the "reversed Napoleon's hat sign" (white arrows). The brim of the hat is formed by the downward sloping transverse processes. The dome is the body of L5.

Management

The goals of treatment of pars defect are aimed at alleviation of pain and facilitation of bone healing. Conservative management with cessation of aggravating activity and spinal bracing for 3–6 months is usually recommended. Surgical treatment for pars defect is generally reserved for patients who fail to respond to conservative treatment.

A direct repair of the pars interarticularis is recommended for adolescents and young adults without significant instability or intervertebral disc degeneration. Several techniques of direct repair have been described including lag screw, cerclage wire, and pedicle screw with rod hook fixation. The fixation construct is often augmented with a bone graft in order to improve healing success. In patients with evidence of significant instability or intervertebral disc degeneration, spinal fusion (in the form of posterolateral and/or interbody fusion) is usually recommended.

Teaching Points

- ▶ L4/L5 and L5/S1 are most frequently affected.
- ▶ Bilateral spondylolysis can be diagnosed on lateral radiographs.
- ▶ Over time a spondylolisthesis can develop in bilateral pars defects.

Further Reading

1. Garcia GM. *Rad Cases: Musculoskeletal Radiology*. New York, NY: Thieme, 2010, pp. 179–180.
2. Li Y and Hresko MT. Radiographic analysis of spondylolisthesis and sagittal spinopelvic deformity. J Am Acad Orthop Surg 2012;20(4):194–205.

Malisa S. Lester, Michelle Naidich, and Mark M. Mikhael

History

▶ A 68-year-old man presents with myelopathic symptoms and neck pain (**Figures 37.1 and 37.2**).

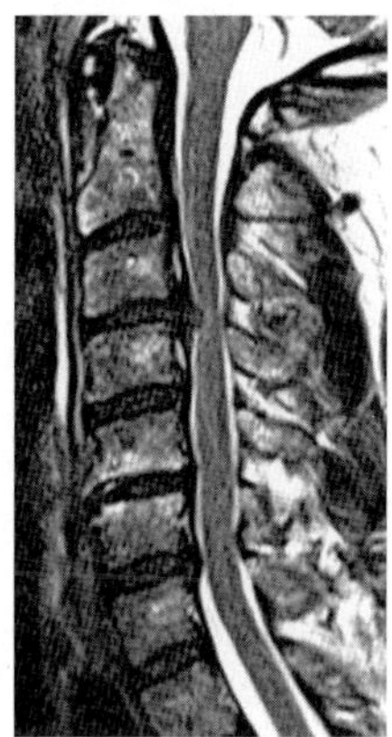

Figure 37.1

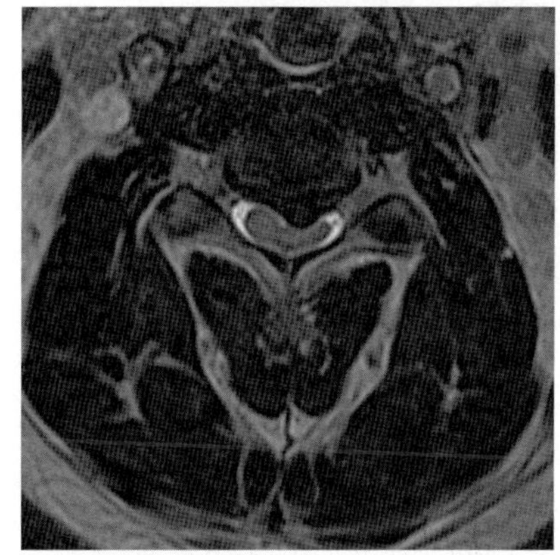

Figure 37.2

Chapter 37 **Cord Compression**

Findings

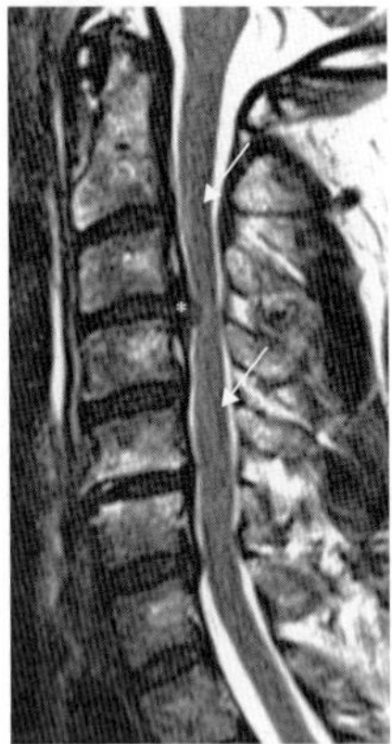
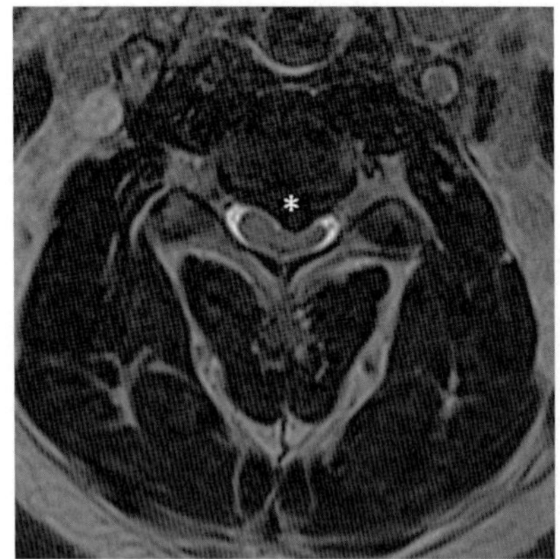

Figure 37.3   Figure 37.4

Cord compression due to degenerative change. A sagittal T2-weighted image (**Figure 37.3**) shows multilevel degenerative disc desiccation, with varying degrees of disc height loss. At C3–C4, there is a disc protrusion (asterisk), which effaces the ventral cervicospinal fluid (CSF) space and compresses the adjacent cervical spinal cord. Mild T2 hyperintense signal is seen within the cervical spinal cord centered at the C3–C4 disc space, corresponding to associated cord edema (arrows). The axial T2 image (**Figure 37.4**) shows the left paracentral disc protrusion (asterisk) deforming and compressing the left aspect of the spinal cord with associated faint hyperintense T2 cord signal.

Differential Diagnosis

▶ Other epidural disease processes in the appropriate clinical setting (e.g., epidural hematoma, abscess, or tumor)

▶ Extramedullary compressing pathology

Discussion

Spinal cord compression can result from any extramedullary pathology. In the setting of degenerative disease, this is usually the result of a disc protrusion/extrusion or an osteophyte. Cord compression results in myelopathy, which may be acute or chronic.

Radiographic Evaluation

MR is the imaging modality of choice for the evaluation of spinal cord compression. MR imaging allows for evaluation of the etiology and degree of spinal canal compromise, as well as the presence of any associated cord edema. Cord edema is represented by hyperintense T2 signal and may be accompanied by cord expansion in the acute setting. CT may be useful in the setting of acute trauma or in patients who are unable to undergo MR imaging. In this latter group, CT myelography may also have a role in the evaluation.

Management

When compression of the spinal cord causes symptoms of myelopathy, such as difficulty with walking and balance, trouble with fine motor skills, or radiculopathy with numbness and tingling in the arms or hands, surgical intervention is typically warranted. The main objective of surgical decompression is to halt any further progressive neurological decline. Full neurological recovery, such as the return of full strength and balance, may not occur despite adequate decompression.

Regardless of the surgical procedure performed, the goal of the operation is to take pressure off the spinal cord and create more space in the spinal canal. When the disease is present at only one or two levels, anterior cervical discectomy and fusion (ACDF) is typically the preferred intervention as it has shown reproducibly favorable outcomes. Posterior decompression, such as laminectomy and fusion or laminoplasty, are typically performed in cases that require multilevel decompression or in cases in which anterior surgery carries increased risk, such as OPLL or a calcified disc causing stenosis. Combined anterior–posterior procedures are sometimes required in cases of spinal cord compression in the setting of excessive cervical kyphosis requiring restoration of lordotic or neutral alignment. In cases of cord compression due to migrated/sequestered fragments behind the vertebral body or compression due to neoplasm in the vertebrae, an anterior vertebral corpectomy and strut graft fusion is performed.

Teaching Points

► MRI is the modality of choice in the evaluation of cord compression.
► In the acute setting, look for an abnormal T2 signal in the cord, which may also be expanded from associated edema.

Further Reading

1. Seidenwurm DJ. Myelopathy. AJNR 2008;29:1032–1034
2. Naidich TB. *Imaging of the Spine*. Philadelphia, PA: Elsevier, 2011.

Chapter 38

Malisa S. Lester, Michelle Naidich, and Mark M. Mikhael

History

▶ A 49-year-old woman presents with low back pain (**Figures 38.1, 38.2, 38.3, and 38.4**).

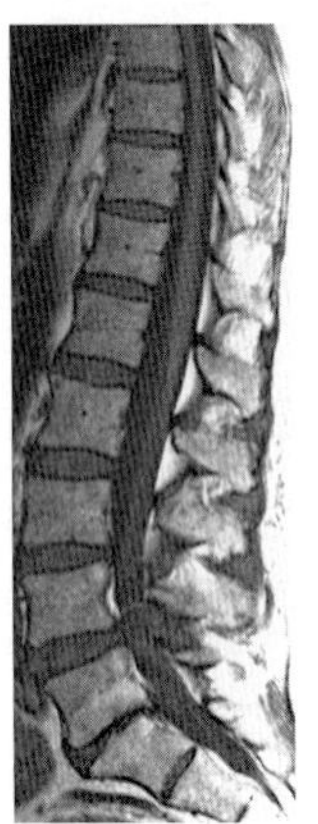

Figure 38.1

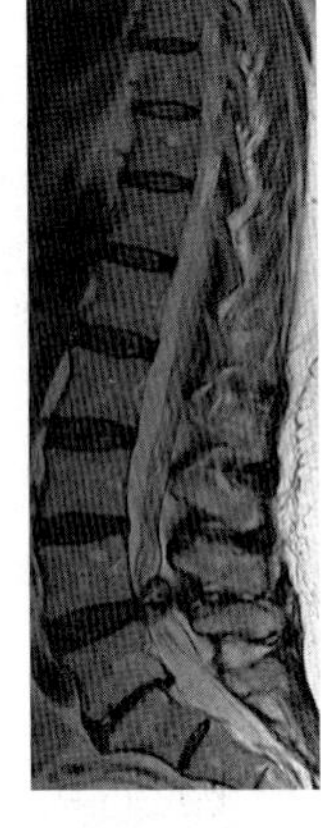

Figure 38.2

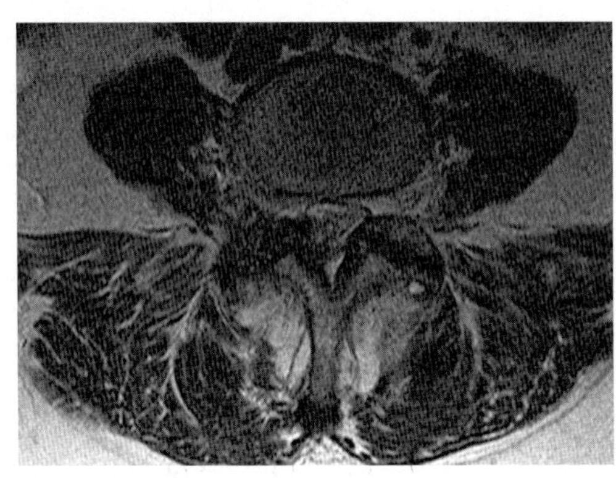

Figure 38.3

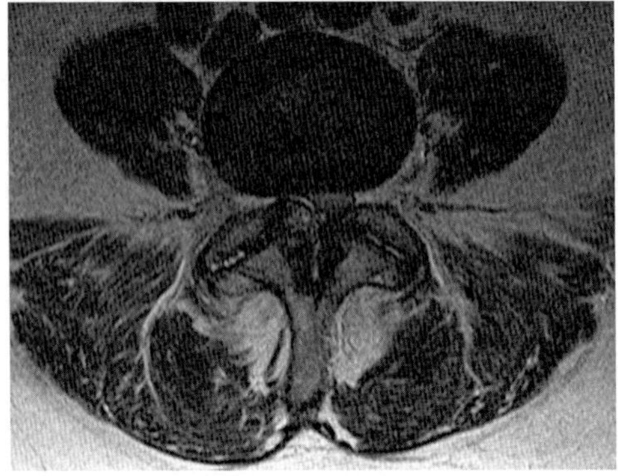

Figure 38.4

Findings

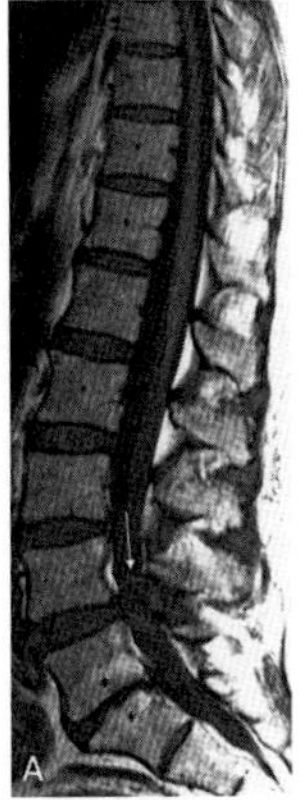
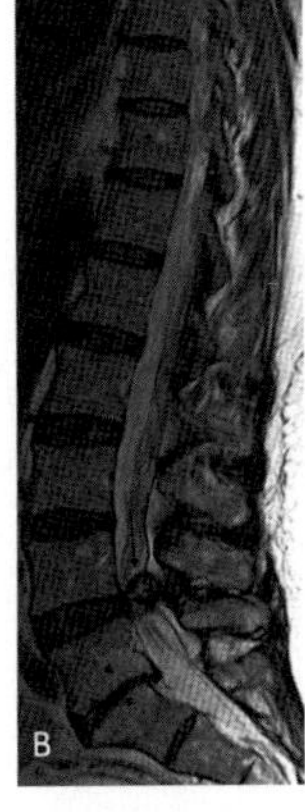

Figure 38.5   Figure 38.6

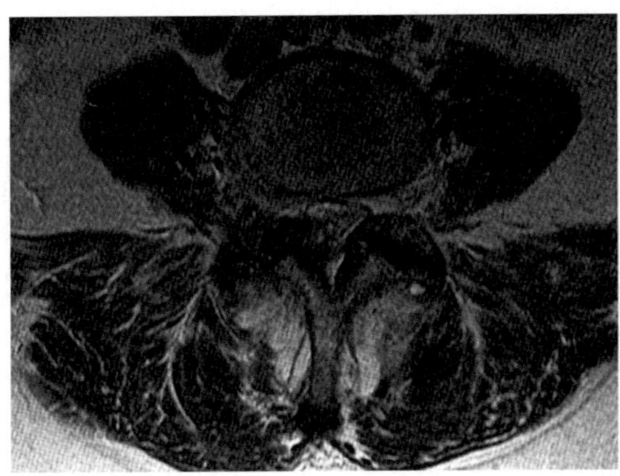

Figure 38.7

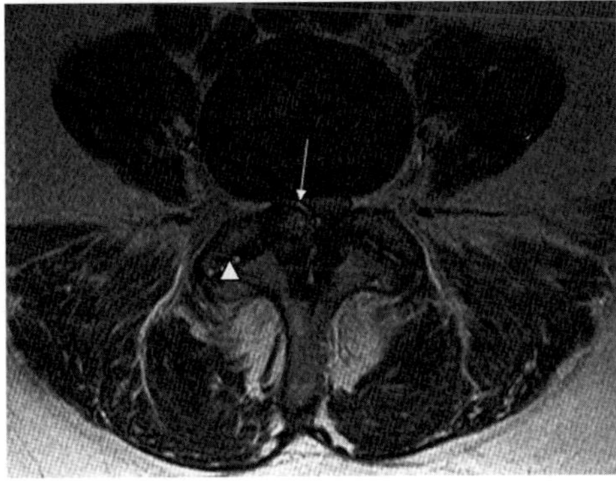

Figure 38.8

Synovial cyst. Sagittal T1-weighted image (**Figure 38.5**) of the lumbar spine shows a rounded area of signal isointense to cerebrospinal fluid (CSF) at the L4–L5 level (white arrow), corresponding to an area of heterogeneous T2 signal (black arrow) with peripheral T2 hypointensity, which appears to float within the central thecal sac on the sagittal T2-weighted images (**Figure 38.6**). Also note the Modic Type 2 endplate changes at L5–S1 on the sagittal T1- and T2-weighted images (asterisks). Contiguous axial T2-weighted images (**Figures 38.7 and 38.8**) at the L4–L5 level demonstrate degenerative facet joint hypertrophy (right greater than left), with joint space narrowing and a small right-sided facet joint effusion (arrowhead). The round area of heterogeneous T2 signal (arrow) is in the right posterolateral epidural space, adjacent to the degenerated facet joint. These findings are compatible with a synovial cyst, which contributes to advanced spinal canal stenosis, right subarticular zone stenosis, and probable compression of the traversing right L5 nerve roots.

Discussion

As the ligamentum flavum degenerates it may develop calcification, cysts, and/or fissures. This weakened ligament, if near a facet joint, may permit herniation of the synovium into the spinal canal. As a result, there is a fluid-filled pocket with a synovial lining arising from the facet joint. A synovial cyst may be seen as a rounded extradural mass when it projects into the spinal canal. Alternatively, a juxtaarticular cyst may form, not extending into the spinal canal. Symptoms result from neural compression. The L4–L5 level is the most commonly reported level involved.

Radiographic Evaluation

An epidural lesion projecting from a facet joint, which is typically degenerated, is the classic appearance of a synovial cyst on MRI or CT. Depending on the contents of the synovial cyst, the central signal intensity may vary. However, commonly, the central signal characteristics follow that of fluid (low signal intensity on T1WI and high signal intensity on T2WI). Synovial cysts may have peripheral hypointense T2 signal. Enhancement is variable.

Management

Neural compression can occur by mass effect of the synovial cyst on the adjacent nerve roots causing radicular pain. In the setting of intractable radicular pain or lower extremity weakness, synovial cysts are often surgically excised through a laminotomy and partial medial facetectomy. Preoperative upright flexion-extension radiographs should be evaluated to rule out possible associated dynamic instability.

Teaching Points

- ▶ Synovial cysts are most common at L4–L5.
- ▶ Look for associated neural compression.

Further Reading

1. Khan AM and Giradi F. Spinal lumbar synovial cysts. Diagnosis and management challenge. Eur Spine J 2006;15(8):1176–1182.
2. Khalatbari K and Ansari H. MRI of degenerative cysts of the lumbar spine. Clin Radiol 2008; 63(3):322–328.

Infections and Inflammatory

Rakesh Mannava, Joseph M. Mettenburg, and Vikas Agarwal

History

▶ A 47-year-old HIV-positive female presents with a 2-month history of unsteady gait and parasthesias in all extremities (**Figures 39.1 and 39.2**).

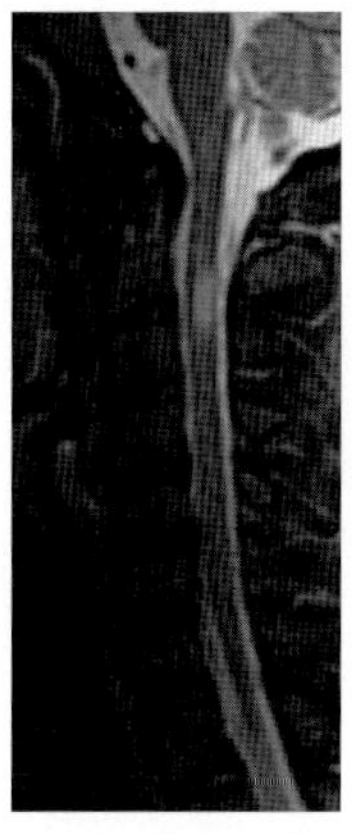

Figure 39.1

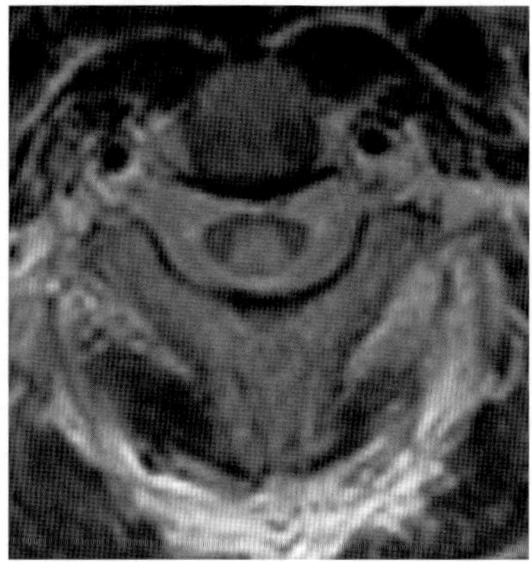

Figure 39.2

Chapter 39 HIV-Associated Myelopathy

Findings

HIV myelitis. Sagittal and axial long TR, long TE images (Figures 39.1 and 39.2) show a nonexpansile area of T2 prolongation within the dorsal spinal cord crossing the midline and spanning a total length of one vertebral segment. There was no enhancement on postcontrast imaging (not shown).

Differential Diagnosis

- ▶ Subacute combined degeneration
- ▶ Multiple sclerosis
- ▶ Demyelination
- ▶ Viral myelitis
- ▶ Tabes dorsalis

Discussion

HIV-associated myelopathy has been found at autopsy in approximately half of all AIDS patients, although only a small fraction manifest symptoms. Vacuolization within the dorsal and lateral white matter tracts is observed by pathology. It is clinically diagnosed based on signs and symptoms of extremity motor and sensory deficits occurring over a span of weeks in the absence of other causes. MRI and somatosensory-evoked potentials corroborate the diagnosis. Early research suggests that intravenous immunoglobulin may improve symptoms.

Radiological Evaluation

In the evaluation of HIV-positive patients with neurological symptoms, MRI is important to exclude treatable processes such as lymphoma, toxoplasmosis, and other opportunistic infections. The most common finding in HIV-associated myelopathy is cord atrophy without cord signal abnormality, typically beginning in the mid to lower thoracic cord and progressing rostral (**Figure 39.3**).

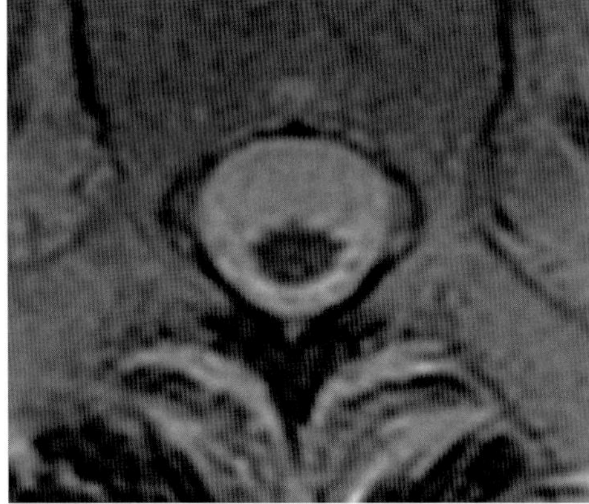

Figure 39.3

HIV-associated myelopathy is seen associated with cord atrophy (Figure 39.3). Cord signal abnormality can, however, be present along the white matter tracts laterally and symmetrically over multiple contiguous vertebral segments. Contrast enhancement is usually absent. Therefore, in a patient with HIV, cord signal abnormality should prompt a diagnostic workup for evaluation of myelitis with HIV-associated myelopathy included in the differential. Subacute combined degeneration (Figure 39.4) from vitamin B_{12} can have a similar pattern of cord signal abnormality and is easily differentiated on the basis of blood tests. Other infectious causes of myelitis, including cytomegalovirus (CMV) and herpes simplex virus type 2 (HSV-2), can cause a similar appearance and should be excluded.

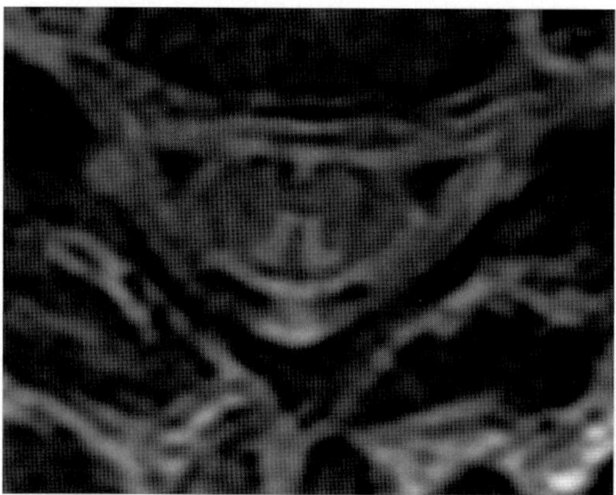

Figure 39.4

Subacute combined degeneration from B$_{12}$ deficiency (Figure 39.4). An axial T2-weighted image through the cord demonstrates increased signal in the posterior columns.

Management

There is no specific treatment for AIDS or HIV-associated myelopathy. However, early research suggests that intravenous immunoglobulin may improve symptoms.

Teaching Points

► HIV-associated myelopathy is a diagnosis of exclusion. The role of MRI is to exclude other pathology and define the extent of cord abnormality.

► Cord atrophy is the most common finding in HIV-associated myelopathy. Cord signal abnormality is less common.

Further Reading

1. Dal Pan GJ, Glass JD, and McArthur JC. Clinicopathologic correlations of HIV-1-associated vacuolar myelopathy: An autopsy-based case-control study. Neurology 1994;44(11):2159–2164.
2. Cikurel K, Schiff L, and Simpson DM. Pilot study of intravenous immunoglobulin in HIV-associated myelopathy. AIDS Patient Care STDS 2009;23(2):75–78.
3. Chong J, Di Rocco A, Tagliati M, et al. MR findings in AIDS-associated myelopathy. AJNR Am J Neuroradiol 1999;20(8):1412–1416.

Chapter 40

Nima Jadidi and Sylvie Destian

History

▶ A 36-year-old male presents with back pain (**Figures 40.1, 40.2, 40.3, and 40.4**).

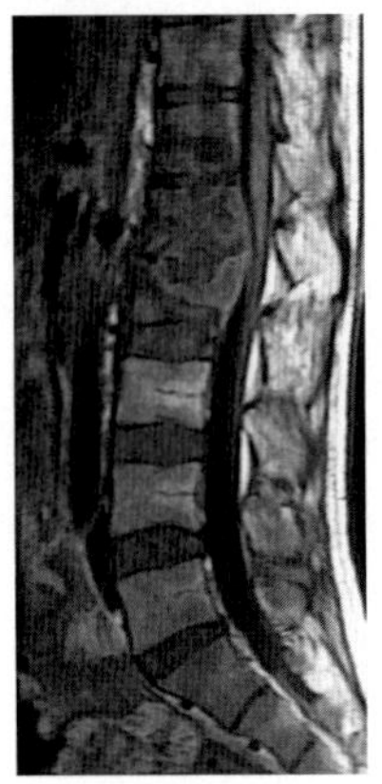

Figure 40.1

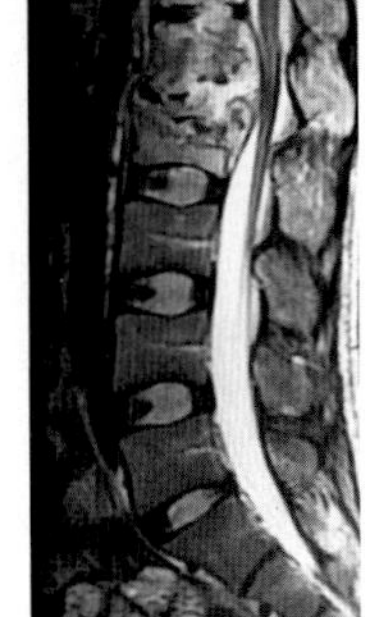

Figure 40.2

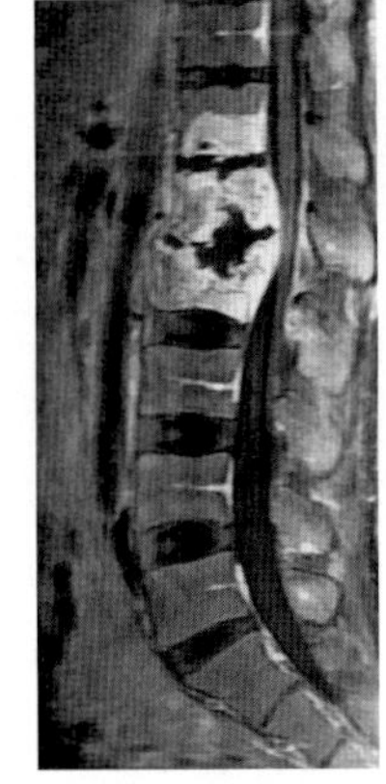

Figure 40.3

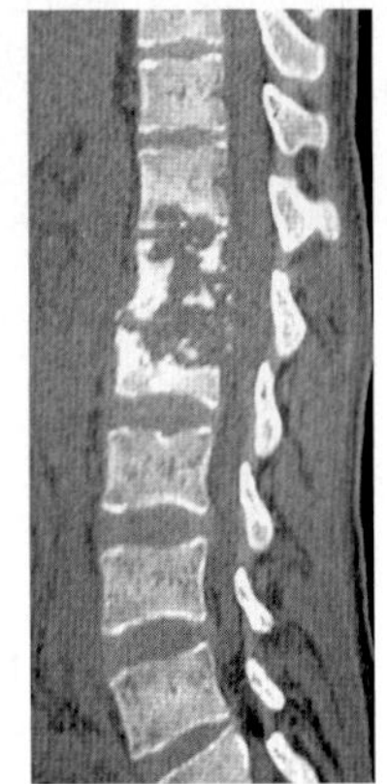

Figure 40.4

Findings

Pott's disease (tuberculosis spondylitis) of the T12–L2 vertebral bodies (Figures 40.1, 40.2, 40.3, and 40.4). Sagittal T1WI (Figure 40.1) demonstrates loss of the normal marrow signal primarily at L1 and L2. There is involvement of the intervening disc space. Sagittal T2WI (Figure 40.2) depicts destruction of the L1 and L2 disc as well as posterior extension into the epidural space with resultant posterior displacement of the conus medullaris. Edema is also noted in the T12 vertebral body, as well as fluid in the abnormal disc spaces. Postcontrast sagittal T1WI (Figure 40.3) depicts intense enhancement of the involved vertebral bodies with an area of necrosis at L1–L2. Sagittal CT reconstruction of the lumber spine (Figure 40.4) shows destruction of the T12–L1 and L1–L2 endplates.

Differential Diagnosis

▶ Pyogenic vertebral osteomyelitis
▶ Multiple compression fractures

Discussion

Although tuberculosis infection of bone is uncommon in the United States, the most common site of skeletal involvement is the spine. Pott's disease or tuberculous spondylitis is a granulomatous infection of the spine caused by *Mycobacterium tuberculosis*. It is an important entity to keep in mind, especially in immunocompromised patients with or without a history of tuberculosis infection.

Tuberculosis is thought to spread hematogenously through Batson's venous plexus, a network of valveless veins that provides a route for the spread of malignancies and infection to the spine and posterior fossa. The infection typically travels to the anterior aspect of the vertebral body and spreads along the anterior longitudinal ligament to involve neighboring vertebral bodies.

Radiological Evaluation

The relative destruction of the anterior aspects of adjacent vertebral bodies can result in a kyphotic (gibbus) deformity similar in appearance to multiple stacked anterior wedge fractures. A gibbus deformity occurs late in the disease process, most commonly at T12–L1. Unlike a bacterial infection, tuberculosis tends to spare the disc spaces early in the disease course. Although CT can demonstrate the bone destruction (Figure 40.4), an MRI is the modality of choice to evaluate the full extent of the disease (Figures 40.5, 40.6, and 40.7). Typical signal characteristics on MRI include decreased signal in the involved area on T1WI and increased signal on T2WI. The disc can be of normal or increased intensity on noncontrast T2-weighted MR imaging but usually enhances with contrast. MRI or CT is also helpful to look for abscess formation either in the spine or in the paraspinal soft tissues. A paraspinal abscess with calcification is highly indicative of tuberculosis spondylitis.

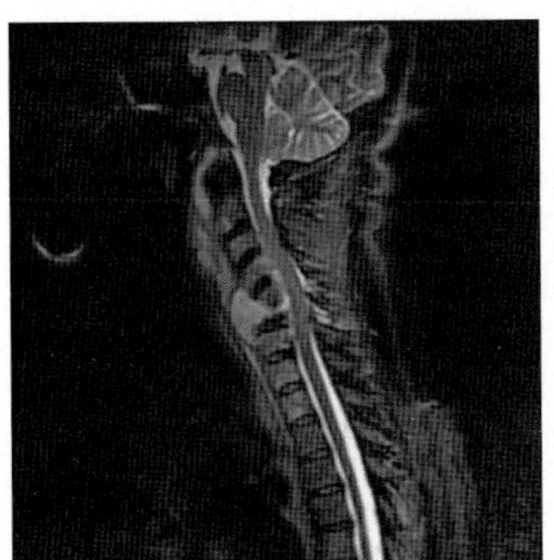

Figure 40.5

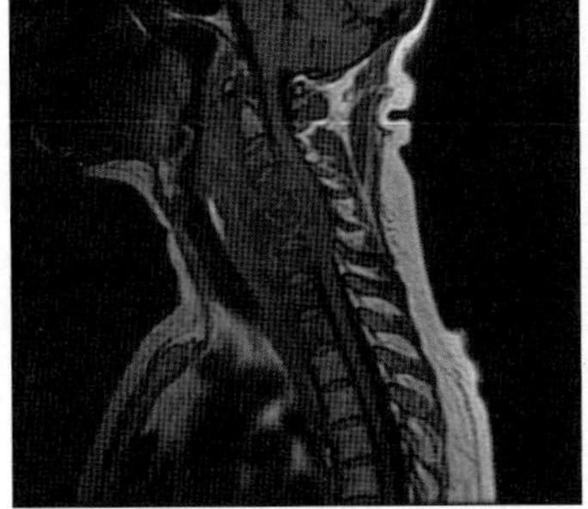

Figure 40.6

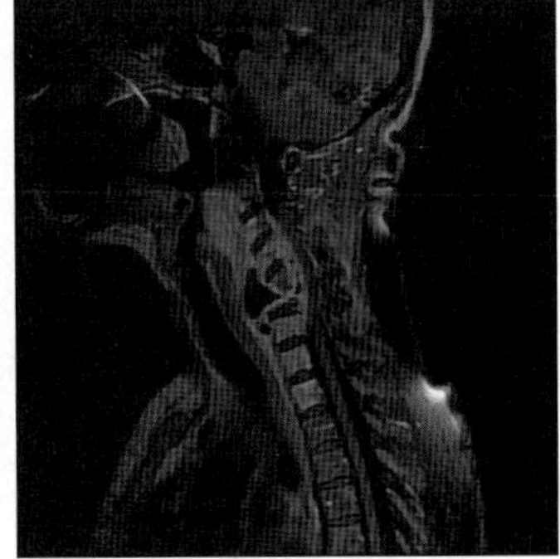

Figure 40.7

Pott's disease in the cervical spine in a 56-year-old female (Figures 40.5, 40.6, and 40.7). Sagittal T2 (Figure 40.5), T1 (Figure 40.6), and postcontrast T1 (Figure 40.7) images demonstrate abnormal alignment at C5–C6 with associated paraspinal and epidural extension of abnormal soft tissue.

Management

The diagnosis is frequently established by biopsy and tissue specimens. Imaging is helpful to confirm clinical suspicion of spinal involvement and to evaluate the extent of the disease. Treatment typically involves antituberculin antibiotics. Depending on the extent of the disease, surgical intervention such as debridement and decompression may be necessary.

Teaching Points

▶ Tuberculosis infection of the spine typically involves the thoracic spine and spreads to adjacent vertebral bodies.

▶ Disc sparing is characteristic of early disease and gibbus deformity is characteristic of late disease.

▶ Always look at the paraspinal soft tissues for disease involvement.

Further Reading

1. Burrill J, Williams CJ, Bain G, et al. Tuberculosis: A radiologic review. Radiographics 2007;27(5):1255–1273.
2. Rivas-Garcia A, Sarria-Estrada S, Torrents-Odin C, et al. Imaging findings of Pott's disease. Eur Spine J 2013;22(Suppl 4):567–578.
3. Harisinghani MG, Mcloud TC, Shepard JA, et al. Tuberculosis from head to toe. Radiographics 2000;20(2):449–470.
4. Brant WE and Helms CA. *Fundamentals of Diagnostic Radiology*. Lippincott, Williams & Wilkins, 2007.

Nima Jadidi and Sylvie Destian

History

▶ A 33-year-old male presents with fever and back pain (**Figures 41.1, 41.2, 41.3, 41.4, 41.5, and 41.6**).

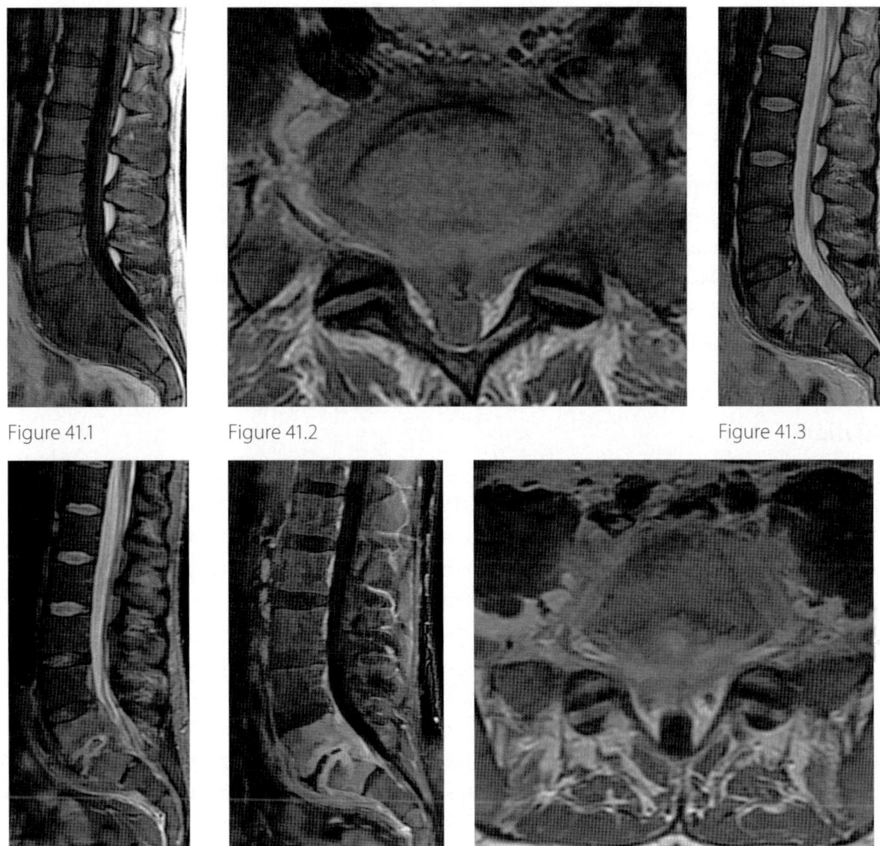

Figure 41.1   Figure 41.2   Figure 41.3

Figure 41.4   Figure 41.5   Figure 41.6

Chapter 41 Discitis/Osteomyelitis

Findings

Osteomyelitis/discitis centered at L5.1 (Figures 41.1, 41.2, 41.3, 41.4, 41.5, and 41.6). Axial and sagittal T1- and T2-weighted images, precontrast and postcontrast, demonstrate destruction of the L5 and S1 vertebral bodies with involvement of the intervening disc space. Corresponding abnormal enhancement is seen on the postcontrast images (Figures 41.3, 41.4, 41.5, and 41.6), with extension of enhancement into the epidural space.

Differential Diagnosis

▶ Pott's disease
▶ Metastatic disease

Discussion

Spondylodiscitis refers to vertebral and disc osteomyelitis. The most common pathogen is *Staphylococcus aureus*; however, tuberculosis is still very prevalent in developing countries. Specific pathogens are also associated with certain conditions, such as sickle cell disease and *Salmonella*. Early diagnosis and treatment are imperative given the significant associated morbidity. Pathogens can reach the spine either via hematogeneous spread or by contiguous spread. In adults, the blood vessels to the vertebra are effectively end arteries. Therefore, bacteria can lodge in the vertebral body and subsequently spread to the disc space and neighboring vertebra. The lumber spine is affected more commonly as it receives more blood flow.

Radiological Evaluation

Plain radiography is not preferred to look for spondylodiscitis as early findings may be absent. Also, coexisting degenerative disease adds an additional hurdle for interpretation. Nevertheless, classic radiographic findings include cortical endplate erosions adjacent to a narrowed disc space. CT is a very sensitive modality to evaluate for osseous involvement (Figures 41.7, 41.8, and 41.9). Although it is not the primary modality, it is excellent at depicting bone changes and paraspinal soft tissue involvement. Findings include disc space gas, erosive bone changes, and epidural and/or paraspinal collections that display variable enhancement.

Although CT myelography may be needed to assess for epidural involvement in some patients, there is a risk of intradural spread from the procedure. MRI is the primary modality as it has excellent sensitivity and specificity. MRI is helpful in evaluating disc involvement, the presence of a paraspinal or epidural abscess, and compression of the spinal cord and/or caudal equina. Unlike an infectious process, neoplastic infiltration usually neglects the intervertebral disc. The classic MRI findings consist of low signal on T1WI, high signal on T2WI, and enhancement of the disc, endplates, and paraspinal and/or epidural soft tissues (Figures 41.1, 41.2, 41.5 and 41.6). Depiction of endplate erosions, bone destruction, loss of disc space height, and paraspinal involvement improves specificity and sensitivity.

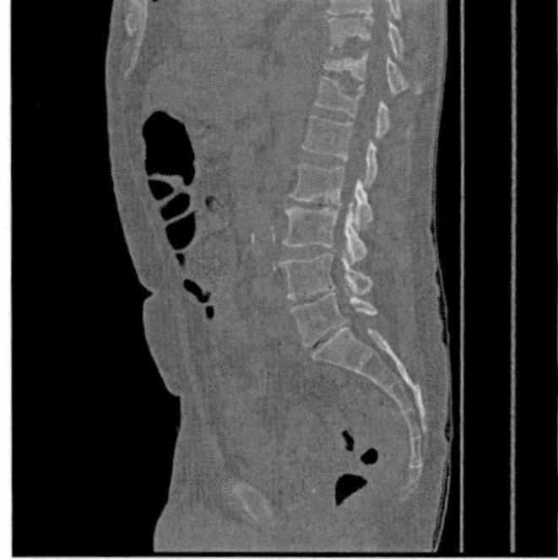

Figure 41.7

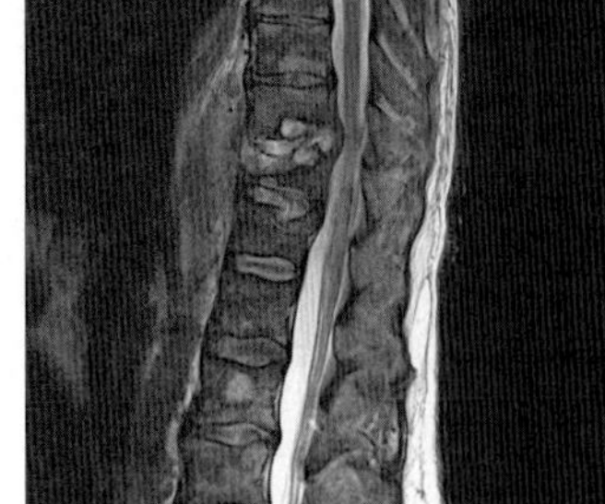

Figure 41.8

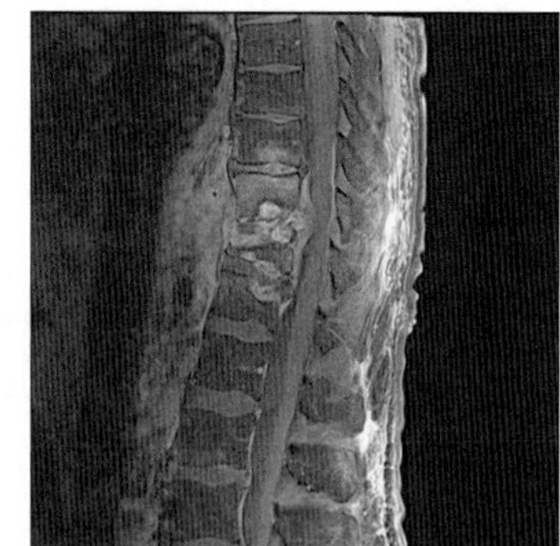

Figure 41.9

A 66-year-old male presents with discitis/osteomyelitis at T10–T12 (**Figures 41.7, 41.8, and 41.9**). A sagittal CT reformation (Figure 41.7) demonstrates osseous destruction mainly of T11, but also with involvement of both T10 and T12. CT poorly characterizes soft tissue involvement, and, therefore, an MRI is suggested. Sagittal T2 (Figure 41.8) and postcontrast T1-weighted images (Figure 41.9) demonstrate the prevertebral and epidural extent of the disease, as well as abnormal enhancement of the involved vertebral bodies and adjacent disc spaces.

Management

Surgical debridement, conservative management, and percutaneous drainage of an abscess are all potential courses of action depending on the particular case. The extent of the disease on imaging as well as the clinical context will dictate the appropriate course of action. In the absence of a progressive neurological deficit, nonoperative management is appropriate. Antimicrobial therapy is typically parenteral and for at least 4–6 weeks, although the exact course of treatment is controversial. MRI is often obtained following treatment to assess the response. Surgical decompression and evacuation of an associated abscess are indicated in cases of severe neurological compression with evident progressive deficit, followed by culture-specific intravenous antibiotics. Debridement of bone and spinal stabilization is indicated in cases of spinal instability due to significant bone destruction.

Teaching Points

► Unlike neoplasm, infection is more likely to affect contiguous vertebrae as well as the endplates and intervening disc space(s).
► MRI is the primary modality as it enables evaluation for an epidural abscess and paraspinal soft tissue involvement.

Further Reading

1. Ledermann HP, Schweitzer ME, Morrison WB, et al. MR imaging findings in spinal infections: Rules or myths? Radiology 2003;228(2):506–514.
2. Dunbar JA, Sandoe JA, Rao AS, et al. The MRI appearances of early vertebral osteomyelitis and discitis. Clin Radiol 2010;65(12):974–981.
3. Oztekin O, Calli C, Adibelli Z, et al. Brucellar spondylodiscitis: Magnetic resonance imaging features with conventional sequences and diffusion-weighted imaging. Radiol Med 2010;115(5):794–803.
4. Hatzenbuehler J and Pulling TJ. Diagnosis and management of osteomyelitis. Am Fam Physician 2011;84(9):1027–1033.
5. Dagirmanjian A, Schils J, Mchenry M, et al. MR imaging of vertebral osteomyelitis revisited. AJR Am J Roentgenol 1996;167(6):1539–1543.

Chapter 42

Sara E. Kingston, Tina Raman, Chia-Shang J. Liu, Bavrina Bigjahan, and Mark S. Shiroishi

History

► A 55-year-old male with a history of intravenous drug use presents with lower back pain and leg weakness (**Figures 42.1, 42.2, 42.3, and 42.4**).

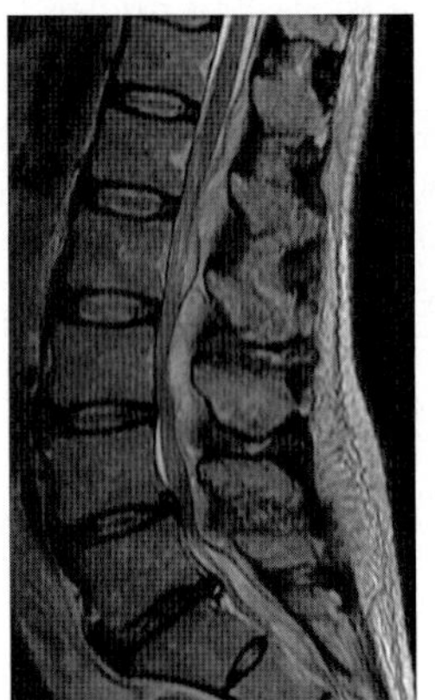

Figure 42.1

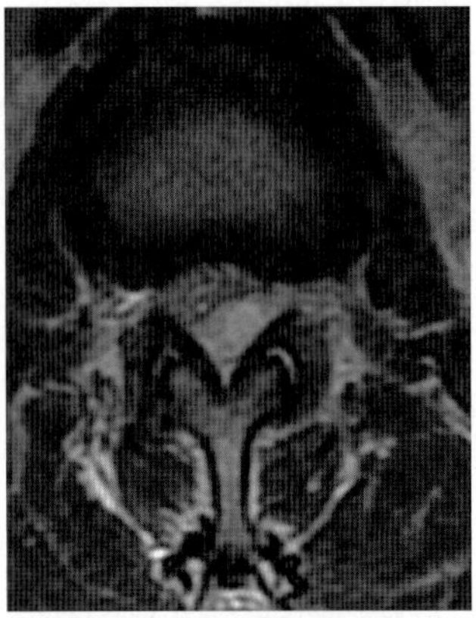

Figure 42.2

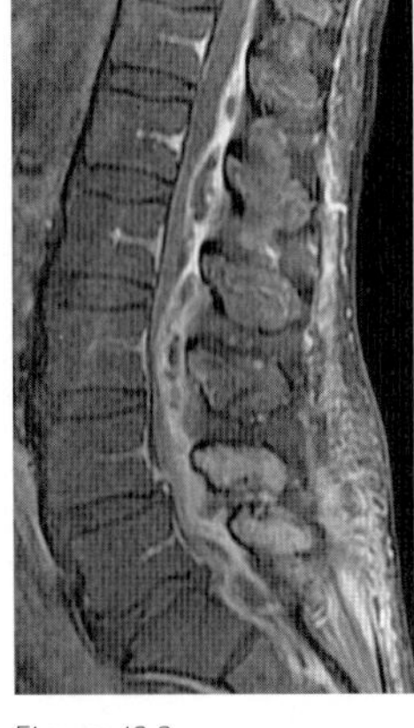

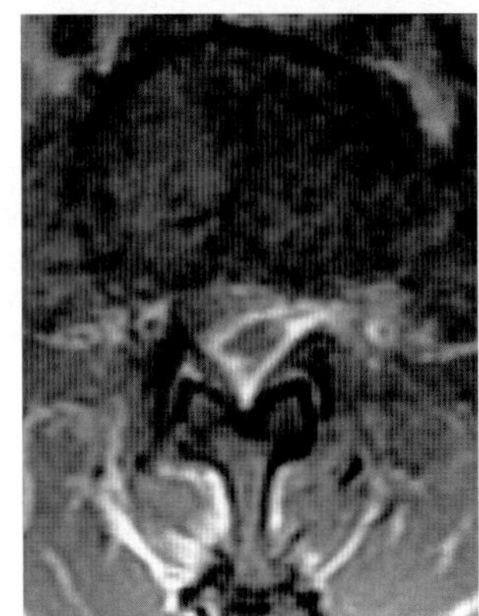

Figure 42.3

Figure 42.4

Findings

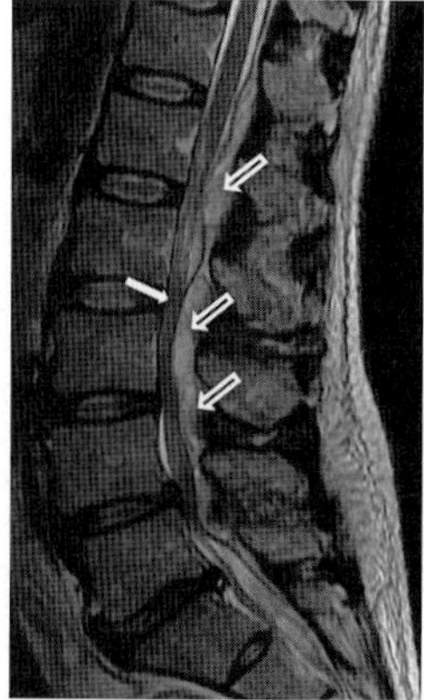

Figure 42.5

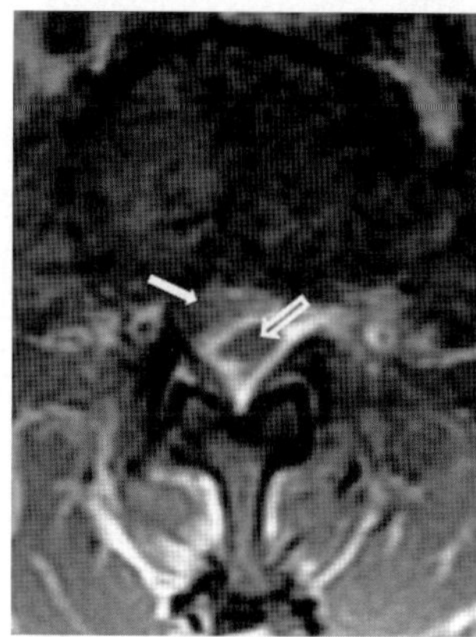

Figure 42.6

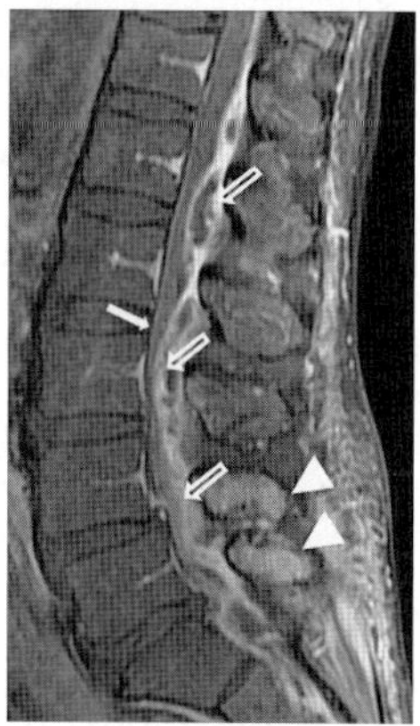

Figure 42.7

Figure 42.8

Epidural abscess (Figures 42.5, 42.6, 42.7, and 42.8). Axial and sagittal T2-weighted (Figures 42.5 and 42.6) and contrast-enhanced T1-weighted images with fat saturation (Figures 42.7 and 42.8) demonstrate an extensive dorsal epidural abscess of the lumbar spine (hollow arrows) with compression of the cauda equina nerve roots (solid white arrows). Contrast enhancement of the L4 and L5 spinous processes (white arrowheads, Figure 42.7) may be related to reactive edema and/or osteomyelitis.

Differential Diagnosis

► Disc extrusion (ventral epidural process)/degenerative disc disease
► Epidural lipomatosis (dorsal epidural process)
► Epidural tumor (metastasis, lymphoma)
► Epidural hematoma
► Pott's disease

Discussion

An epidural abscess describes a bacterial infection of the spine in which purulent fluid or infected tissue tracks through the epidural space at one or more spinal segments. This deleterious pathology is closely accompanied by high risk for neurological sequelae and thus classic teaching dictates urgent surgical intervention.

Direct Extension
  Vertebral body osteomyelitis
  Local soft tissue infections
    Paravertebral
    Retropharyngeal
    Psoas
Hematogenous Spread
  Skin and soft tissue infections
  Respiratory tract
  Genitourinary tract
  Abdominal viscera
  Oral cavity
  Infective endocarditis
Iatrogenic Inoculation
  Spinal surgery
  Percutaneous spinal procedures
  Epidural catheterization
  Central nerve block

Although spinal epidural abscesses (SEAs) are uncommon, they are associated with a relatively high associated morbidity and mortality, particularly with a delay in treatment. They occur when purulent contents accumulate between the dura matter and osseoligamentous structures within the vertebral canal. Bacteria may gain access to the epidural space through direct extension, hematogenous spread, or iatrogenic inoculation (Table 42.1). *Staphylococcus aureus* is the most common causative agent while other causes include *Streptococcus* species, gram-negative bacilli, anaerobes, fungi, *Mycobacterium tuberculosis*, and rarely parasitic organisms. Risk factors include conditions of impaired immunity (e.g., HIV infection, diabetes mellitus, end-stage renal disease, alcoholism, cancer), chronic corticosteroid use, intravenous drug abuse, distant infections, and spinal procedures. No obvious risk factors are found in about 20% of cases.

Epidural abscesses most commonly occur posterior to the spinal cord and this propensity is attributable to the anatomy of this region. Ventrally, the dura is closely applied to the posterior longitudinal ligament from C1 to S2.3. Dorsally, the epidural space begins to appear at C7 and is present the entire length of the canal, in varying depths, signifying a true space.

The classic clinical triad includes back pain, fever, and neurological deficits that may manifest as limb weakness, paralysis, sensory disturbances, and fecal/urinary incompetence. The succession of stages can be rapid, occurring over the course of 7–10 days, thus further contributing to the urgency in diagnosis. Supportive laboratory evidence includes leukocytosis and elevated erythrocyte sedimentation rate (ESR) and C-reactive protein (CRP). CRP levels may be useful for monitoring the response to surgical intervention and antibiotics.

Radiological Evaluation

Though spinal radiographs do not aide in detecting spinal epidural abscesses, they should still be obtained as the initial study as vertebral discitis/osteomyelitis may be associated with SEA. Emergent contrast-enhanced MRI is considered the diagnostic modality of choice to diagnose SEAs. SEAs appear hyperintense on T2-weighted imaging (Figures 42.1, 42.2, 42.5, and 42.6) and isointense or hypointense on T1-weighted imaging. Abscesses will display rim enhancement (Figures 42.3, 42.4, 42.7, and 42.8) while phlegmon will demonstrate homogeneous enhancement. CT cannot reliably exclude early signs of epidural abscess formation and is therefore not generally recommended (**Figures 42.9, 42.10, 42.11 and 42.12**). If MRI is contraindicated, CT myelography may be useful in identifying the location and extent of extradural compression, seen as partial or complete obstruction to cerebrospinal fluid (CSF) flow with associated mass effect on adjacent neural elements. However, CT-myelography findings are not specific for SEAs and must be distinguished from other lesions compressing the thecal sac.

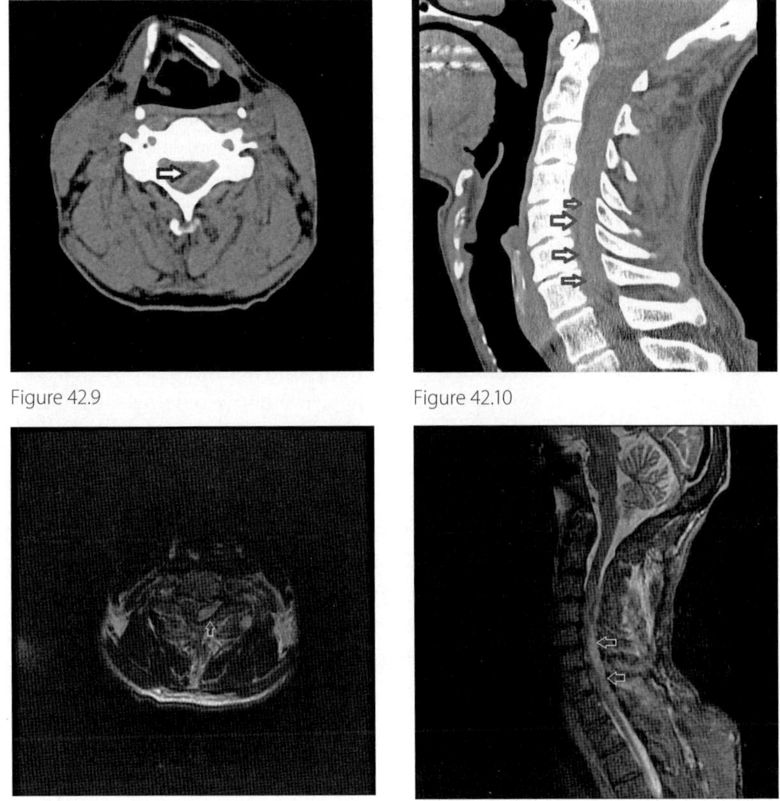

Figure 42.9

Figure 42.10

Figure 42.11

Figure 42.12

Epidural abscess in a patient with progressive neurological decline over 24 hours (**Figures 42.9, 42.10, 42.11, and 42.12**). Non-contrast enhanced axial (Figure 42.9) and sagittal (Figure 42.10) CT images were initially obtained in this patient. There is suggestion of a subtle abnormality within the spinal canal (white arrows, Figures 42.9 and 42.10). This is significantly better appreciated on axial (Figure 42.11) and sagittal (Figure 42.12) T2-weighted MR images. The patient was taken to the OR and found to have an epidural abscess. Due to its limited evaluation of the spinal canal, CT is generally not used in the initial evaluation of patients suspected of having an epidural abscess.

Management

An epidural abscess with neurological deficit is a surgical emergency and requires expedient intervention. When the time to surgical intervention falls within 24 hours of the onset of neurological symptoms, good results can be obtained 50–80% of the time.

The goals of surgery are eradication of the infection and all devitalized tissue and stabilization of the spine. In the most common setting of a posterior epidural abscess, a posterior approach is undertaken with a laminectomy performed for decompression. All visualized purulent fluid and tissues should be removed via suction and irrigation. Ideally, facet joints are left intact to prevent further destabilization. At the time of the debridement, the spine should be stabilized by instrumentation and fusion if there is evidence of instability due to infection or extensive resection.

Intravenous antibiotics are a critical adjunctive to surgery after cultures are taken to ensure an organism-specific approach. Antibiotic therapy is typically enacted for a period of 4–6 weeks.

As has been described throughout the literature, early identification is the key for treatment of an epidural abscess. The prognosis for recovery is closely correlated with the duration of the neurological deficit preoperatively and the degree of compression of the thecal sac. Complete paralysis and/or sensory loss prior to operative intervention are poor prognostic factors. Unfortunately, many of the conditions that are risk factors for the disease, as mentioned earlier, are also associated with poorer recovery.

A few studies have shown that an SEA without neurological deficit, or evidence of sepsis, has the potential to be treated with 4–8 weeks of intravenous antibiotics alone. In this scenario, close monitoring would be imperative with admission to an ICU setting and serial examinations and inflammatory markers. The prevailing consensus, however, is that medical management should be limited to those for whom surgery carries an unacceptable high risk for mortality. Studies have shown that most patients fail medical management and ultimately require emergent decompression, with a higher risk of neurological sequelae due to the delay. A recent retrospective review identified four risk factors that were predictive of failure of medical management for cervical spinal epidural abscess: diabetes mellitus, leukocytosis greater than $12.5 \times 10^3/\mu L$, positive blood cultures, and CRP greater than 115 mg/L with an 8.5% risk of failure of medical management with no risk factors present, 35.4% with one risk factor, 40.2% with two risk factors, and 76.9% with three or more risk factors. Additionally, other studies have found methicillin-resistant *Staphylococcus aureus* (MRSA) infection and age greater than 65 years to be predictive of failed antibiotic management alone for SEA.

Teaching Points

▶ Emergent contrast-enhanced MRI is the diagnostic imaging modality of choice to diagnose a SEA.

▶ An epidural abscess with neurological deficit is a surgical emergency and requires decompressive laminectomy, debridement, and stabilization with instrumentation and fusion as needed.

▶ In select patients with medical comorbidities precluding surgery, in whom neurological deficit is absent or stable, medical management may be successful with close monitoring of clinical status.

▶ The prognosis for recovery is closely correlated with the duration of the neurological deficit preoperatively and with the degree of compression of the thecal sac.

Further Reading

1. Tompkins M, Panuncialman I, Lucas P, and Palumbo M. Spinal epidural abscess. J Emerg Med 2010;39(3):384–390.
2. Pradilla G, Nagahama Y, Spivak AM, et al. Spinal epidural abscess: Current diagnosis and management. Curr Infect Dis Rep 2010;12(6):484–491.
3. Diehn FE. Imaging of spine infection. Radiol Clin North Am 2012;50(4):777–798.
4. Bluman M, Palumbo A, and Lucas R. Spinal epidural abscess in adults. J Am Acad Orthop Surg 2004;12(3):155–163.
5. Herkowitz HN, Garfin SR, Eismont FJ, et al. (Eds.). *The Spine*, 6th ed. Philadelphia, PA: W.B. Saunders, 2011, pp. 1688–1702.
6. Dimar, J, Crawford CH, and Smith C. Spinal epidural abscess: A review of diagnosis and treatment. Curr Orthopaed Pract 2014;25:29–33.
7. Winn RH, Tubb RS, Pugh JA, and Oakes JW. *Youmans Neurological Surgery*, 6th ed. Philadelphia, PA: Saunders, 2011, pp. 1918–1927.
8. Darouiche RO. Spinal epidural abscess. N Engl J Med 2006;355:2012–2020.
9. Chapman JR, Lee MJ, Bellabarba C, et al. Is there a difference in neurologic outcome in medical versus early operative management of cervical epidural abscesses? Spine J 2015;15:10–17.
10. Chapman JR, Bellabarba CB, Lee MJ, et al. Spinal epidural abscesses: Risk factors, medical versus surgical management, a retrospective review of 128 cases. Spine J 2014;14(8):1673–1679.
11. Harris MB, Bono CM, Wood KB, et al. Independent predictors of failure of nonoperative management of spinal epidural abscesses. Clin Orthop Relat Res 2005;439:56–60.

Daniel S. Treister, Anandh Rajamohan, Daniel Helmy, and Mark S. Shiroishi

History

▶ A 34-year-old female with history of prior arachnoid cyst resection presents for follow-up MRI (**Figure 43.1**).

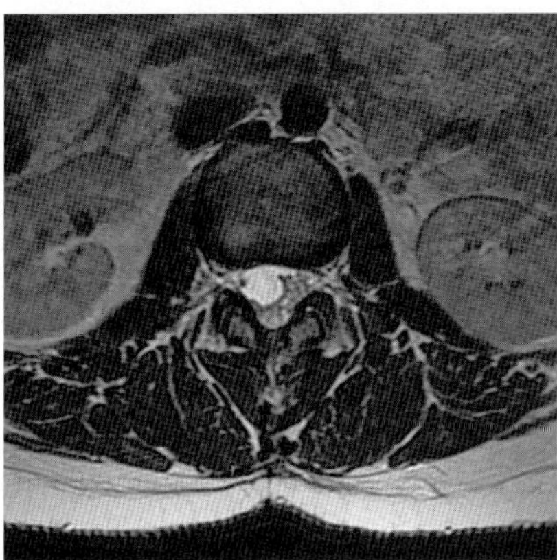

Figure 43.1

Chapter 43 **Arachnoiditis**

Findings

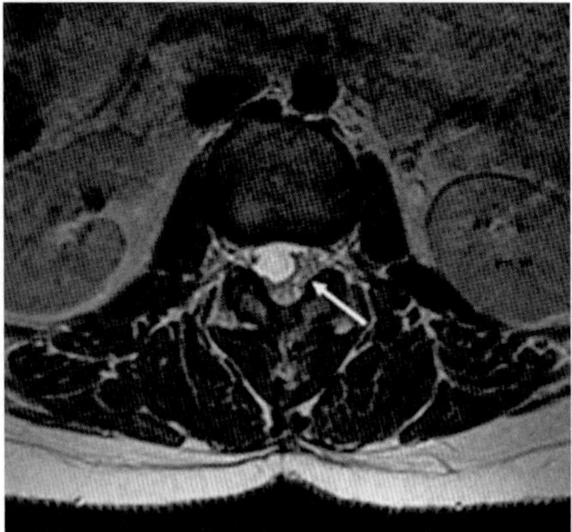

Figure 43.2

Arachnoiditis (**Figure 43.2**). Axial T2-weighted MRI of the lumbar spine demonstrates clumping and peripheral displacement of the cauda equina nerve roots posteriorly and to the left in the region previously containing an arachnoid cyst (arrow).

Differential Diagnosis
▶ Carcinomatous meningitis
▶ Infectious meningitis
▶ Lymphoma
▶ Lumbar spine stenosis
▶ Cauda equina tumor
▶ Guillain-Barré disease

Discussion

Spinal arachnoiditis is a nonspecific inflammatory condition of the arachnoid layer of the spinal meninges or cauda equina. The inflammation may be associated with infectious processes or be the result of a noninfectious insult to the arachnoid membrane such as surgery, trauma, or contamination of the subarachnoid space (**Table 43.1**). Infectious causes were the most common cause of arachnoiditis in the first half of the twentieth century; however, noninfectious causes, such as surgery, are now more commonly associated with it. Chronic inflammation results in progressive scarring of the arachnoid and the formation of adhesions between the arachnoid mater, pia mater, dura mater, and spinal nerve roots. The presentation is often nonspecific. Involvement of the spinal nerve roots may result in the clinical symptomatology of arachnoiditis, which includes burning pain in the lower back and/or legs. Arachnoiditis has also been associated with paravertebral muscle spasms, limited range of motion of the trunk, hypoesthesias, and bowel/bladder dysfunction. Many patients with arachnoiditis may also be asymptomatic with the diagnosis discovered as an incidental finding on radiographic studies.

Infectious

Bacterial/viral

Syphilis

Parasitic infections

Fungal
Tuberculosis

Noninfectious

Trauma

Noniatrogenic injury

Surgery or other instrumentation

Epidural injection

Contamination

Contrast agents (oil-based > water-soluble; water-soluble ionic > water-soluble nonionic)
Steroids
Anesthetics

Other intrathecal medications
Intrathecal hemorrhage
Neoplasms
Lymphoma/leukemia
Metastatic disease
Cauda equina neoplasms
Other
Spinal stenosis
Degenerative disc disease
Arthritis (particularly ankylosing spondylitis)

Radiological Evaluation

Arachnoiditis is best evaluated with CT myelography or MRI with the latter preferable because it is noninvasive and requires no ionizing radiation. In the past, intrathecal injection of a contrast agent required for CT myelogram could potentially exacerbate preexisting arachnoid inflammation. However, the development of water-soluble spinal contrast agents has resulted in a reduction of contrast-related arachnoiditis, which was classically seen with older oil-based agents. The myelographic appearance of arachnoiditis is variable and is likely related to the stage of disease. Myelography in arachnoiditis may demonstrate prominent cauda equina nerve roots, loss of root-sleeve filling, and subarachnoid filling defects with shortening and narrowing of the thecal sac. **Figure 43.3** is an axial and sagittal CT myelogram with peripheral clumping of nerve roots (arrows) leading to an "empty sac" appearance. Three patterns of arachnoiditis have been described on axial MRI, which correlate with increasing disease severity:

1. Central nerve root clumping. See **Figure 43.4**, an axial T2-weighted MRI that demonstrates central clumping of nerve roots (arrow).
2. Peripheral nerve root clumping resulting in an "empty sac" appearance
3. Replacement of subarachnoid space with a soft-tissue mass.

Calcification of the arachnoid may result in a condition known as arachnoiditis ossificans, which is visible on CT or MRI. See **Figure 43.5**, a noncontrast CT of the lumbar spine, shows calcifications with the thecal sac along the nerve roots (arrows), consistent with arachnoiditis ossificans.

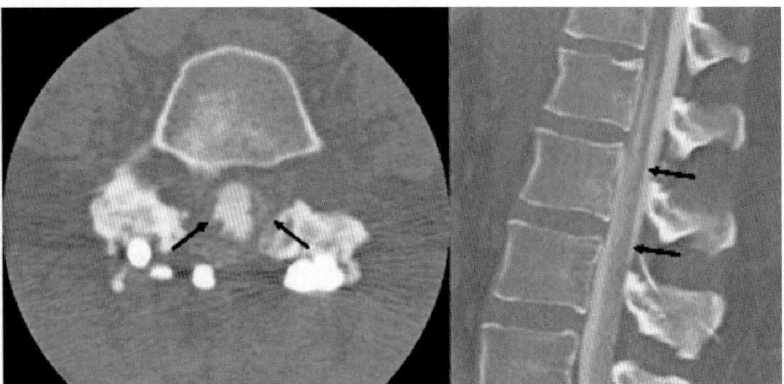

Figure 43.3

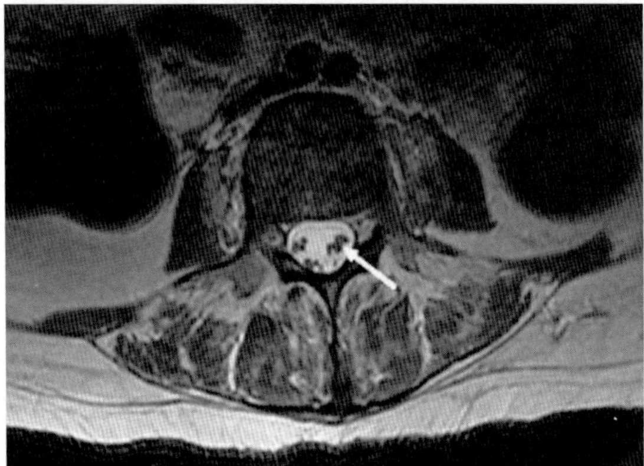

Figure 43.4

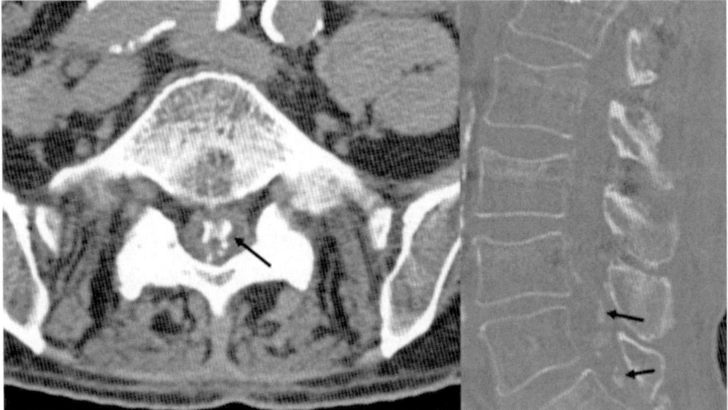

Figure 43.5

Management

There is currently no definitive curative treatment for spinal arachnoiditis. Pain management in these patients can consist of narcotics, steroids, or spinal cord stimulation. The role of surgery is controversial and is considered only in severe cases of pain or some kind of progressive neurological deficit, which is rare. It is important to rule out infectious causes of arachnoiditis because these cases are potentially treatable.

Teaching Points

▶ Arachnoiditis is best visualized with CT myelography and MRI.
▶ Three patterns of arachnoiditis on MRI have been described, which correlate with increasing disease severity.

Further Reading

1. Heary RF and Mammis A. Arachnoiditis. In *Spine Surgery,* 3rd ed. (Benzel EC, ed.). Philadelphia, PA: Elsevier Health Sciences, 2012, pp. 1869–1873.
2. Jorgensen J, Hansen PH, Steenskov V, and Ovesen N. A clinical and radiological study of chronic lower spinal arachnoiditis. Neuroradiology 1975;9(3):139–144.
3. Ross JS, Masaryk TJ, Modic MT, et al. MR imaging of lumbar arachnoiditis. AJR Am J Roentgenol 1987;149(5):1025–1032.

Chapter 44

Philip Dougherty and Kathleen R. Fink

History

► A 57-year-old patient presents with bilateral weakness (**Figures 44.1 and 44.2**).

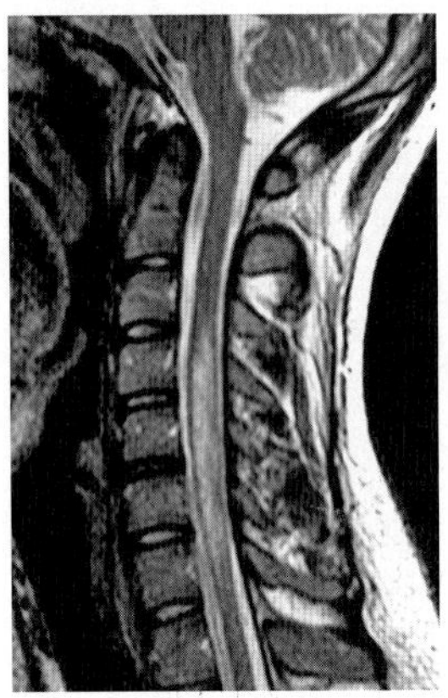

Figure 44.1

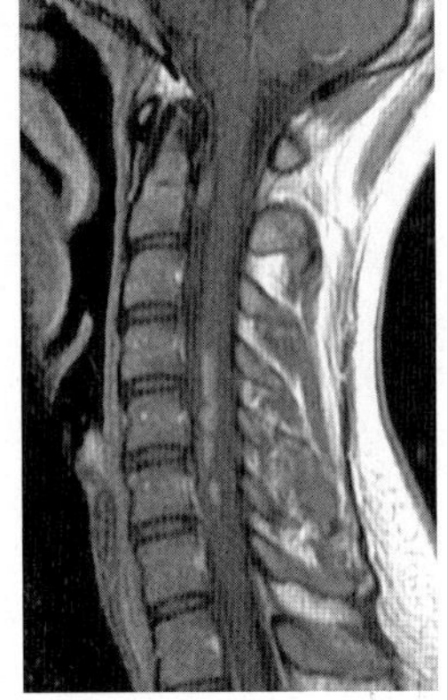

Figure 44.2

Findings

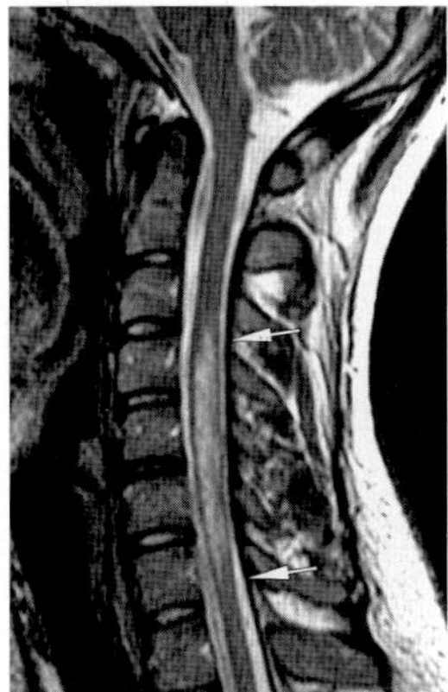 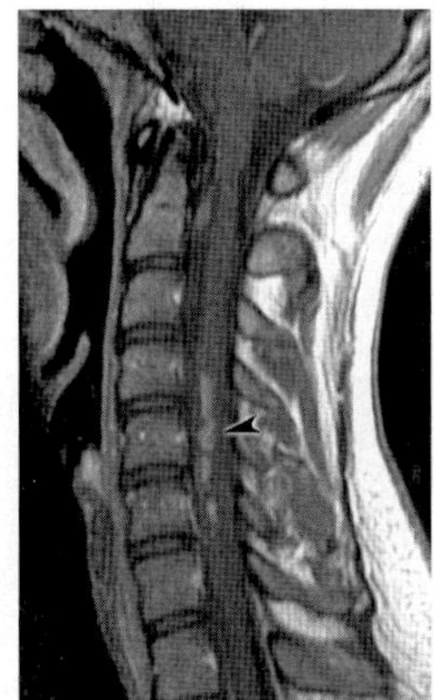

Figure 44.3   Figure 44.4

Transverse myelitis. Sagittal T2 (Figure 44.3) and contrast-enhanced T1 (Figure 44.4) MRI show focal cord expansion with edema spanning C4 to C7 vertebral body levels (white arrows). There is associated enhancement (arrowhead).

Differential Diagnosis

- ▶ Idiopathic myelitis
- ▶ Viral myelitis
- ▶ Acute disseminated encephalomyelitis (ADEM)
- ▶ Multiple sclerosis (MS)
- ▶ Neuromyelitis optica (NMO)
- ▶ Cord infarct
- ▶ Cord neoplasm

Discussion

Transverse myelitis (TM) results from a focal inflammatory process of the spinal cord, often involving motor, sensory, and autonomic tracts at one level. TM can be divided into acute complete and acute partial forms. There are multiple causes, including viral infection, mycoplasma, vaccinations, demyelination, collagen-vascular disease, and paraneoplastic syndromes; but many cases are idiopathic. MS can present initially as TM, usually of the acute partial subtype, but in general MS is more likely to cause shorter segment lesions with relative sparing of motor symptoms.

In addition to imaging, serological analysis is helpful to exclude lupus, HIV, B_{12} deficiency, and NMO, and cerebrospinal fluid (CSF) analysis is helpful to evaluate for MS. Brain MRI is used to look for concomitant white-matter lesions that would suggest the diagnosis of MS. Associated optic neuritis should suggest a diagnosis of NMO.

Transverse myelitis commonly begins with back or radicular pain followed by the abrupt onset of bilateral lower extremity paresthesias progressing to paraplegia. Bowel and bladder dysfunction are common. Progression is rapid with maximal neurological impairment within days. Prognosis is variable after treatment with one-third of patients experiencing a good, fair, or poor recovery.

Radiological Evaluation

Contrast-enhanced MRI is the imaging study of choice, and should include axial and sagittal T1- and T2-weighted sequences. Proton density, STIR, and DWI images are also often useful.

Imaging findings include smooth spinal cord expansion associated with centrally located T2/STIR hyperintensity. The signal abnormality typically involves more than two-thirds of the axial cross-sectional area (Figure 44.5) and extends over three vertebral bodies or more in length (Figure 44.3). A central isointensity or "dot" may be present, representing the gray matter being squeezed by surrounding edema.

Contrast enhancement is variable, occurring approximately half the time. When present, enhancement usually occurs at the periphery of the T2 abnormality in a focal nodular or diffuse pattern (Figure 44.6). The mid-thoracic cord is the most common segment involved.

It is important to differentiate TM from an intramedullary tumor. Tumoral enhancement typically involves the entire cross-sectional area of the cord and is associated with heterogeneous areas of hemorrhage and necrosis. Definitive diagnosis is difficult and biopsy may be required.

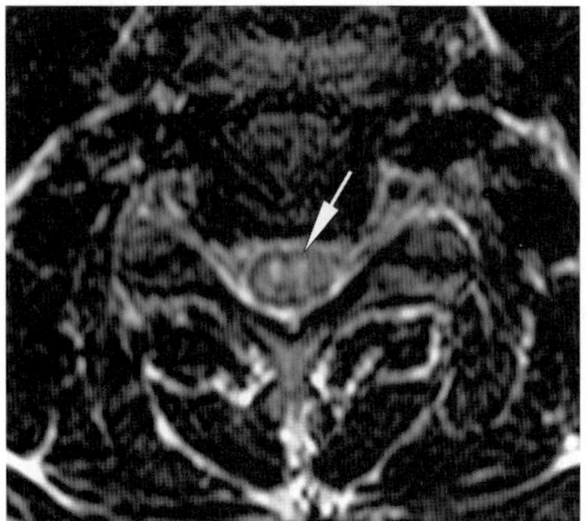

Figure 44.5

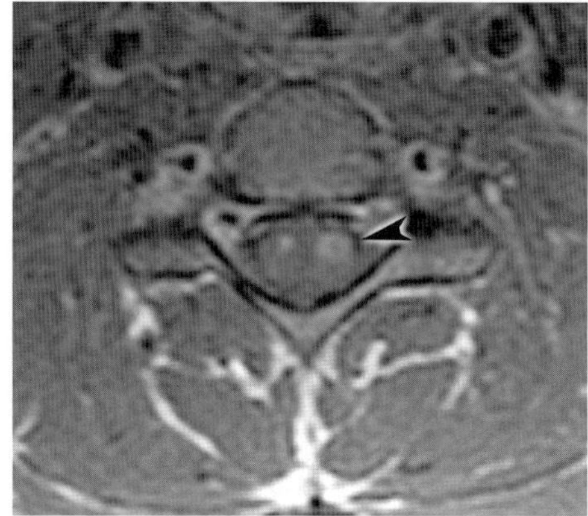

Figure 44.6

Transverse myelitis (**Figures 44.5 and 44.6**). An axial T2-weighted MRI (Figure 44.5) shows involvement of a significant portion of the cross-sectional area of the spinal cord (arrow). A contrast-enhanced T1-weighted MRI (Figure 44.6) shows nodular enhancement (arrowhead).

Management

Management of TM depends on the underlying cause. While there is no effective cure for TM, high-dose corticosteroids are used to decrease inflammation and blunt the autoimmune response. Specific therapies vary based on the underlying etiology. Rehabilitation therapies are typically employed for cases with significant neurological injury and/or deficit.

Teaching Points

▶ Transverse myelitis is a clinical diagnosis with many possible etiologies. Clinical history, examination, imaging findings, and serological and CSF analysis all contribute to making the diagnosis. Despite extensive workup, many cases are idiopathic.

▶ MRI findings of TM include T2/STIR hyperintensity involving more than two-thirds of the axial area of the cord and extending over three or more vertebral bodies in length. Contrast enhancement is variable, but is most commonly peripheral enhancing.

Further Reading

1. Choi KH, Lee KS, Chung SO, et al. Idiopathic transverse myelitis: MR characteristics. AJNR Am J Neuroradiol 1996;17(6):1151–1160.
2. Scott TF, Frohman EM, De Seze J, et al. Evidence-based guideline: Clinical evaluation and treatment of transverse myelitis: Report of the Therapeutics and Technology Assessment Subcommittee of the American Academy of Neurology. Neurology 2011;77:2128–2134.

History

▶ A 6-year-old female presents with localized back pain (**Figure 45.1**).

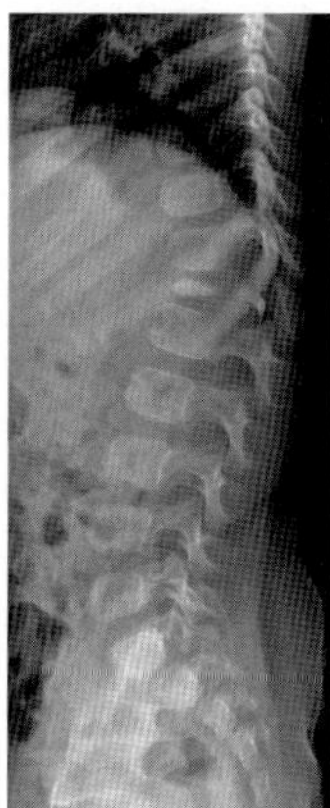

Figure 45.1

Chapter 45   Langerhans Cell Histiocytosis of the Spine

Findings

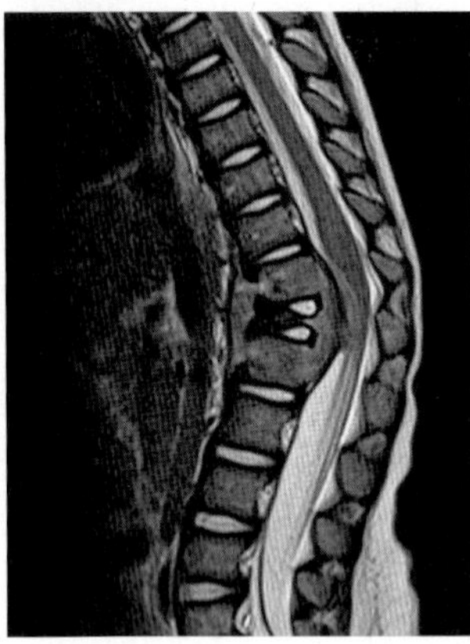

Figure 45.2

Histiocytosis of the spine (Figure 45.1 and Figure 45.2). Lateral X-ray of the thoracolumbar spine (Figure 45.1) demonstrates T12 vertebra plana, with associated focal kyphotic deformity. A sagittal FSE T2 image of the thoracolumbar spine (Figure 45.2) best demonstrates the "dumbbell" appearance of the associated soft tissue component anteriorly and posteriorly, with the intracanal component of Langerhans cell histiocytosis (LCH) having a mass effect upon the conus of the spinal cord.

Differential Diagnosis

In a pediatric patient, the differential for a vertebra plana includes the following:
- Metastasis
- Lymphoma
- Leukemic infiltration
- Ewing sarcoma
- Osteomyelitis
- Tuberculosis
- Langerhans cell histiocytosis

Discussion

LCH is a disorder characterized by an abnormal accumulation of histiocytes throughout the body. It is primarily a disease of childhood, with an annual incidence of 4.6 per million in children under the age of 14 years. However, it can occur in any age group, and rarely can be seen in adults. Males are more commonly affected than females.

The skeleton is a most frequently affected tissue in children, seen in 75–80% of patients, with unifocal involvement more common than multifocal disease. Spinal disease accounts for approximately 6.5–25% of all bony LCH, with the thoracic spine being the most common area of involvement, followed by the lumbar and cervical spine. Recently, it has been suggested that cervical spinal involvement is more common than thoracic involvement.

Of patients 80% present with pain, with this typically localized to the site of disease with a tendency for progressive symptoms over time. Radicular pain (with or without sensory loss) usually occurs in the setting of cervical or lumbosacral spinal involvement. Other clinical features include restricted spinal movement (with torticollis/neck stiffness common in those with cervical spinal disease), spinal deformity, and neurological deficits. Neurological deficits are uncommon; however, adult patients are more likely to present in this manner than children.

Radiological Evaluation

The radiology of spinal LCH reflects the pathological process of these lesions typically destroying and replacing the normal bony architecture. The majority appear osteolytic, with the appearance in pediatric disease similar to that for multiple myeloma in adults. In children, it typically involves the vertebral bodies, with relative sparing of the posterior elements. This pattern of involvement can result in a pathological compression fracture, leading to the classical "vertebra plana" appearance (Figure 45.1). This appearance is uncommon in those presenting in adulthood. Radiography and bone scintigraphy are used to establish the extent of disease, with CT best at demonstrating the bony destructive features, and MRI optimal at characterizing the associated soft tissue disease and possible intracanal/foraminal extension.

On MRI, most lesions are low to intermediate signal on T1-weighted imaging, typically hyperintense on T2-weighted imaging, and demonstrate marked homogeneous enhancement after administration of gadolinium. A classical "dumbbell" appearance is a typical feature of pediatric spinal involvement (Figure 45.2). Newer imaging modalities, such as PET-CT, may play a role in disease workup. The diagnosis of spinal LCH depends on a combination of clinical, radiographic, and pathological features, with tissue diagnosis often required, especially in those presenting in adulthood, with specific histological and immunohistochemical staining features seen for LCH.

Management

Treatment depends on the extent and severity of the disease. Many patients undergo spontaneous resolution of their disease. The need for surgery or adjuvant therapy is usually reserved for those having specific issues, such as neurological manifestations, progressive spinal deformity, or persisting/progressive pain despite conservative management.

Teaching Points

► Spinal LCH in the pediatric patient classically presents as a "vertebra plana."
► Although classically considered a disease of childhood, LCH can occur in adulthood with imaging typically demonstrating an osteolytic lesion of the vertebra. Diagnosis often requires biopsy.

Further Reading

1. Huang WD, Yang XH, Wu ZP, et al. Langerhans cell histiocytosis of spine: A comparative study of clinical, imaging features, and diagnosis in children, adolescents, and adults. Spine J 2013;13:1108–1117.
2. Khung S, Budzik JF, Amzallag-Bellenger E, et al. Skeletal involvement in Langerhans cell histiocytosis. Insights Imaging 2013;4:569–579.
3. Sapkas G and Papadakis M. Vertebral Langerhans cell histiocytosis in an adult patient: Case report and review of the literature. Acta Orthop Belg 2011;77:260–264.

Chapter 46

Quynh Nguyen and Nupur Verma

History

▶ A 33-year-old male patient presents to the Emergency Department with complaints of new onset severe buttock pain and difficulty urinating for one day. A physical examination revealed bilateral lower extremity weakness, saddle anesthesia, and a distended urinary bladder by ultrasound evaluation (**Figures 46.1 and 46.2**).

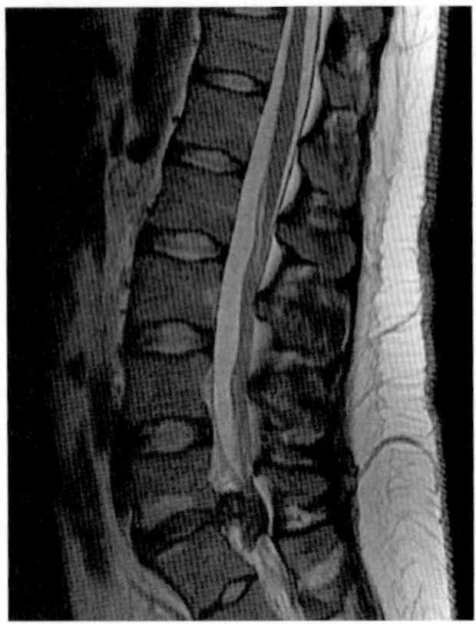

Figure 46.1

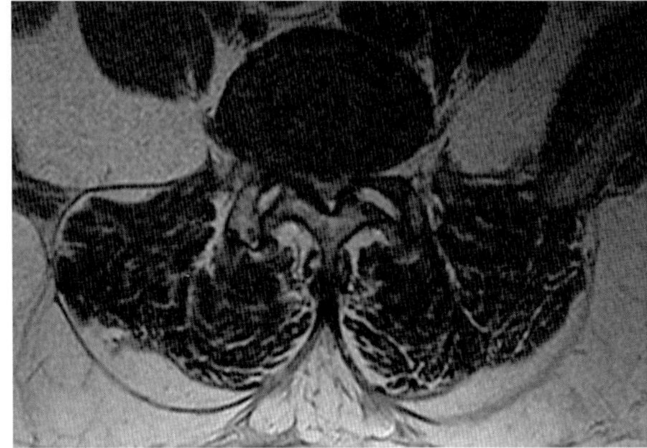

Figure 46.2

Findings

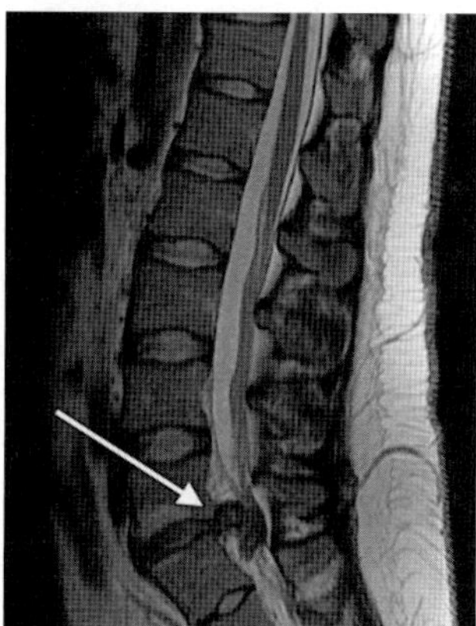

Figure 46.3

Cauda equina syndrome, high-grade stenosis at L4–5 with a clinical presentation of bilateral lower extremity weakness, saddle anesthesia, and urinary retention (due to a disc extrusion) (Figures 46.2 and 46.3). Axial T2 (Figure 46.2) and sagittal (Figure 46.3) images demonstrate a large L4–5 disc extrusion, with a possible free fragment, resulting in severe central stenosis at L4–5. There is complete effacement of the cerebrospinal fluid and compression of the nerve roots.

Discussion

Although disk herniation and stenosis are a relatively common finding on cross-sectional imaging, cauda equina syndrome is only seen in 0.12% of patients with these imaging findings. However, because of the morbidity that may result from prolonged compression of the nerve roots, including permanent loss of bowel, bladder and sexual function, patients are commonly screened for high-grade stenosis with MRI. MR findings of severe stenosis of the cauda equina roots anywhere from the conus medullaris through the coccygeal nerves support the diagnosis of cauda equina syndrome in the clinical setting of bladder, bowel, or sexual dysfunction and/or saddle anesthesia. Lumbar spondylosis, including disc herniations, are the most common etiology for a high grade stenosis however, other etiologies such as epidural hematoma, epidural abscess and tumor can also cause a high grade stenosis leading to cauda equina syndrome.

The most common symptom of cauda equina is urinary retention with some degree of paresthesias, or dysesthesias in the lower extremities. Intractable low back and lower extremity pain are also suggestive of cauda equina syndrome.

Physical examination findings may reveal decreased sensation and motor strength of the lower extremities, hyporeflexia of the lower extremities, saddle anesthesia, bladder distention with overflow incontinence, incomplete voiding with high postvoid residual urine, and/or decreased sphincter tone.

Radiological Evaluation

MRI is the gold standard for evaluating stenosis of the spinal column due to its excellent soft tissue resolution allowing for visualization of the disc, ligamentum flavum, or other compressive lesions (abscess, hematoma, masses). For patients who cannot undergo MRI (e.g., patients with a noncompatible pacemaker, metallic foreign objects, claustrophobia, or hardware from prior spine surgeries), CT myelography provides a reasonable alternative method of evaluating for potential extrinsic factors compressing the neural structures of the spinal canal.

Management

Surgical decompression with removal of the offending agent is the first line of treatment. Surgery within the first 24–48 hours after the onset of symptoms is recommended to maximize the potential for neurological recovery. Incontinence of stool is recognized as a poor prognostic factor.

Teaching Points

- ► Cauda equina syndrome should always be in the differential diagnosis of patients presenting with urinary retention, lower extremity paresthesias, or intractable pain.
- ► MRI is the imaging modality of choice to identify compression of the thecal sac.
- ► Urgent surgical decompression supports the best chance for neurological recovery.

Further Reading

1. Small SA, Perron AD, and Brady WJ. Orthopedic pitfalls: Cauda equina syndrome. Am J Emerg Med 2005;23:159–163.
2. American College of Radiology. ACR Appropriateness Criteria'. Clinical Indication Back Pain, Variant 6. Date Accessed 1/2/2014. http://www.acr.org/~/media/ACR/Documents/AppCriteria/Diagnostic/LowBackPain.pdf
3. Ahn UM, Ahn NU, Buchowski JM, et al. Cauda equina syndrome secondary to lumbar disc herniation: A meta-analysis of surgical outcomes. Spine 2000;25:1515–1522.

Section 5

Metabolic and Demyelinating

Anant Krishnan and Richard Silbergleit

History

▶ A 32-year-old female presents with progressive sensory myelopathy (**Figures 47.1, 47.2, 47.3, and 47.4**).

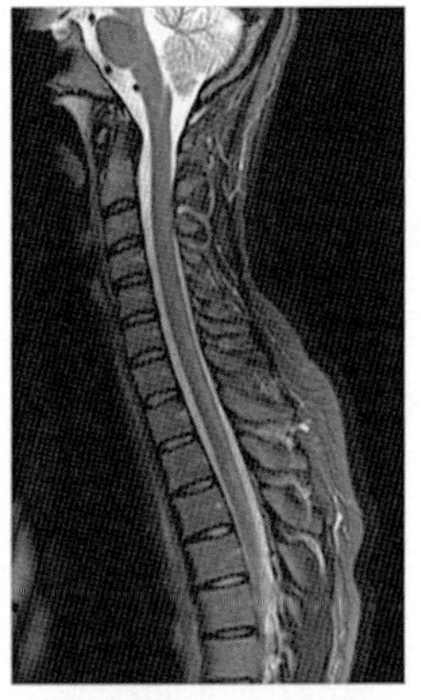

Figure 47.1

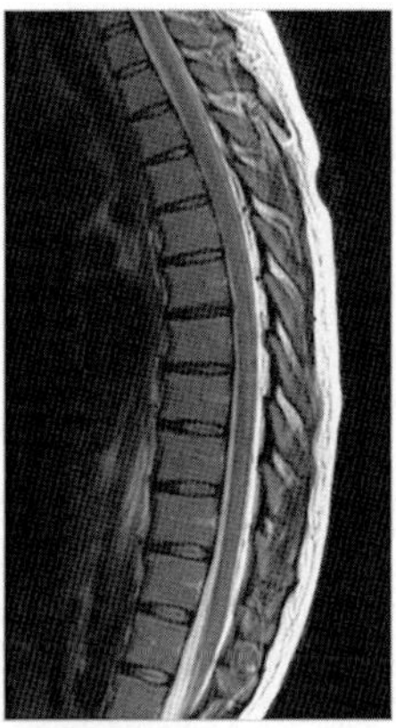

Figure 47.2

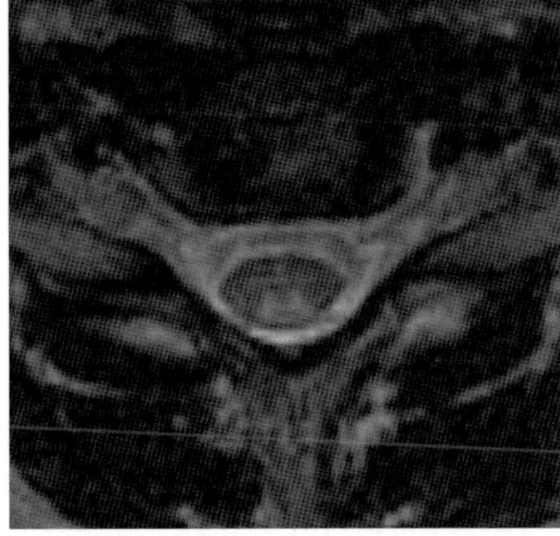

Figure 47.3

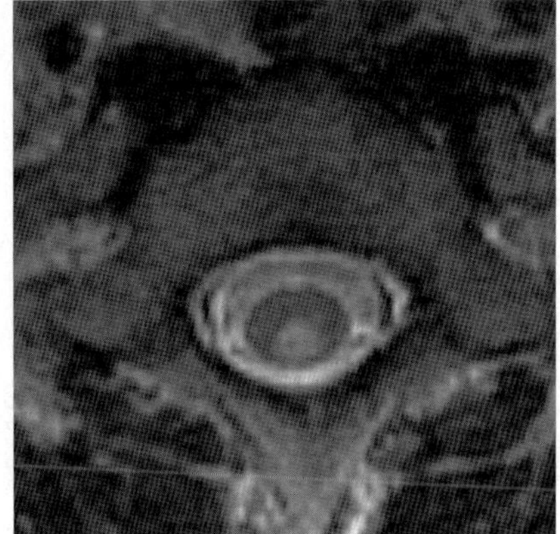

Figure 47.4

Chapter 47   Subacute Combined Degeneration of the Spinal Cord

Findings

Subacute degeneration of the spinal cord (SCD) from B_{12} deficiency. Sagittal T2-weighted images (**Figures 47.5 and 47.6**) and axial T2-weighted images (**Figures 47.7 and 47.8**) of the cervical and thoracic spine demonstrate a T2 hyperintense signal (arrows) extending craniocaudally along the dorsal aspect of the spinal cord. On the axial views, bilateral involvement of the dorsal columns of the spinal cord is seen.

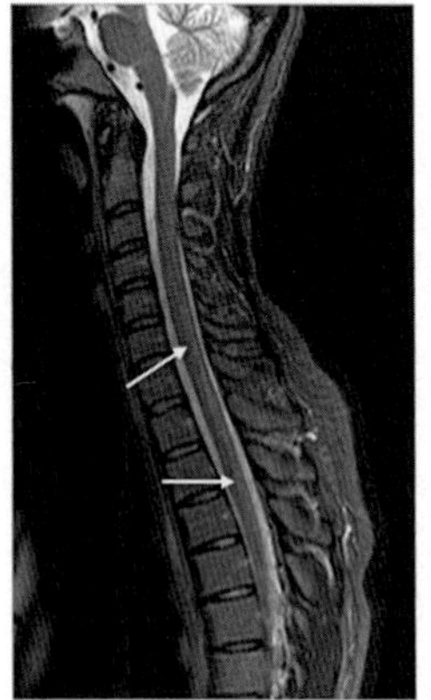

Figure 47.5

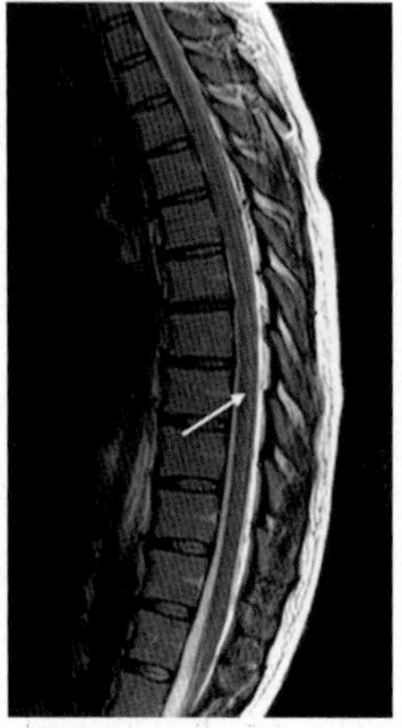

Figure 47.6

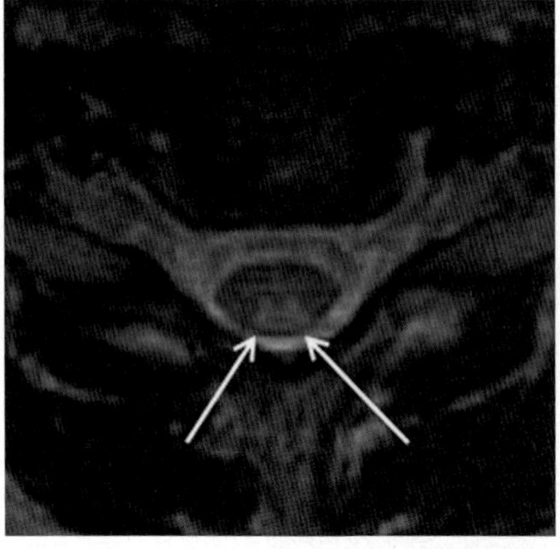

Figure 47.7

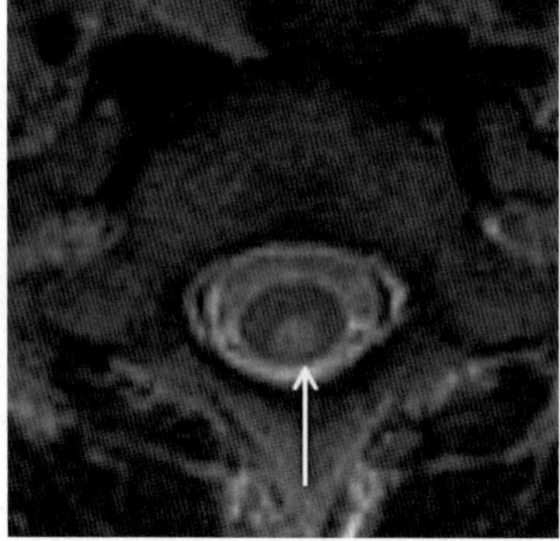

Figure 47.8

A workup was performed demonstrating abnormally low serum B_{12} levels of 103 pg/ml (normal range = 271–870 pg/ml) and elevated serum methylmalonic acid of 10.63 μmol/L (normal range ≤ 0.4). Mean corpuscular volume (MCV) was high and red blood cell count (RBC) was decreased at 3.4 Tril/L. On this basis, a diagnosis of vitamin B_{12}-deficient SCD was made.

Differential Diagnosis

▶ Other causes of SCD such as nitrous oxide inhalation have similar imaging features. A clinical history of nitrous oxide inhalation during surgery, dental work, or from recreational reasons, and related laboratory findings help separate this entity.

▶ HIV vacuolar myelopathy can closely mimic SCD imaging, but may also be associated with cord expansion. A potential cause is viral interruption of the methylation pathway leading to a similar clinical, radiological, and pathological end result. Cerebrospinal fluid (CSF) testing and blood work are also helpful in HIV and other infectious etiologies.

▶ Copper deficiency myeloneuropathy. Copper deficiency is a cause of neurological dysfunction and can present with sensory ataxia, myelodysplastic syndrome, and anemia. Some patients demonstrate imaging findings very similar to SCD including dorsal column T2 hyperintensity in the cervical spinal cord. Causes for copper deficiency include excess zinc ingestion (denture creams) or treatment, malabsorption, gastric bypass surgery (including bariatric), and total parenteral nutrition; in some patients there is a presumed defect in copper transport.

▶ Demyelinating disease (especially multiple sclerosis). T2 hyperintensities are not restricted to the dorsal or lateral columns, rarely extend greater than 2 vertebral lengths, and are discontinuous. Imaging findings in the brain and clinical history are additional differentiating features. Other causes such as transverse myelitis and neuromyelitis optica involve a larger cross-sectional area of the cord and have additional clinical and CSF findings.

▶ Spinal cord ischemia. Clinical features are distinct and isolated dorsal column involvement is less likely.

Discussion

Described in detail in 1900 by Russell and colleagues but identified even earlier in the nineteenth century (Lichtheim in 1887 described it in relation to pernicious anemia), subacute combined degeneration of the spinal cord refers to the gradually progressive myelopathy accompanying combined demyelination of the posterior and lateral columns of the spinal cord. The microscopic findings are of demyelination of these specific tracts with initially swelling and later vacuolation of the myelin sheath.

B_{12} deficiency is the primary source of SCD. In the United States, dietary deficiency is only rarely the cause and the most common cause is pernicious anemia, which is an immune-mediated destruction of the gastric parietal cells leading to atrophic gastritis and decreased availability of intrinsic factor. Other causes include malabsorption from intestinal infections, tropical sprue, and surgical procedures such as gastric bypass. B_{12} is involved in the methylation as demonstrated in **Figure 47.9** (B_{12} pathway; MTHF, methyltetrahydrofolate).

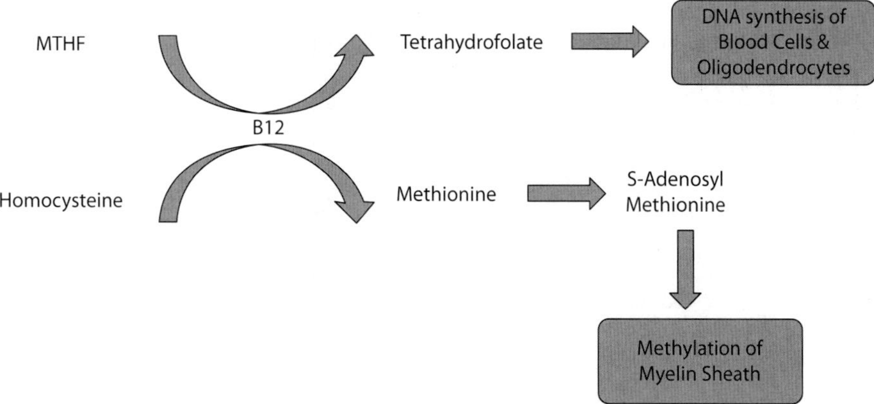

Figure 47.9

An effective B_{12} deficiency can also be caused by nitrous oxide, which can oxidize B_{12} leading to its excretion. As a result, patients with borderline B_{12} deficiency can manifest clinically after nitrous oxide exposure. The imaging findings are identical to other causes of B_{12} deficiency (**Figures 47.10 and 47.11**), as discussed below.

An 18-year-old female presents with paresthesia following nitrous oxide exposure (Figures 47.10 and 47.11). Sagittal and axial T2-weighted images demonstrate T2 hyperintensity in the dorsal columns (case courtesy of Dr Stephen Kilanowski).

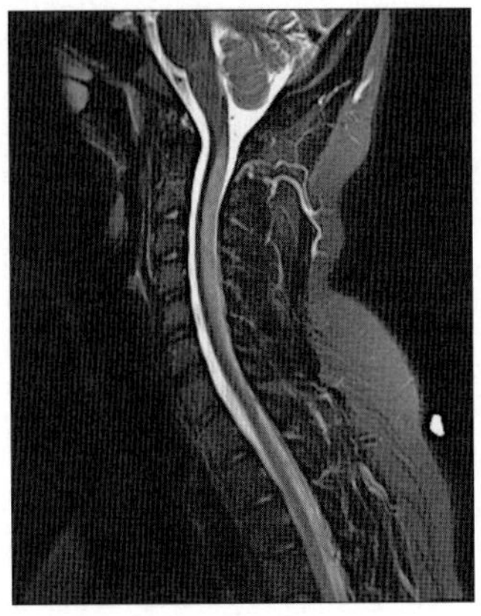

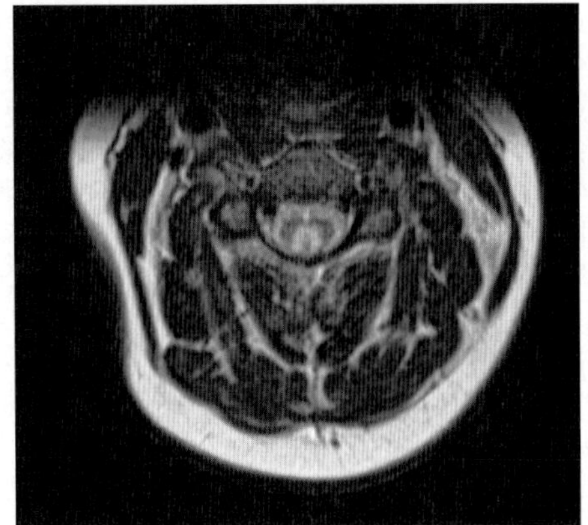

Figure 47.10

Figure 47.11

Biochemical analysis of patients with suspected SCD includes identification of decreased serum B_{12} levels and elevated serum methylmalonic acid levels (B_{12} is involved in the metabolism of methylmalonic coenzyme A to succinyl coenzyme A; a deficiency of B_{12} can cause excess methylmalonic acid).

Radiological Evaluation

Imaging findings correspond to the clinical and pathological location of involvement, primarily affecting the dorsal columns in the lower cervical and upper thoracic regions. On sagittal T2-weighted images, symmetric vertically oriented hyperintensities can be seen along the dorsal columns (Figures 47.5, 47.6, and **47.12**). On axial images, this has been likened to "inverted V" or "inverted rabbit ears" (Figures 47.7 and **47.13**). Occasionally lateral column involvement may be seen, though in some cases, despite the clinical evidence of lateral column involvement, MRI may fail to demonstrate findings. Enhancement has also been rarely described.

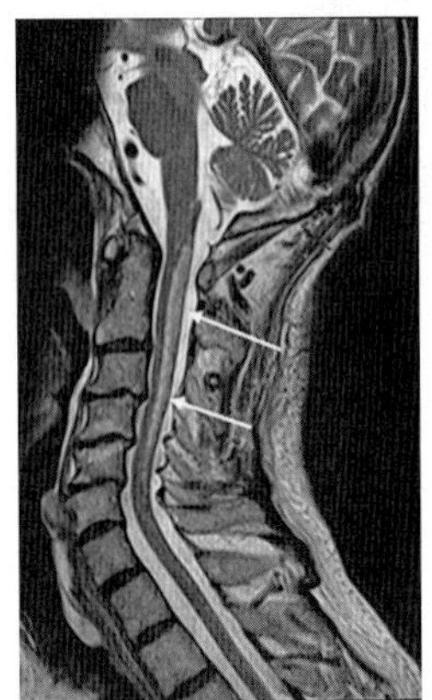

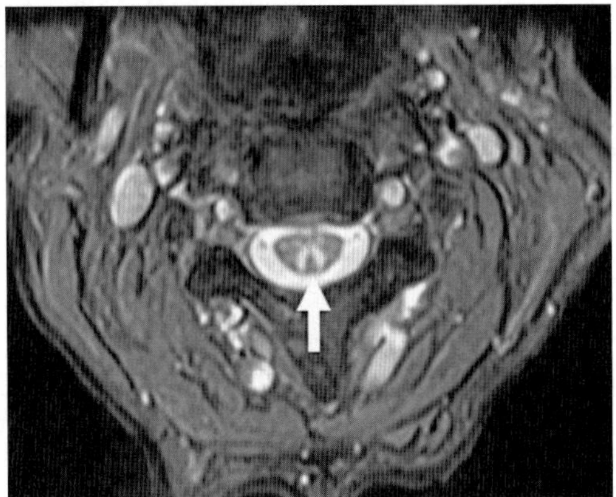

Figure 47.12

Figure 47.13

A 79-year-old male presents with imbalance and difficulty walking over 1 to 2 weeks and bilateral upper extremity paresthesias (**Figures 47.12 and 47.13**). Sagittal T2 (Figure 47.12) demonstrates longitudinal T2 hyperintensity (arrows) extending along the posterior aspect of the spinal cord. An axial gradient T2* image (Figure 47.13) demonstrates an "inverted V" morphology from involvement of the bilateral posterior columns (thick arrow).

Management

B_{12} supplementation early in the disorder can reverse symptoms and MRI findings.

Teaching Points

▶ Bilateral dorsal column T2 hyperintensity is very suggestive of subacute combined degeneration.

▶ Similar imaging findings can be seen after exposure to nitrous oxide and also in HIV patients.

Further Reading

1. Renard D, Dutray A, Remy A, et al. Subacute combined degeneration of the spinal cord caused by nitrous oxide anaesthesia. Neurol Sci 2009;30:75–76.
2. Naidich M and Ho S. Subacute combined degeneration. Radiology 2005;237:101–105.
3. Ravina B, Loevner L, and Bank W. MR findings in subacute combined degeneration of the spinal cord: A case of reversible cervical myelopathy. AJR 2000;174:863–865.
4. Goodman BP, Chong BW, Patel AC, et al. Copper deficiency myeloneuropathy resembling B12 deficiency: Partial resolution of MRI findings with copper supplementation. AJNR 2006;27:2112–2114.
5. Surtees R. Biochemical pathogenesis of subacute combined degeneration of the spinal cord and brain. J Inher Metab Dis 1993;16:762–770.

Chapter 48

Megha Nayyar, Lakshmanan Sivasundaram, Alexander Lerner, and Mark S. Shiroishi

History

▶ A 30-year-old female presents with parasthesias, blurred vision, and urinary incontinence (**Figure 48.1**).

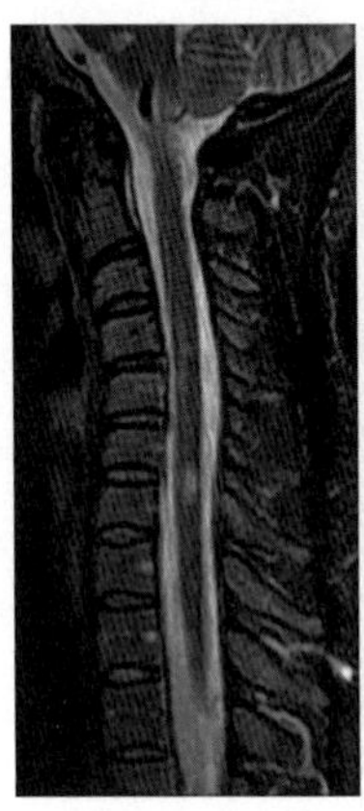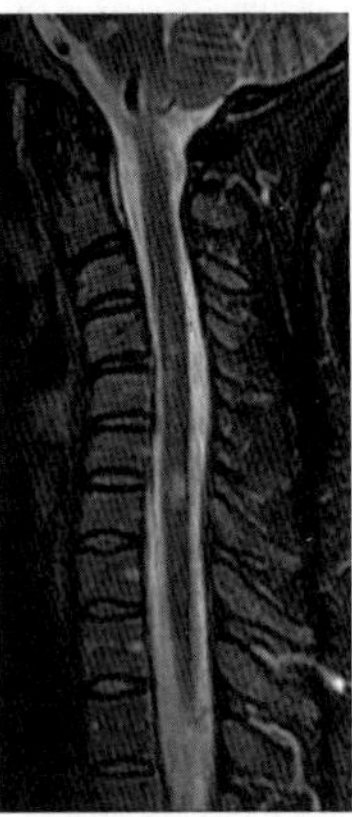

Figure 48.1

Findings

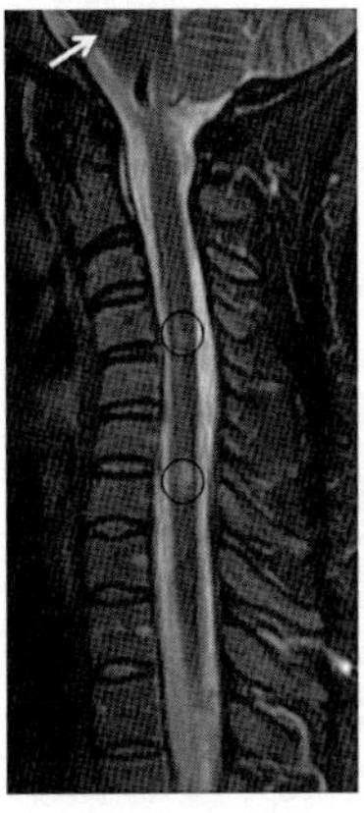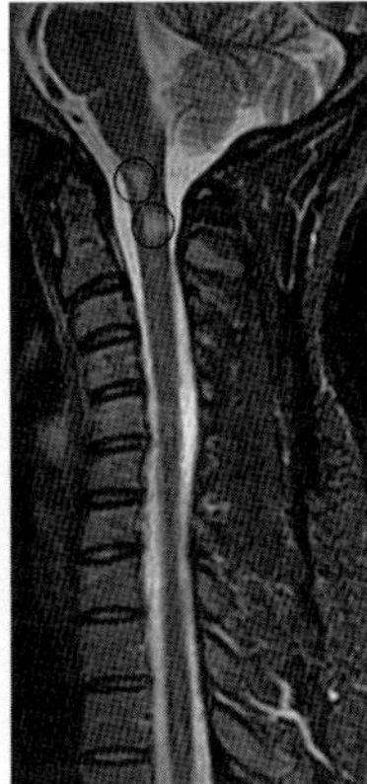

Figure 48.2

Multiple sclerosis with spinal involvement **(Figure 48.2)**. Sagittal STIR [Short Tau Inversion Recovery] MRI shows hyperintense demyelinating lesions (black circles) within the cervical spinal cord that are less than two vertebral segments in length. A lesion is also seen within the inferior pons (arrow).

Differential Diagnosis

► Idiopathic transverse myelitis
► Spinal cord neoplasms
► Spinal cord infarction
► Neuromyelitis optica
► Acute disseminated encephalomyelitis

Discussion

Multiple sclerosis (MS) is an autoimmune inflammatory demyelinating disease of the central nervous system with lesions that are disseminated in space and time. It occurs more commonly in women than men and the mean age of onset is between 20 and 40 years. Genetic susceptibility as well as environmental factors play a role in the pathogenesis of multiple sclerosis, including a geographic association with higher prevalence further north of the equator. The most common symptoms include sensory disturbance in the limbs, partial or complete loss of vision, motor dysfunction of the limbs, diplopia, and gait abnormality. The four clinical phenotypes of MS are relapsing remitting, secondary progressive, primary progressive, and progressive relapsing. Integration of imaging, clinical, and laboratory features is needed to establish a diagnosis of MS.

Radiological Evaluation

Neuroimaging is a crucial element in the diagnosis and management of MS. Most patients with MS will demonstrate focal imaging abnormalities within the spinal cord. The cervical segment of the cord is most commonly affected and the lesions typically involve less than half the cross-sectional area of the cord **(Figures 48.2 and 48.3)**. They also usually extend less than two vertebral segments in length, may cross the gray-white matter boundary of the cord, and often involve the dorsolateral aspect of the cord. Lesions typically appear hyperintense on T2-weighted and STIR images. Unlike in the brain, the lesions often do not appear hypointense on T1-weighted images. Contrast enhancement can be seen in the subacute or acute phase and may mimic an enhancing cord tumor **(Figure 48.4)**. Atrophy of the cord is usually seen in late-stage disease. Chronic and acute lesions may be seen within the cord at the same time.

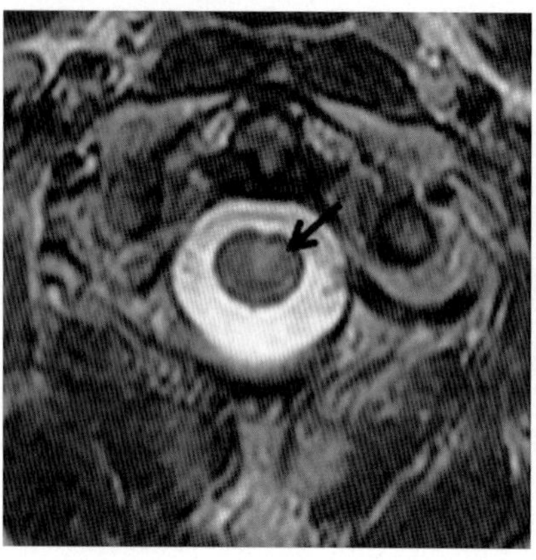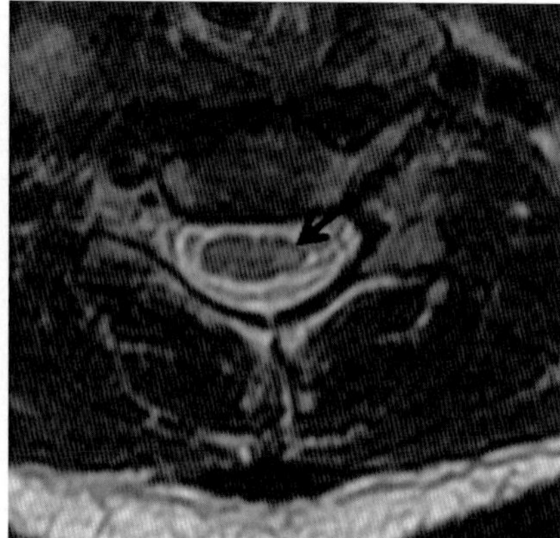

Figure 48.3

MS in the spine (**Figure 48.3**). Axial T2-weighted images demonstrate hyperintense lesions (arrows) that involve both gray and white matter and occupy less than half the cross-sectional area of the cord. A lesion also shows a dorsolateral location (right-sided image).

There is a high incidence of associated brain lesions and so a brain MRI should also be obtained to confirm the diagnosis and to determine the extent of disease (Figures 48.4 and 48.5). Spinal cord abnormalities, especially of the upper cervical cord, have been correlated with clinical disability in MS. Thus, assessing the spinal cord of patients with MS is an important aspect of management.

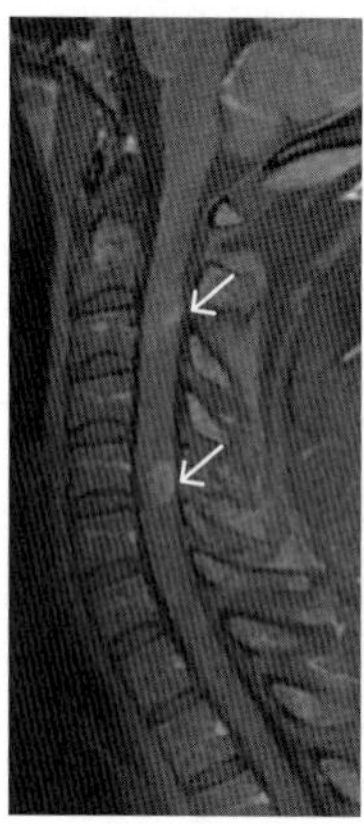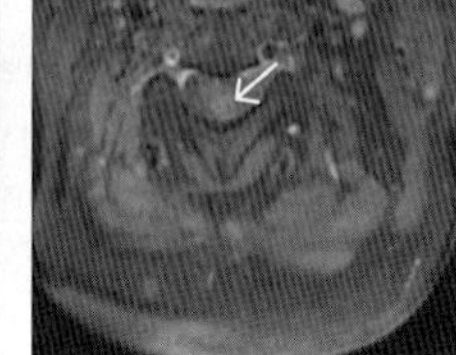

Figure 48.4

MS in the spine (**Figure 48.4**). Sagittal (left) and axial (right) fat-saturated contrast-enhanced T1-weighted images demonstrate enhancing lesions (arrows) within the cervical cord.

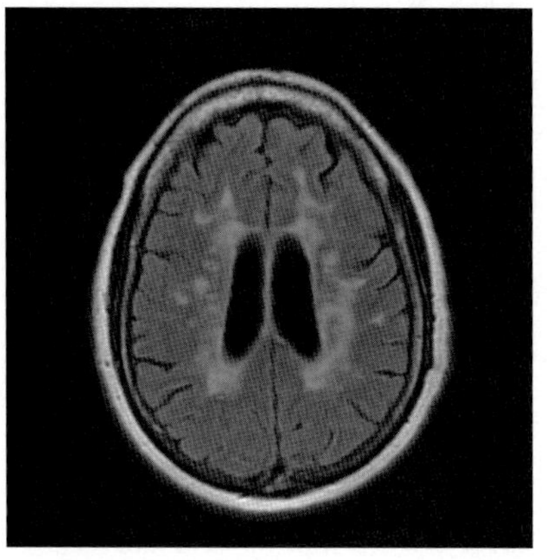

Figure 48.5

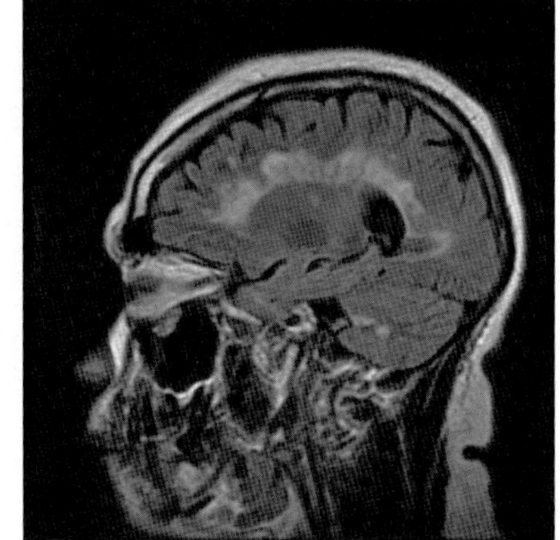

Figure 48.6

Brain lesions seen in MS (**Figures 48.5 and 48.6**). Axial and sagittal T2/FLAIR images of the brain demonstrate the typical periventricular lesions seen in MS.

Management

There is currently no cure for MS. Acute exacerbations of MS are managed with corticosteroids and plasmapheresis. Agents that can be used to modify progression include interferon-beta, mitoxantrone, and glatiramer acetate.

Teaching Points

▶ Integration of imaging, clinical, and laboratory features is needed to establish a diagnosis of MS.
▶ A brain MRI should also be obtained because there is a high incidence of associated brain lesions.
▶ Acute spinal cord MS lesions may enhance and mimic an enhancing cord tumor.

Further Reading

1. Stuve O and Oskenberg J. Multiple sclerosis overview. In *GeneReviews*® [Internet] (Pagon RA, Adam MP, Ardinger HH, et al., eds.). Seattle,WA: University of Washington, 1993–2014.
2. Chen MZ. Multiple sclerosis, spinal cord. In *Diagnostic Imaging. Spine* (Ross JS, Brant-Zawadzki M, Moore KR, et al., eds.). Philadelphia, PA: Amirsys Inc., 2007, pp. III-2-20–III-2-23.
3. Lerner A, Mogensen MA, Kim PE, Shiroishi MS, Hwang DH, Law M Clinical applications of diffusion tensor imaging. World Neurosurg 2014;82(1–2):96–109. (Figure 48.3 reprinted with permission from Elsevier.)

Chapter 49

H. Kate Lee

History

▶ A 79-year-old male presents with atraumatic neck pain for 2 days (**Figures 49.1 and 49.2**).

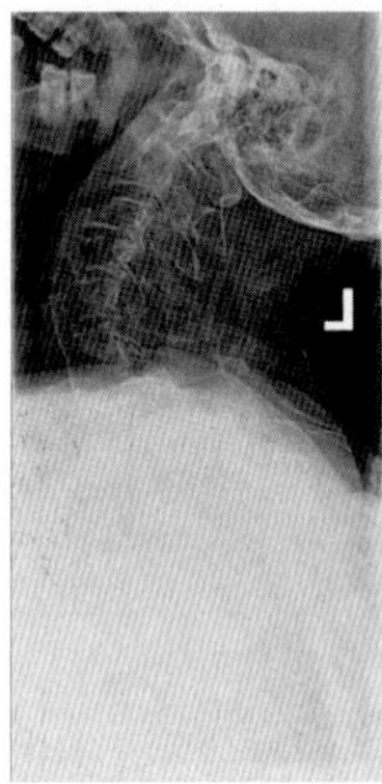

Figure 49.1

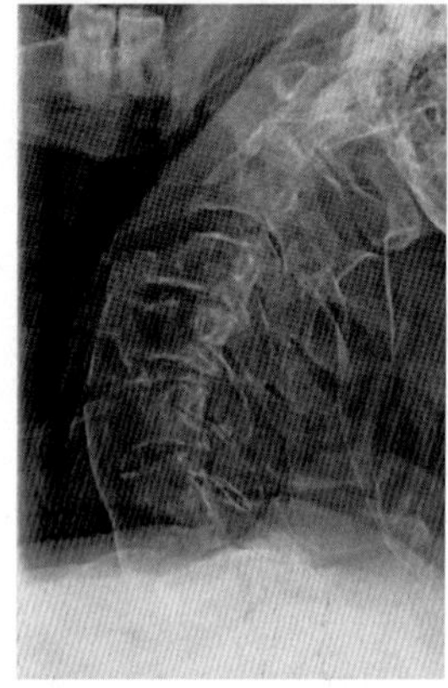

Figure 49.2

Findings

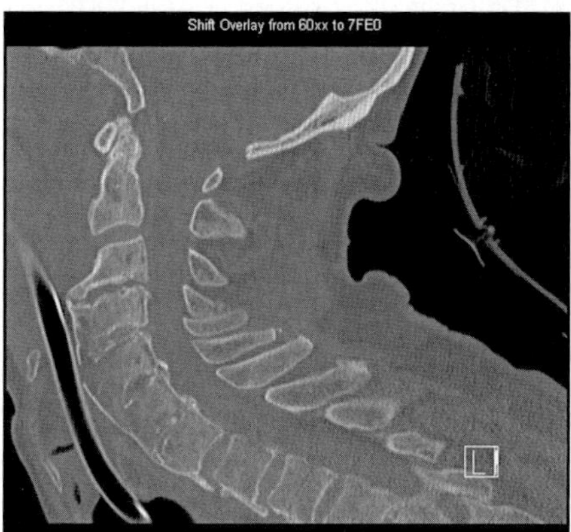

Figure 49.3

Diffuse idiopathic skeletal hyperostosis (**Figures 49.1, 49.2, and 49.3**). Lateral radiographs of the cervical spine (Figures 49.1 and 49.2) demonstrate flowing ossifications anterior to more than four contiguous cervical vertebral bodies indicating DISH. Figure 49.2 (magnified) better demonstrates a cortical discontinuity at the C4–C5 level, consistent with a fracture. Sagittal CT reconstruction (Figure 49. 3) shows fractures at the C4–C5 ossification and C4 spinous process as well as widening of the C4–C5 disc space, indicating a hyperextension mechanism.

Differential Diagnosis

► Spondylosis deformans
► Ankylosing spondylitis (AS)
► Reactive arthritis
► Psoriatic arthritis
► Fluorosis

Discussion

Diffuse idiopathic skeletal hyperostosis (DISH) (also known as Forestier disease) is a condition commonly seen in up to 10% of elderly white males (sixth to seventh decades). It is an enthesopathy in which there is reactive bone proliferation at the tendinous and ligamentous insertions.

The main differential diagnosis of spinal DISH includes spondylosis deformans, ankylosing spondylitis, reactive arthritis, and psoriatic arthritis. In spondylosis deformans or degenerative disease, osteophytes typically form only at the corners of the vertebral bodies with associated disc space narrowing and endplate sclerosis and/or irregularity.

Fusion of the facet joints, costovertebral joints, and sacroiliac joints is characteristic of ankylosing spondylitis and helps to exclude DISH. Syndesmophytes in AS tend to form thinner ossifications along the outer fibers of the annulus fibrosus. Fluorosis may produce osteophytes, whiskering, and ligamentous ossification, but all bones are typically uniformly increased in density.

Patients with thoracic or lumbar DISH typically present with back stiffness or pain while patients with large cervical DISH can present with obstructive symptoms such as dysphagia. Due to the stiffness, patients with DISH are prone to hyperextension injury and spinal fractures with complications including nonunion, deformity, neurological injury, and death.

Radiological Evaluation

Plain films and CT show a thick, laminated "flowing ossification" along the anterior or right anterolateral aspects of at least four contiguous vertebrae. The left thoracic aorta is typically spared due to aortic pulsation. The disc spaces are preserved unless there is a superimposed degenerative change. Although the thoracic spine is most commonly involved, the cervical and lower lumbar spine are also frequently involved. Pathological features include focal and diffuse calcification and ossification of the anterior longitudinal ligament, paraspinal connective tissue, and annulus fibrosis; degeneration in the peripheral annulus fibrosis fibers; anterolateral extensions of fibrous tissue; hypervascularity; chronic inflammatory cellular infiltration; and periosteal new bone formation on the anterior surface of the vertebral bodies.

DISH is associated with hyperostosis frontalis interna, ossification of the posterior longitudinal or vertebral arch ligament, enthesopathy (iliac crests, ischial tuberosities, greater trochanters), and spur formation in the appendicular skeleton (olecranon and calcaneus). Patients have a higher risk of osseous trauma (Figure 49.4).

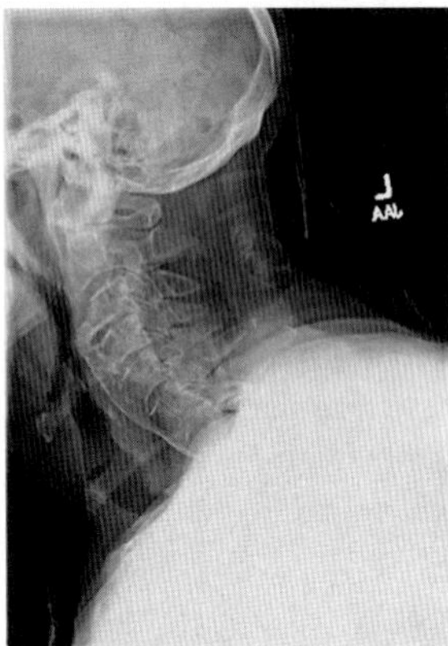

Figure 49.4

Acute fracture at C4–C5 in a 56-year-old patient with DISH (**Figure 49.4**). A lateral radiograph demonstrates an acute fracture through C4–C5, including involvement of the anterior ossification.

Management

Nonoperative treatment aimed at reducing pain and stiffness and preventing complications is a mainstay and includes activity modification, physical therapy, brace wear, nonsteroidal antiinflammatory drugs (NSAIDs), and steroid injections. Because of the relationship between DISH and conditions such as obesity, insulin resistance, and Type II diabetes mellitus, treating those conditions may slow or halt the progression of DISH. In DISH complicated by fractures (such as spinal canal stenosis, myelopathy, or spinal deformity), spinal decompression and stabilization can be performed. Cervical spine traction is to be used with caution as it may result in excessive distraction due to lack of ligamentous structures. Three column fractures following trauma are common given the rigidity of the spine, and can be highly unstable with a potential for serious neurological injury. Patients who experience difficulty swallowing due to DISH may need surgery to remove the anterior cervical bone mass.

Teaching Points

► DISH is a common bone-forming disorder of the spine.
► Although mostly asymptomatic, DISH can cause symptoms such as dysphagia, pain, stiffness, and possibly symptoms related to vascular compression.
► DISH can render patients vulnerable to spinal fractures even after minor trauma, especially related to a hyperextension mechanism.

Further Reading

1. Cammisa M, De Serio A, and Guglielmi G. Diffuse idiopathic skeletal hyperostosis. Eur J Radiol 1998;27(Suppl 1):S7–11.
2. Taljanovic MS, Hunter TB, Wisneski RJ, et al. Imaging characteristics of diffuse idiopathic skeletal hyperostosis with an emphasis on acute spinal fractures: Review. AJR Am J Roentgenol 2009;193(3 Suppl):S10–19, Quiz S20–24.
3. Resnick D. Diffuse idiopathic skeletal hyperostosis. In *Diagnosis of Bone and Joint Disorders*, 4th ed. (Resnick D, ed.). Philadelphia, PA: Saunders, 2002, pp. 1476–1503.
4. Paley D, Schwartz M, Cooper P, et al. Fractures of the spine in diffuse idiopathic skeletal hyperostosis. Clin Orthop Relat Res 1991;(267):22–32.
5. Sreedharan S and Li YH. Diffuse idiopathic skeletal hyperostosis with cervical spinal cord injury––a report of 3 cases and a literature review. Ann Acad Med Singapore 2005;34(3):257–261.
6. Resnick D and Niwayama G. Radiographic and pathologic features of spinal involvement in diffuse idiopathic skeletal hyperostosis (DISH). Radiology 1976;119:559–568.

Chapter 50

David Rodriguez and Vikas Agarwal

History

▶ A 79-year-old male presents with an incidental finding on CT scan for trauma (**Figures 50.1, 50.2, and 50.3**).

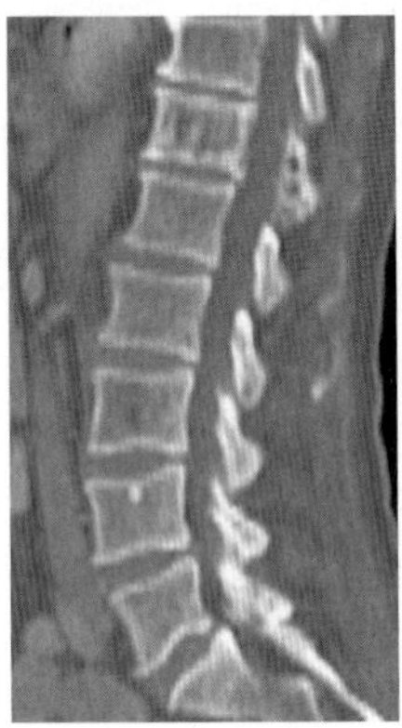

Figure 50.1

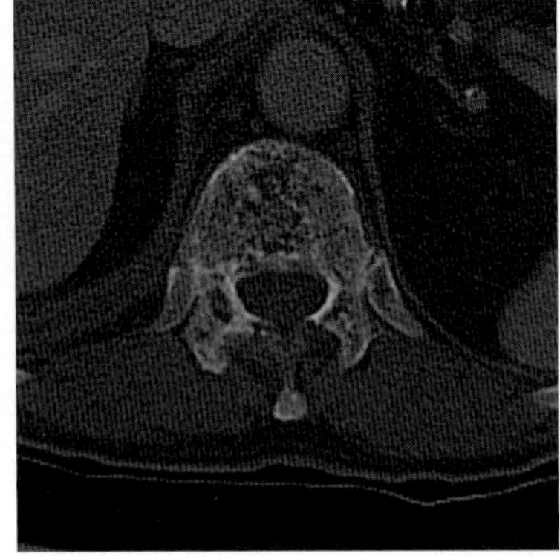

Figure 50.2

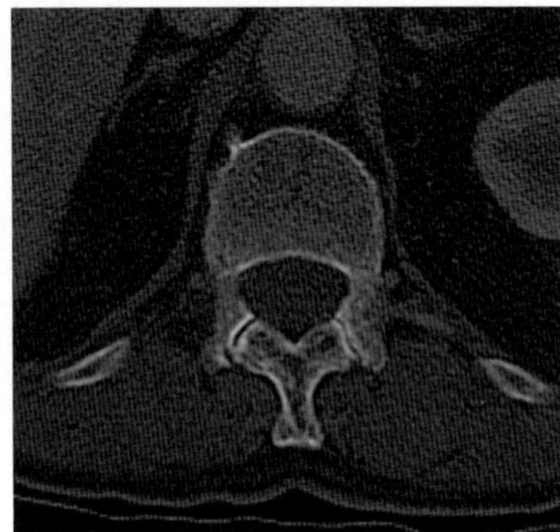

Figure 50.3

Findings

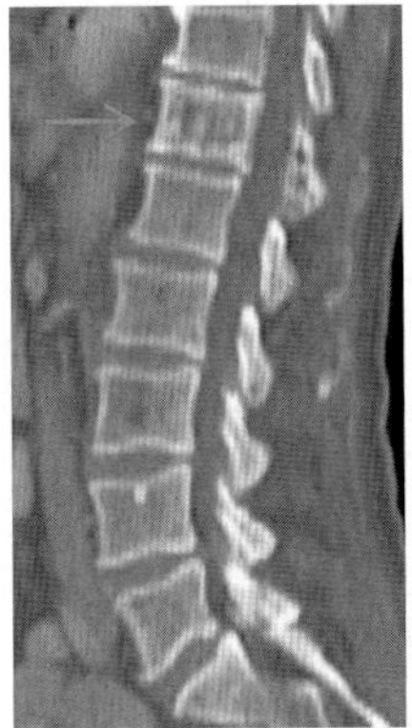

Figure 50.4

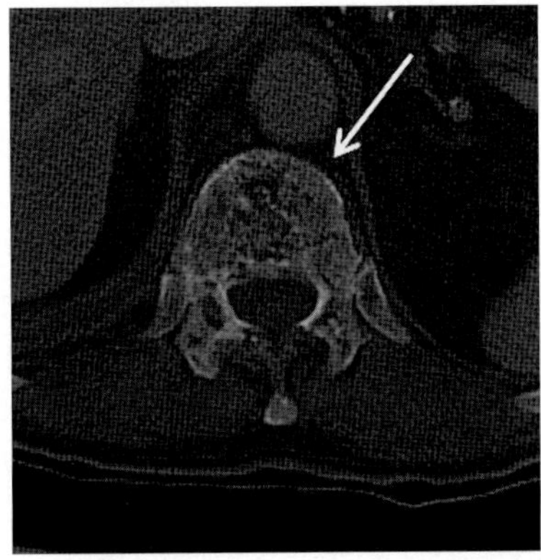

Figure 50.5

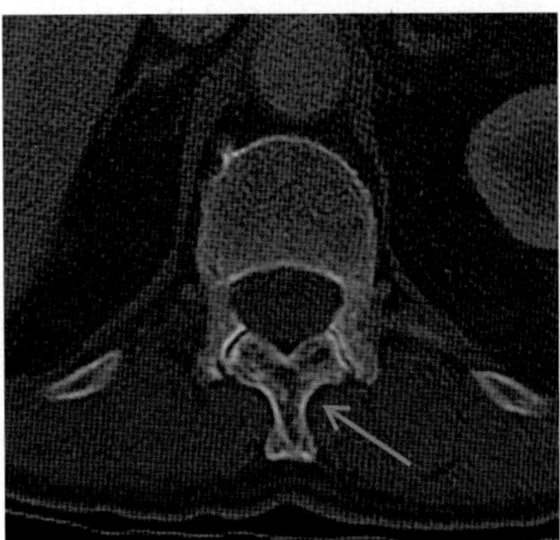

Figure 50.6

Paget disease on CT. A sagittal CT image (**Figure 50.4**) demonstrates thickened sclerotic borders of the T12 vertebrae in a "picture frame" appearance. Axial CT images (**Figures 50.5 and 50.6**) demonstrate a mixed lytic and sclerotic appearance of the T12 vertebrae, with the appearance of coarsened trabeculae, consistent with Paget disease of bone.

Differential Diagnosis

▶ Sclerotic metastasis
▶ Fibrous dysplasia
▶ Multiple myeloma

Discussion

Paget disease is seen in 3–4% of the population over 40 years of age. In this entity, there is excessive and abnormal remodeling of bone. There are three phases: the lytic phase (incipient-active), the mixed phase (active), and the blastic phase (late-inactive). Paget disease of the spine can usually be distinguished from other pathologies by its characteristic coarsened trabeculae and enlargement of the vertebral body (2). Spinal involvement is seen in 30–75% of cases.

The most important complication is sarcomatous transformation, occurring in approximately 1% of cases. On imaging, look for focal bone destruction beyond the cortex with an associated soft-tissue mass. There can be additional nonneoplastic sequelae including osseous weakening with bowing of the appendicular skeleton, fractures, secondary osteoarthritis, cranial nerve compression, spinal canal and neural foraminal stenosis, and basilar invagination.

Radiological Evaluation

Paget disease can have a varied appearance depending on the stage of the disease:
▶ Lytic phase:
  ▪ Thinned and lucent cortex
▶ Mixed phase:
  ▪ Mixed lytic and sclerotic
  ▪ Coarsened and thickened trabeculae
▶ Blastic phase:
  ▪ Bony sclerosis and enlargement

Lack of clinical symptoms does not preclude a diagnosis of Paget disease, as it can often be asymptomatic. Due to the potential for future clinical symptoms or even malignant transformation, it is important to recognize the appearance of Paget disease when reviewing spinal examinations. Findings can be typical but subtle, with bony enlargement and coarsened trabeculae seen as typical of Paget disease.

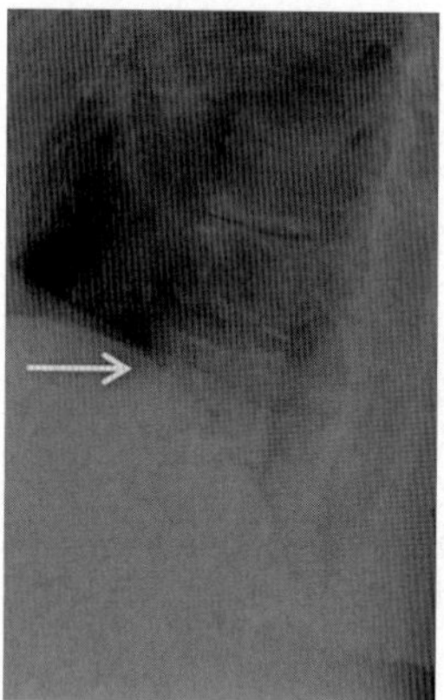

Figure 50.7

Paget disease of T12 (**Figure 50.7**). Coned down view from a lateral thoracic spine radiograph depicts enlargement of the T12 vertebral body with coarsened trabeculae that is typical of Paget disease.

Radiographs and CT are the mainstay for diagnosing Paget disease. However, vertebral bodies affected by Paget disease can have, depending on the stage of disease, increased marrow fat and a heterogeneous "speckled" appearance on MRI (**Figure 50.8**). A bone scan is a cost-effective way to search for Paget involvement throughout the entire skeleton (**Figures 50.9 and 50.10**).

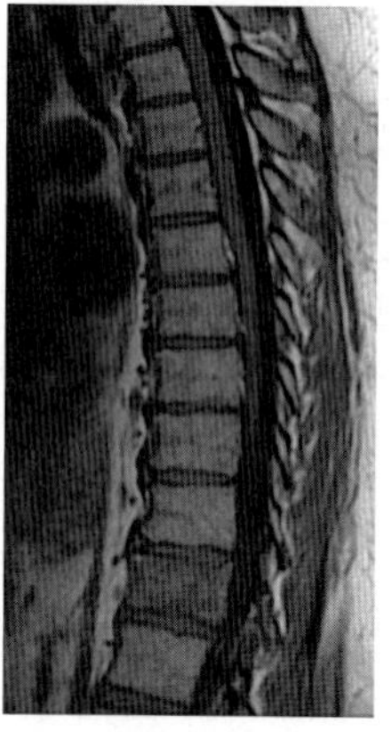

Figure 50.8

Paget disease on MRI (Figure 50.8). A T1-weighted sagittal image of the thoracic spine demonstrates a heterogeneous and "speckled" appearance of the T12 vertebrae typical of Paget disease.

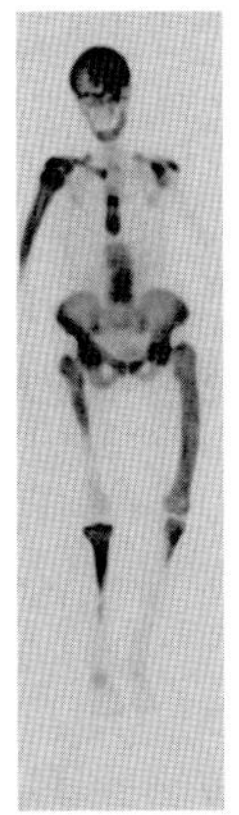 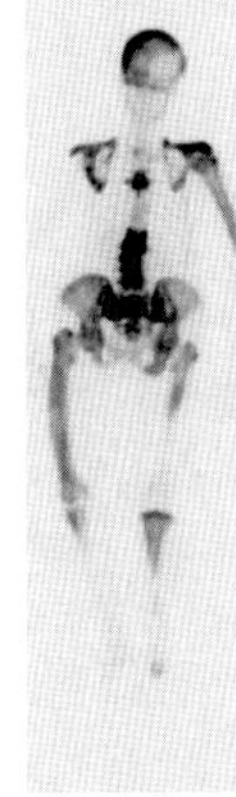

Figure 50.9   Figure 50.10

Paget disease on nuclear medicine imaging (Figures 50.9 and 50.10). An 82-year-old female presents with multifocal bone pain. Frontal and posterior whole body bone scan images demonstrate increased uptake with a suggestion of bony enlargement of several thoracic and lumbar vertebrae, consistent with Paget disease (there is also Paget disease affecting the skull, pelvis, humerus, scapula, femur, tibia, and hindfoot).

Management

If asymptomatic, no treatment may be necessary. For symptomatic cases, bisphosphonates can be used to decrease bone turnover.

Teaching Points
- ► Learn to recognize the appearance of Paget disease as many patients may be asymptomatic.
- ► Paget disease can be polyostotic, so look for involvement throughout the body.
- ► Mixed phase of Paget disease is the most common encountered by radiologists.
- ► There is a small, but significant, predisposition for malignant transformation.

Further Reading
1. Whitehouse RW. Paget disease of bone. Semin Musculoskel Radiol 2002;6(4):313–322.
2. Dell'Atti C, Cassar-Pullicino VN, Lalam RK, et al. The spine in Paget disease. Skeletal Radiol 2007;36:609–626.
3. Smith SE, Murphy MD, Motamedi K, et al. From the archives of the AFIP. Radiologic spectrum of Paget disease of bone and its complications with pathologic correlation. Radiographics 2002;22:1191–1216.

Chapter 51

Shamir Rai, Ismail Tawakol Ali, and Savvas Nicolaou

History

► A 5-year-old child presents with stunted growth, short neck, mental retardation, and coarse facial features (prominent supraorbital rims bilaterally) with facial asymmetry, cardiac compromise, corneal clouding, stiffness of joints and a history of recurrent respiratory infections (**Figures 51.1 and 51.2**).

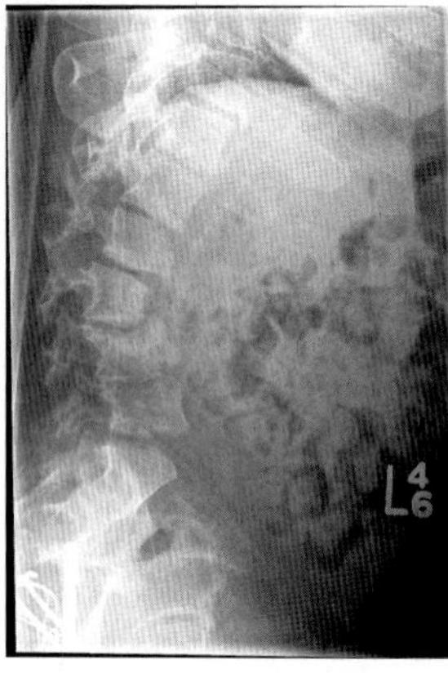 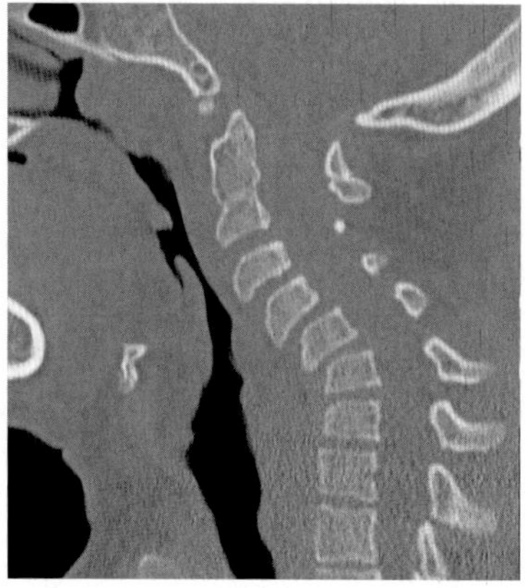

Figure 51.1

Figure 51.2

Chapter 51 Hurler Syndrome/Mucopolysaccharidoses Type I

Findings

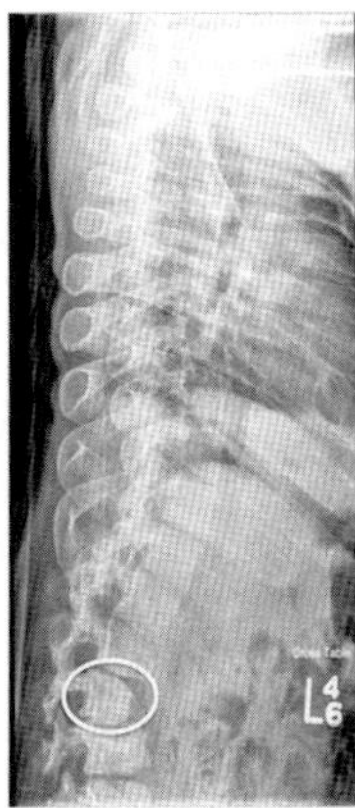 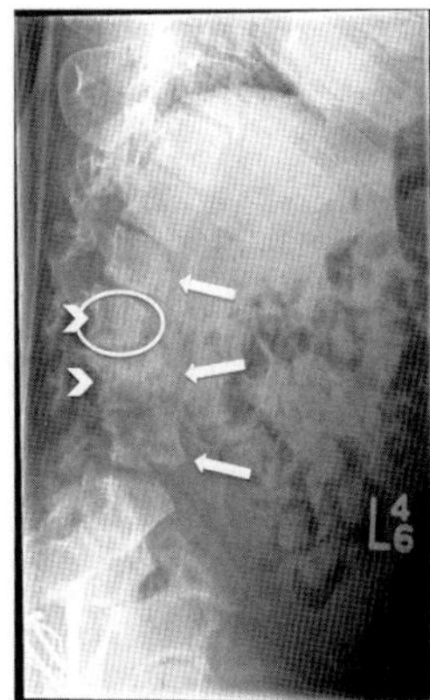

Figure 51.3

Hurler syndrome [mucopolysaccharidoses (MPS) Type I] (**Figure 51.3**). Lateral views of the thoracolumbar spine demonstrate characteristic hypoplastic rounded vertebral bodies (circle). "Anterior beaking" (arrows) with posterior scalloping (arrowheads) is present. Additionally, broadened "paddle-shaped" ribs are present, with the ribs being broadened distally and narrowed at the takeoff from the vertebral bodies. Findings are consistent with dystosis multiplex seen in MPS.

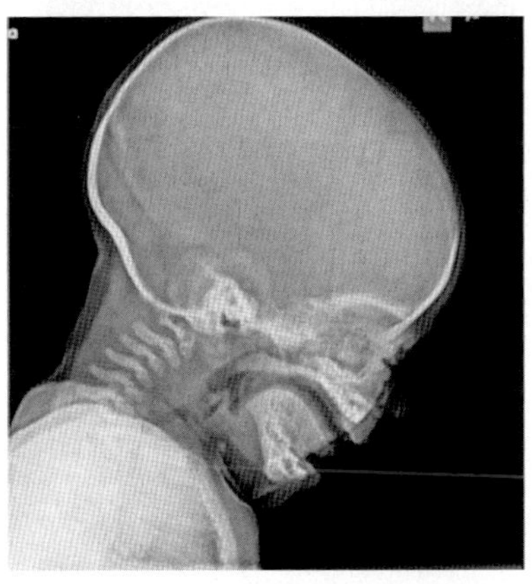 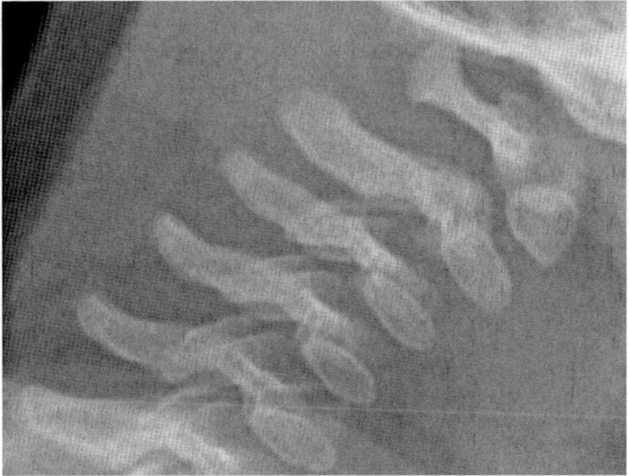

Figure 51.4

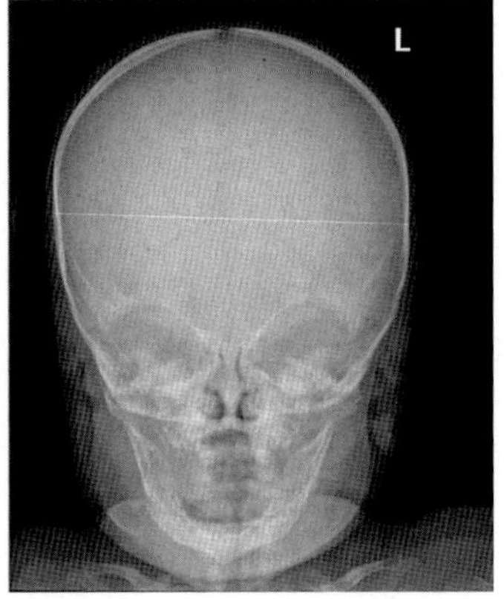

Figure 51.5

The upper portion of the odontoid is separated from the body of C2 (os odontoideum); however, no subluxation is visible (**Figures 51.4 and 51.5**). The orbits are mildly dysmorphic with superior elevation of the lateral orbital margins (harlequin orbits).

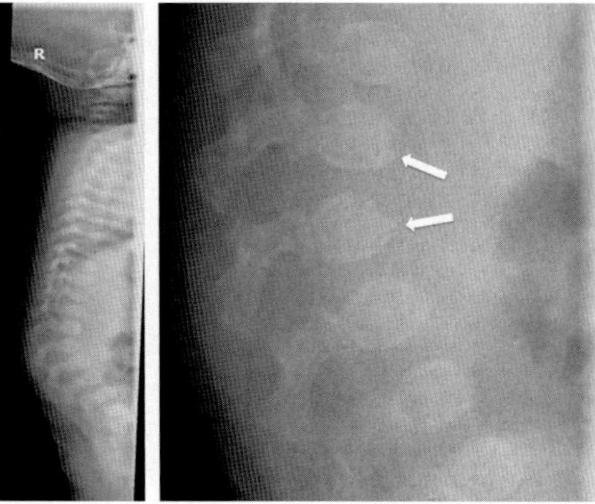

Figure 51.6

Focal kyphosis is present at the lumbosacral junction, which measures approximately 40 degrees (**Figure 51.6**). Anterior vertebral body beaking is present at the L2 and L3 vertebral bodies (arrows).

Sagittal CT demonstrates odontoid process dysplasia with a characteristic triangular-shaped configuration in MPS (**Figure 51.7**). A prominent cervical kyphotic deformity is present. "Anterior beaking" (arrows) is noted along with a loss of vertebral height.

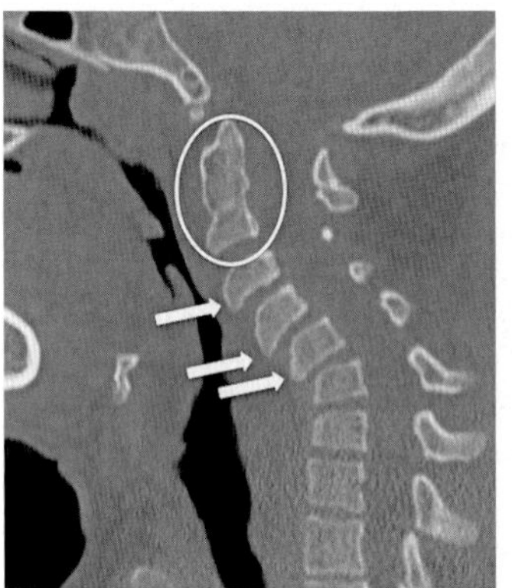 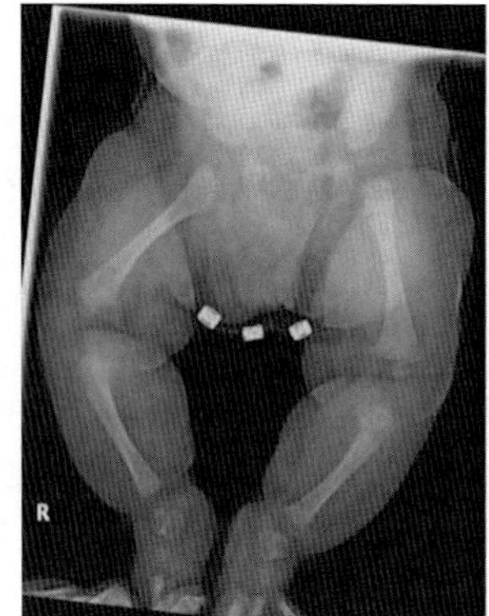 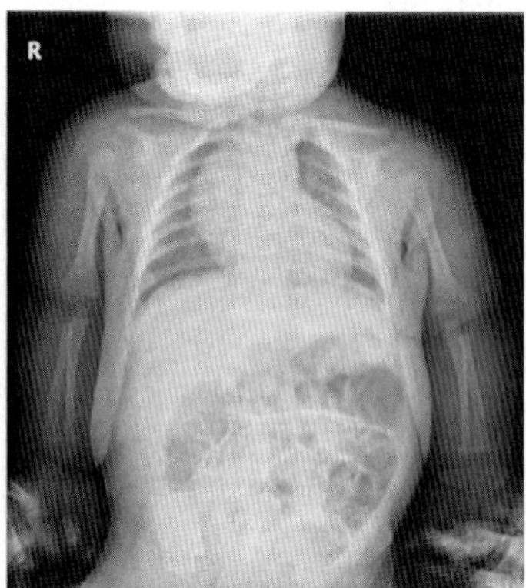

Figure 51.7   Figure 51.8

The humeri and femuri appear to be disproportionally short (**Figure 51.8**). The long bones appear undertubulated. The acetabular angles are minimally increased.

Differential Diagnosis

Mucopolysaccharidoses, which has a very characteristic constellation of radiological findings known as dystosis multiplex.

Discussion

MPS consists of a heterogeneous group of 11 clinically distinct heritable lysosomal storage disorders that are caused by a deficiency in glycosaminoglycan-degrading enzymes. MPS is classified on the basis of the specific deficient enzyme. All MPS disorders are characterized by skeletal involvement. Undegraded glycosaminoglycans (GAGs) accumulate in tissues and lead to progressive damage of various tissues including the heart, respiratory system, bones, joints, and central nervous system. The overall incidence of all types of

MPS is 1 in 25,000. Transmission occurs in an autosomal recessive fashion, with the exception of MPS II, which is X-linked. The typical manifestations encountered in the majority of MPS include organomegaly, short stature, coarse facial features, mental retardation, and developmental delay. Other manifestations include otitis media, airway obstruction, impaired vision (secondary to corneal clouding and photophobia), and cardiovascular involvement (myocardial hypertrophy, systolic dysfunction, cor pulmonale, valve dysfunction, and heart failure). The clinical manifestations are diverse, however, most patients exhibit a constellation of radiological findings known as dystosis multiplex, which will be described in more detail below.

The focus of this section will be on MPS I, which is a deficiency of the enzyme alpha-L-iduronidase in lysosomes with an incidence of 1/100,000. MPS I includes Hurler, Hurler-Scheie, and Scheie syndromes, which represent a spectrum of severity. The focus here will be on Hurler syndrome, which is the most severe form. Most children born with Hurler syndrome appear nearly normal at birth; however, if left untreated they show a progressive mental and physical decline. Patients typically present between 6 months and 2 years of age with developmental delay, recurrent respiratory infections, chronic nasal discharge, and coarse facial features (wide nasal bridge and flattened midface). The commonly encountered manifestations of Hurler syndrome are corneal clouding, dystosis multiplex, organomegaly, heart disease, mental retardation, and death in early childhood.

Issues involving the cervical spine are very common in MPS and can be life-threatening. Atlantoaxial instability with resultant myelopathy and spastic quadriparesis have been described. GAG accumulation behind the odontoid process may result in stenosis and compression, although not as common in Hurler syndrome (MPS I). Atlantoaxial instability has been noted in children with severe MPS I.

Radiological Evaluation

Skeletal abnormalities are an early prominent feature of most MPS disorders. Regular imaging of the cervical, thoracic, and lumbar spine, hips, and lower spine is recommended, typically with plain radiographs. The cervical spine should be monitored with lateral flexion and extension views. The degree of skeletal involvement varies between subtypes. A characteristic constellation of radiographic abnormalities, known as dystosis multiplex, is classically seen in MPS resulting from defective endochondral and membranous growth throughout the body.

Findings include the following:

- There are hypoplastic vertebral bodies that are flattened and rounded, which can result in scoliosis with or without kyphotic deformity. Anterior beaking with posterior scalloping of the vertebral bodies may be present with a loss of vertebral height.
- Thoracolumbar kyphosis, especially dorsal kyphosis ("gibbus deformity"), is a hallmark orthopedic feature of Hurler syndrome, occurring in nearly all children.
- Atlantoaxial instability, stenosis, and compression of the spinal cord at the craniovertebral junction (C1–C2 joint most commonly) are seen.
- Odontoid process dysplasia–hypoplasia ranges from total aplasia to a triangular-shaped configuration with a loss in vertical height and broad-based tip.
- Periodontoid tissue and ligament thickening occur.
- There is hip dysplasia with shallow acetabula and coxa valga.
- Knees are in a valgus position (genu valgum).
- There is enlargement of the skull with a thick calvarium and a J-shaped sella turcica (characteristic, but not diagnostic by itself).
- There is a lack of pneumatization of the mastoid process cell and of paranasal cavities.
- There is broadening of the clavicles and ribs ("paddle-shaped" or "oar-shaped").
- Rounding of the iliac wings with inferior tapering of the ilium occurs.
- Hypoplastic epiphyses are in the extremities with a thickened diaphysis.
- There is a curved distal radius toward a hypoplastic ulna ("Madelung's deformity").

Management

Definitive diagnosis is made through measuring enzyme activity in cultured fibroblasts or leukocytes. The course of MPS is variable with an average expected life span of 1 or 2 decades with severe forms. In slow progressing forms, patients are able to reach adulthood. In Hurler syndrome (severe form) the average age at death is 5 years, with very few making it to 10 years of age. The treatment mainly consists of symptomatic and supportive care. New therapies have been developed in recent years aimed at enzyme replacement, substrate inhibition, and hematopoietic cell transplantation that have significantly improved the duration and quality of life of patients with Hurler syndrome.

Contrary to popular belief, there is no clinical evidence to support the use of bracing as a stand-alone treatment for both kyphosis and scoliosis; it is typically reserved only for young children with progressive deformity who are not candidates for surgery. A kyphosis greater than 70 degrees or scoliosis greater than 50 degrees is a relative indication for surgery. The presence of myelopathy is a clear indication for surgery. Delaying surgery if possible is suggested to allow maximal growth of the spine and further development of the already osteopenic, small, and dysplastic bones.

Because of the associated atlantoaxial instability, all children with MPS should avoid high-risk activity such as contact sports.

Teaching Points

▶ MPS I (Hurler syndrome) is an autosomal recessive lysosomal storage disorder caused by a deficiency in glycosaminoglycan-degrading enzymes.
▶ GAGs accumulate and cause damage in various tissues including the heart, respiratory system, bones, joints, and central nervous system.
▶ Symptoms encountered in the majority of MPS include organomegaly, short stature, coarse facial features, mental retardation, and developmental delay.
▶ A definitive diagnosis is made through measuring enzyme activity in cultured fibroblasts or leukocytes.
▶ Most patients exhibit a constellation of radiological findings known as dystosis multiplex.
▶ Regular imaging of the cervical, thoracic, and lumbar spine, hips, and lower spine is recommended, typically with plain radiographs.

Further Reading

1. Cleary MA and Wraith JE. The presenting features of mucopolysaccharidosis type IH (Hurler syndrome). Acta Paediatr 1995;84:337.
2. Rasalkar DD, Chu WCW, Hui J, et al. Pictorial review of mucopolysaccharidosis with emphasis on MRI features of brain and spine. Br J Radiol 2011;84:469–477.
3. Lala-Gitteau E, Majzoub S, Labarthe F, et al. Ophthalmologic signs in mucopolysaccharidoses: Two case reports. J Fr Ophtalmol 2007;30(2):165–169.
4. Malm G, Lund AM, Mansson JE, et al. Mucopolysaccharidoses in the Scandinavian countries: Incidence and prevalence. Acta Paediatr 2008;97:1577.
5. Muenzer J. The mucopolysaccharidoses: A heterogeneous group of disorders with variable pediatric presentations. J Pediatr 2004;144(5):S27–S34.
6. Palmucci S, Attina G, Lanza ML, et al. Imaging findings of mucopolysaccharidoses: A pictorial review. Insights Imaging 2013;4:443–459.
7. Zafeiriou DI and Batzios SP. Brain and spinal MR imaging findings in mucopolysaccharidoses: A review. Am J Neuroradiol 2013;34(1):5–13.

History

▶ A middle-aged patient presents with chronic, generalized pain (**Figures 52.1 and 52.2**).

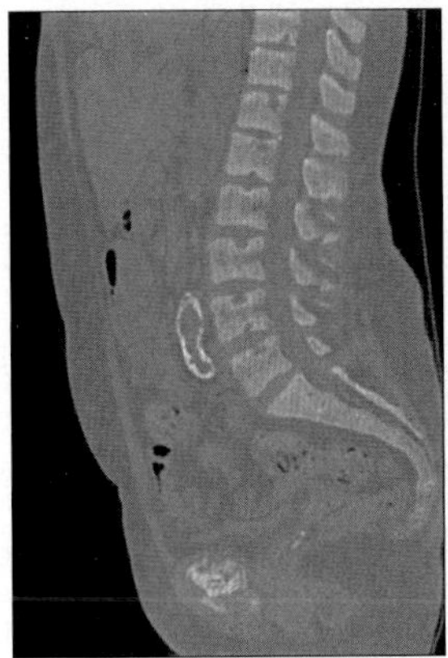

Figure 52.1

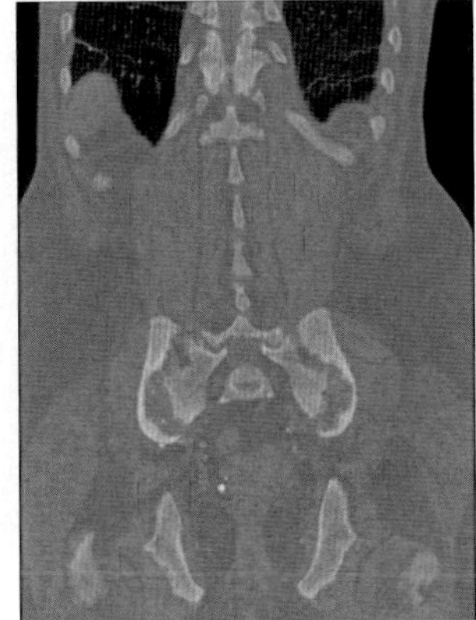

Figure 52.2

Chapter 52 **Renal Osteodystrophy and Secondary Hyperparathyroidism**

Findings

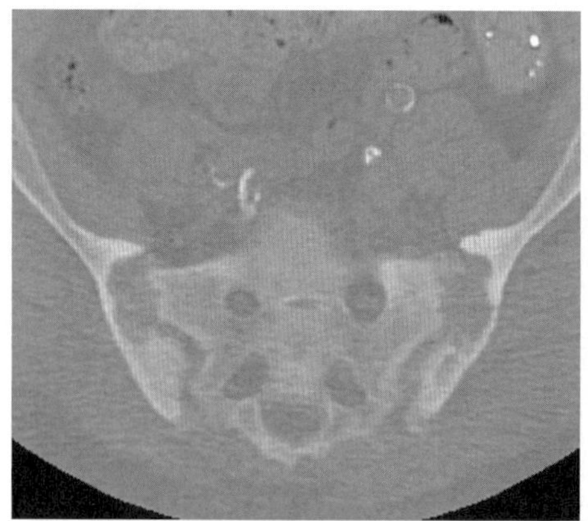

Figure 52.3

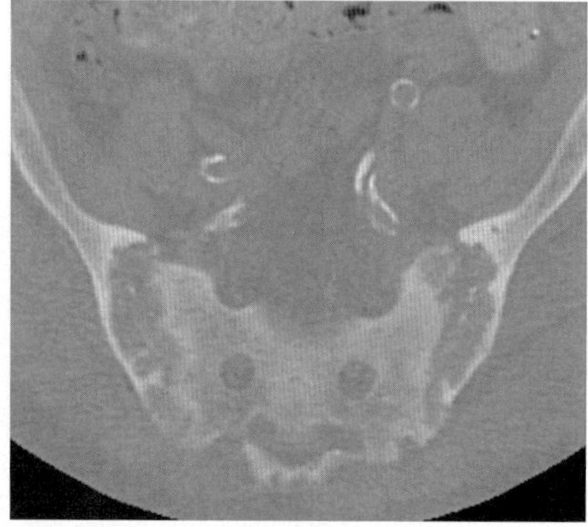

Figure 52.4

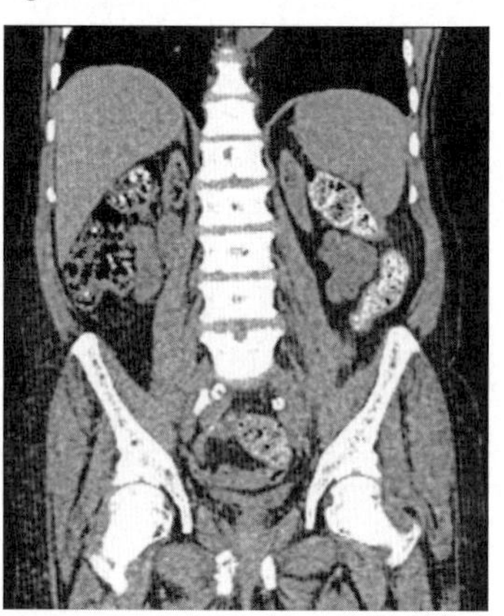

Figure 52.5

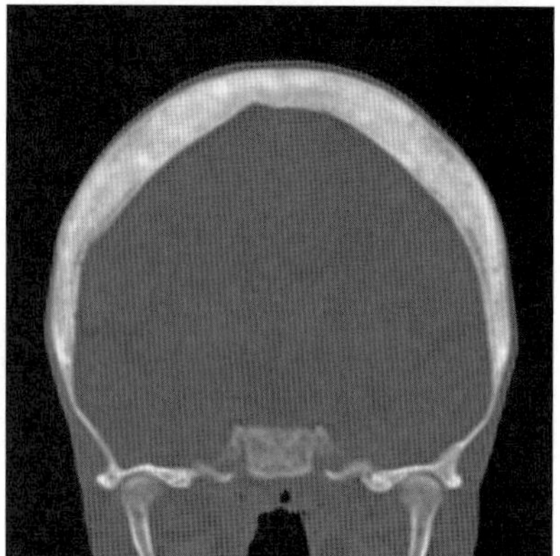

Figure 52.6

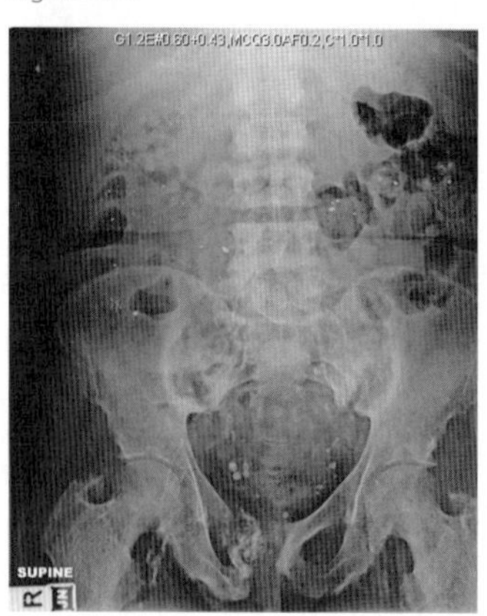

Figure 52.7

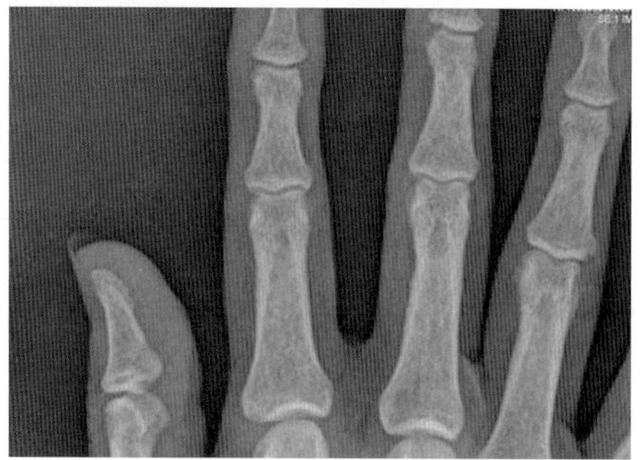

Figure 52.8

Renal osteodystrophy and secondary hyperparathyroidism (**Figures 52.3, 52.4, 52.5, 52.6, 52.7, and 52.8**). A sagittal CT reconstruction (Figure 52.1) shows increased subendplate densities at multiple contiguous levels to produce an alternating dense-lucent-dense appearance ("rugger jersey" spine). An anteroposterior (AP) abdominal radiograph (Figure 52.2) demonstrates irregular widening of the pubic symphysis and thinning of the medial femoral cortex indicative of subperiosteal resorption. Coronal CT reconstruction (Figure 52.3) shows atrophic kidneys in the same patient on hemodialysis. Coronal and sagittal CT images (Figures 52.4 and 52.5) demonstrate irregular widening of both sacroiliac joints indicating subperiosteal resorption. A coronal CT image (Figure 52.6) shows diffusely increased bone density in the skull. A magnified posterior-anterior (PA) radiograph of the hand (Figure 52.7) demonstrates thinning of the radial aspect of the middle phalanges of the hand pathognomonic for subperiosteal reaction in hyperparathyroidism. An axial CT image (Figure 52.8) shows a round lucent lesion in the left iliac bone proven to be an osteoclastoma or brown tumor in the same patient.

Differential Diagnosis

► Osteomalacia
► Rheumatoid arthritis
► Seronegative spondyloarthropathy
► Neoplasm (multiple myeloma, metastasis) mimicking brown tumor or
► Pigmented villonodular synovitis (PVNS) or synovial chondromatosis mimicking amyloid deposition
► Infection

Discussion

Renal osteodystrophy is a constellation of musculoskeletal abnormalities associated with chronic renal insufficiency featuring some combination of osteomalacia (adults), rickets (children), secondary hyperparathyroidism, osteosclerosis, and soft tissue and vascular calcifications. Secondary hyperparathyroidism (HPTH) results from an inability of the kidneys to adequately excrete phosphate leading to hyperplasia of parathyroid chief cells and an excess of parathyroid hormone.

Radiological Evaluation

Due to more sophisticated diagnostic methods and more efficient treatment classical radiographic features of secondary hyperparathyroidism and osteomalacia/rickets are now less frequently seen. Radiological investigations may play an important role in the early diagnosis and follow-up of the renal bone disease. Although new imaging modalities have been introduced in clinical practice (scintigraphy, CT, MRI, quantitative imaging), plain film radiography, especially fine quality hand radiographs, still represents the most widely used examination.

Imaging manifestations of HPTH include brown tumors, periosteal new bone formation, chondrocalcinosis, as well as subperiosteal, cortical, subchondral, trabecular, endosteal, and subligamentous bone resorption. One of the most common imaging manifestations is osteosclerosis (up to 34%) where there is diffusely increased, chalky bone density (Figure 52.6) with dense endplates ("rugger jersey spine") in the thoracolumbar spine (Figure 52.1). A pathognomonic radiographic sign of HPTH is subperiosteal bone resorption, typically seen on the radial aspect of the middle phalanges of the hand (Figure 52.7), the medial aspect of the proximal tibia and femoral neck (Figure 52.2), at the sacroiliac joints (Figures 52.2, 52.4, and 52.5), and at the distal clavicle. Brown tumors or osteoclastomas (Figure 52.8) were once said to be more common in primary HPTH but are now more commonly associated with secondary HPTH due to the overwhelming prevalence of patients with secondary disease. If the underlying HPTH is treated, the subperiosteal resorption may disappear before the brown tumor does.

Another imaging feature of renal osteodystrophy is the presence of soft tissue calcifications (Figure 52.9). Periarticular calcinosis (solitary or multiple painless, periarticular masses) can be seen bilaterally and can also involve the ligaments. It is important to be aware that there are no radiological or histological differences between the lesions seen in renal osteodystrophy and the lesions of tumoral calcinosis.

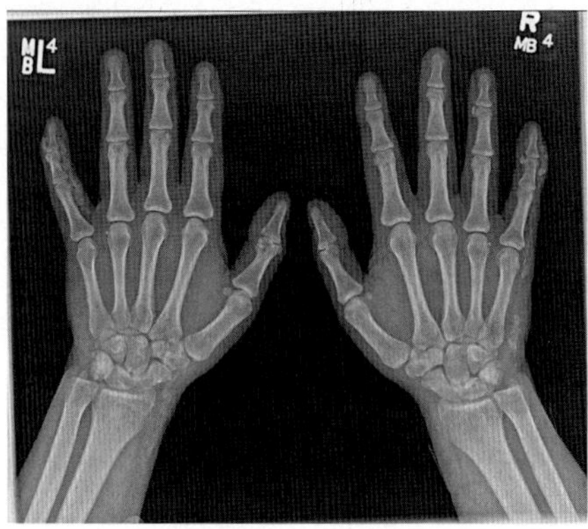

Figure 52.9

Periarticular calcifications (**Figure 52.9**). In this patient on long-term dialysis, soft tissue calcifications are evident without significant underlying erosive change of the bones. The most frequent case of a calcified periarticular mass is chronic renal failure, but correlation with the patient's history and serum chemistry levels is necessary.

Amyloid deposition can be seen in renal osteodystrophy. One important feature of maintenance hemodialysis performed for chronic renal disease is the development of hemodialysis-associated amyloidosis. Dialysis-related amyloidosis occurs secondary to the deposition of β_2-microglobulin and most commonly involves the lower segment of the cervical spine. Radiographs mimic an infectious process and can have a wide variety of features ranging from lytic lesions to erosions. CT imaging further delineates the degree of osteolytic areas and osseous sclerosis. MRI is often helpful as it optimally depicts the intraosseous, periarticular, and soft-tissue involvement. In the spine, a destructive spondyloarthropathy is often low signal on both T1- and T2-weighted images, helping to distinguish it from discitis/osteomyelitis (Figures 52.10, 52.11, and 52.12). Over time, collapse of the vertebral bodies may occur, with potential spinal cord compromise.

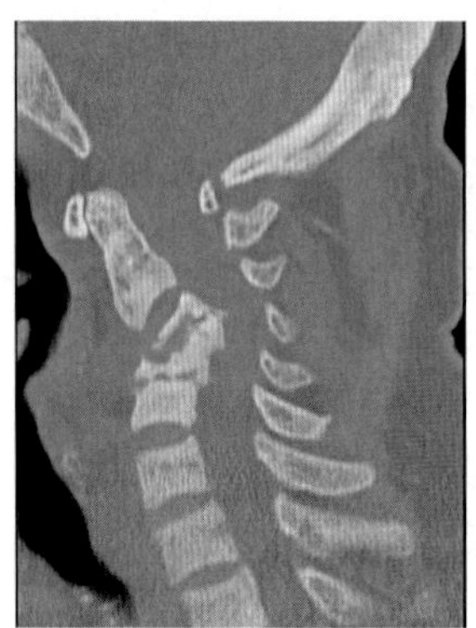

Figure 52.10

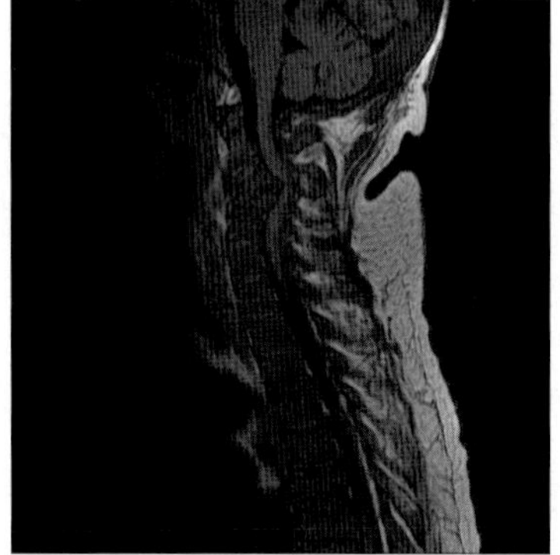

Figure 52.11

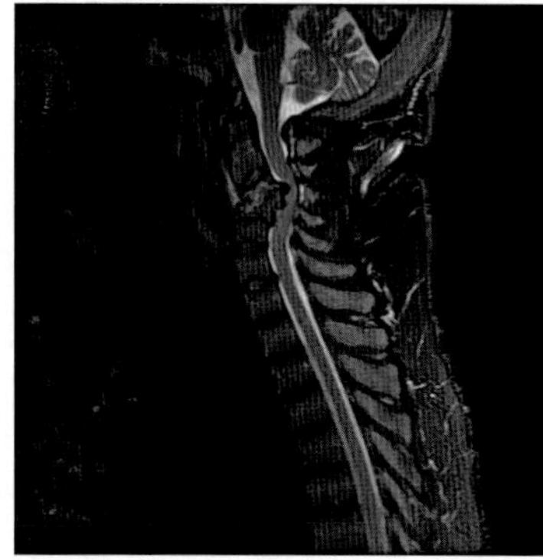

Figure 52.12

Hemodialysis-associated spondyloarthropathy (**Figures 52.10, 52.11, and 52.12**). A sagittal CT reconstruction (Figure 52.10) demonstrates diffuse sclerosis of the vertebral bodies and calvarium. There is associated collapse and deformity at the upper cervical spine, which projects into the spinal canal. Sagittal T1 FLAIR (Figure 52.11) and T2 fat-saturated (Figure 52.12) images demonstrate resultant central canal stenosis. Marrow signal changes are predominantly low signal on both T1- and T2-weighted images with the exception of some marrow edema within the C3–C4 collapsed body.

It is often impossible to distinguish renal osteodystrophy from other entities without additional clinical or radiographic information as erosive changes attributable to secondary hyperparathyroidism may be easily confused with rheumatoid arthritis, seronegative spondyloarthropathies, infection, or even malignancy. Brown tumors and amyloid deposition can easily be mistaken for a neoplastic process.

Management

Medical management is typically indicated in the treatment of patients with chronic renal failure and secondary hyperparathyroidism. This includes phosphate-binding agents to decrease phosphorus absorption in bowel and vitamin D_3 administration (if vitamin D resistance predominates). Arterial and cardiac valve calcifications are serious complications that can adversely affect cardiovascular hemodynamics in these patients. Recently phosphate-binding agents that do not contain calcium, new vitamin D analogues, and calcimimetic compounds have been advocated to help offer therapeutic alternatives for managing renal osteodystrophy while limiting the risks of excessive soft tissue and vascular calcifications. Parathyroidectomy can be performed for tertiary or autonomous hyperparathyroidism.

Teaching Points

▶ Chronic renal insufficiency/failure, hemodialysis/peritoneal dialysis, renal transplantation, and administration of various medications are associated with complex biochemical disturbances of the calcium–phosphate metabolism, resulting in a wide spectrum of bone and soft tissue abnormalities.

▶ Renal osteodystrophy encompasses secondary hyperparathyroidism, osteomalacia/rickets, osteoporosis, and soft tissue/vascular calcification.

▶ Complications arising from renal osteodystrophy and the associated treatment including long-term hemodialysis and renal transplantation include amyloid deposition, destructive spondyloarthropathy, osteonecrosis, and musculoskeletal infection.

▶ Due to more sophisticated diagnostic methods and more efficient treatment, classical radiographic features of secondary hyperparathyroidism and osteomalacia/rickets are now less frequently seen.

▶ Radiological investigations may play an important role in the early diagnosis and follow-up of renal osteodystrophy. Although numerous newer imaging modalities have been introduced in clinical practice, plain film radiography still represents the most widely used examination.

Further Reading

1. Naidich T, Castillo M, Cha S, et al. *Imaging of the Spine*. Philadelphia, PA: Saunders, 2011.
2. Jevtic V. Imaging of renal osteodystrophy. Eur J Radiol 2003;46(2):85–95.
3. Tigges S, Nance EP, Carpenter WA, and Erb R. Renal osteodystrophy: Imaging findings that mimic those of other diseases. AJR Am J Roentgenol. 1995;165(1):143–148.
4. Goodman W. Medical management of secondary hyperparathyroidism in chronic renal failure. Nephrol Dial Transplant 2003;18(Suppl 3):iii2–iii8.

Chapter 53

Manpreet Bajwa, Shivani Gupta, Ismail Tawakol Ali, and Savvas Nicolaou

History

► An 83 year old female with low back pain (**Figures 53.1 and 53.2**).

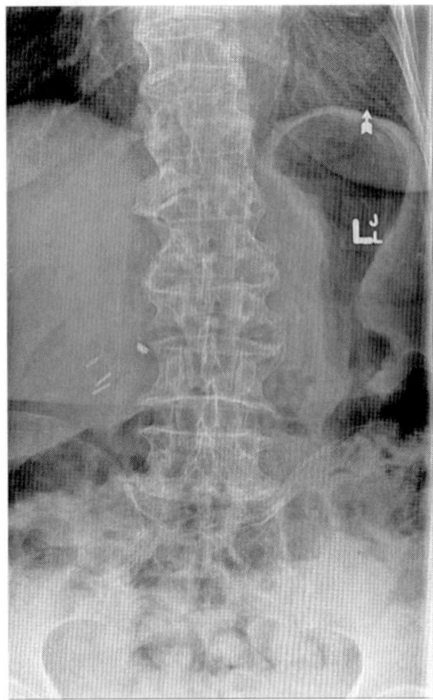

Figure 53.1

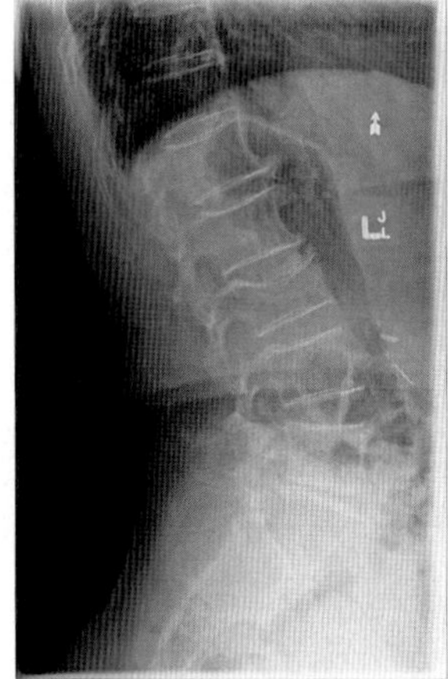

Figure 53.2

Findings

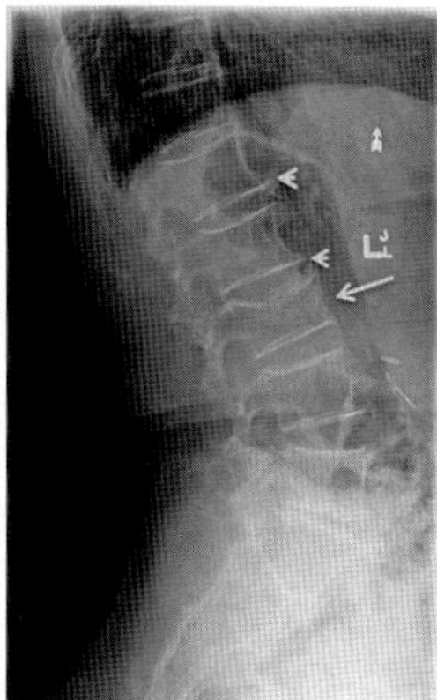

Figure 53.3

Osteopenia secondary to osteoporosis (**Figures 53.1 and 53.3**). Anteroposterior (AP) (Figure 53.1) and lateral (Figure 53.3) upright plain lumbar radiographs of an 83-year-old female with known osteoporosis show generalized severe osteopenia along with increased radiolucency of vertebral bodies and radiodensity of the cortical rim (arrowhead). The well-demarcated cortical rim gives the impression of a "picture frame" or an "empty box." An anterior wedge compression fracture deformity of the L3 vertebral body (arrow) is noted with approximately 20% loss of vertebral height.

Differential Diagnosis

Osteopenia can be seen secondary to several different pathologies (see Discussion).

Discussion

Osteoporosis is the reduction in bone mass and microarchitectural deterioration of bone tissue that results in increased bone fragility and increased susceptibility to fractures. Bone mass has been proven to decrease after the fourth or fifth decade in universally all populations. Osteoporosis predisposes to fractures of the hip, pelvis, distal forearm (Colles' fracture), humerus, and the vertebrae.

There are several etiologies resulting in osteoporosis:

► Anemia
► Dietary deficiency (malnutrition, calcium deficiency)
► Drugs (steroids, heparin)
► Congenital (osteogenesis imperfecta)
► Metabolic (pregnancy, postmenopausal, senile, Cushing's disease, acromegaly, diabetes mellitus, hyperparathyroidism)
► Chronic liver disease
► Alcoholism
► Disuse (most common after a traumatic osseous injury requiring immobilization)
► Congenital (neuromuscular disease, glycogen storage disease)

Large vertebral bodies result in a lower compression force of the spine; therefore persons with smaller vertebral bodies are more likely to experience a fracture.

Elderly women experience vertebral fractures from normal activities such as lifting rather than falling.

Hip osteoporotic fractures are associated with more deaths, disabilities, and medical costs than the collective amount of all other osteoporotic fractures. In addition to its effects on health, osteoporotic fractures have an impact economically, costing the United States $17.9 billion and the United Kingdom £1.7 billion per annum.

Calcium and vitamin D are essential for bone growth in children and a decrease in bone loss in adults.

Radiological Evaluation

Signs of osteoporosis are often seen on imaging. The most common imaging finding is osteopenia (increased radiolucency of bone). Osteopenia, however, is not diagnostic of osteoporosis, as other entities can also result in osteopenia (for example, osteomalacia, hyperparathyroidism, and neoplasm such as multiple myeloma). On radiographs, osteopenia can be difficult to diagnose. At least 30–50% of bone mass must be lost before it is visualized on radiographs. Cortical thinning can be seen, including loss of the normal trabeculae.

Bone densitometry is the best tool to predict the risk of an osteoporotic fracture. Imaging techniques such as dual-energy X-ray absorptiometry (DXA) and quantitative CT can help determine the degree of bone loss.

Complications of osteoporosis can be assessed on various imaging modalities, including CT and MR (Figures 53.3, 53.4, 53.5, 53.6, and 53.7). Compression fractures in the spine (refer to Chapter 4) are best assessed on MRI to determine acuity.

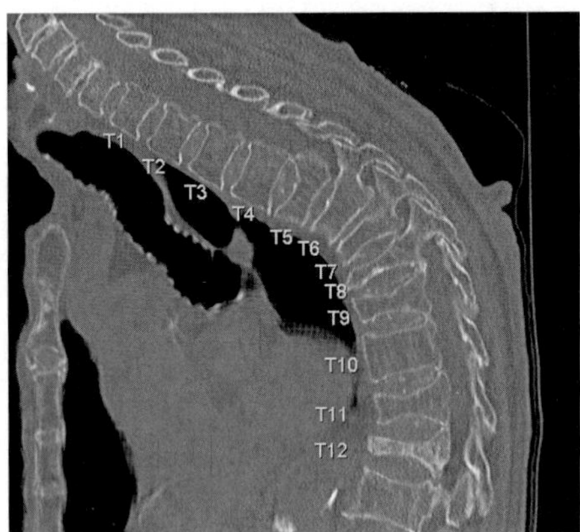

Figure 53.4

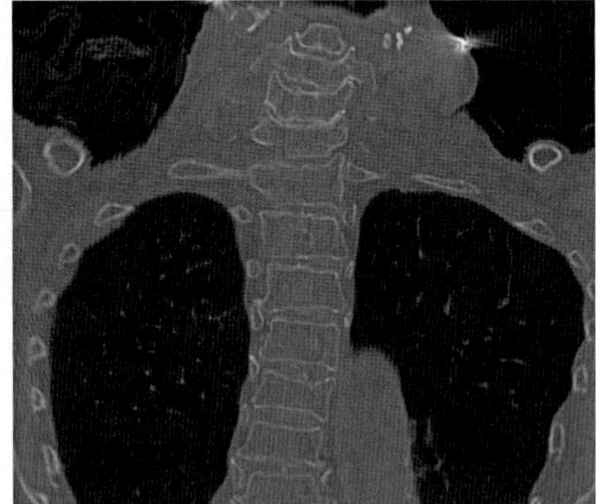

Figure 53.5

Multiple osteoporotic compression fractures (**Figures 53.4 and 53.5**). Sagittal noncontrast CT (Figure 53.4) of the thoracic spine in a 93-year-old female demonstrates multilevel osteoporotic insufficiency fractures of the thoracic vertebral bodies. There is generalized severe osteopenia along the thoracic spine. There is approximately 40% loss of vertebral height centrally at T5 and 35% loss of vertebral height at T6. There is near complete vertebral body height loss at T7 and T8. An anterior wedge compression fracture is noted at T9 with approximately 60% loss of vertebral height. There are also compression fractures at T11 and T12 with approximately 75% loss of vertebral body height, most pronounced centrally. A coronal noncontrast CT of the thoracic spine (Figure 53.5) again demonstrates multilevel osteoporotic insufficiency fractures of the thoracic vertebral bodies.

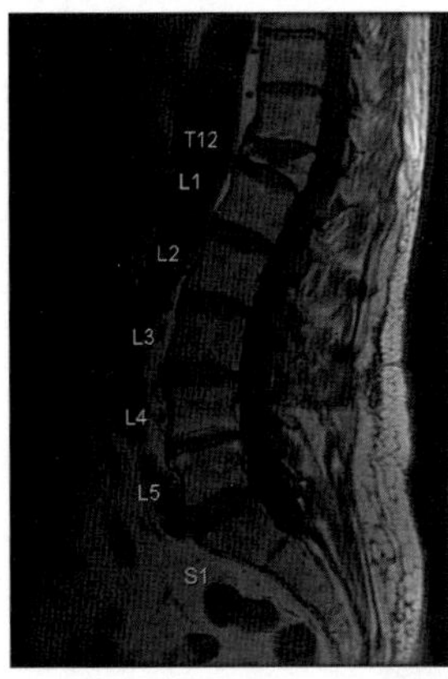

Figure 53.6

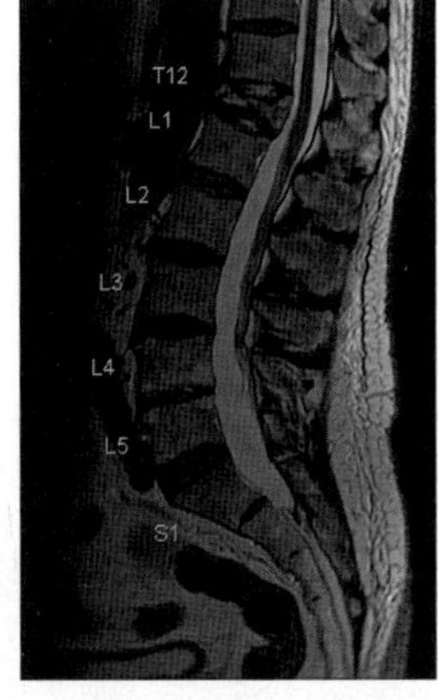

Figure 53.7

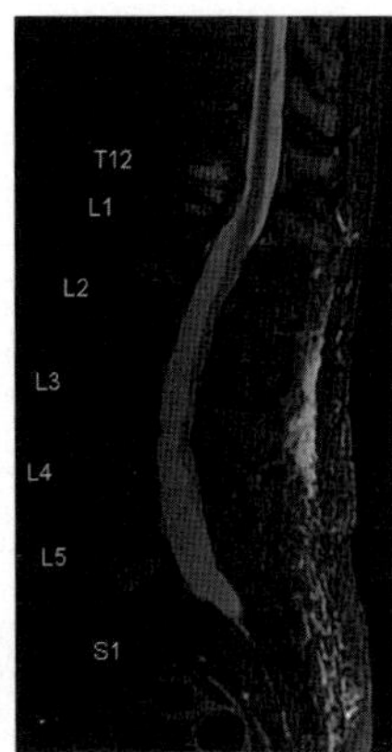

Figure 53.8

MR evaluation of osteoporotic fractures (**Figures 53.6, 53.7, and 53.8**). Sagittal T1 (Figure 53.6), T2 (Figure 53.7), and STIR (Figure 53.8) magnetic resonance lumbar spine images demonstrate severe compression of the T12 vertebral body with approximately 70% height loss in a 64-year-old male with known osteoporosis. The T12 vertebral body demonstrates some high STIR signal within the body centrally as well as within the discs above and below in keeping with edema. There is a diffuse heterogeneous appearance to the marrow, most pronounced at the L4 and L5 levels, in keeping with the diagnosis of osteoporosis.

Management

Prevention of osteoporosis is most important and begins early. Diet and physical activity should be optimized to augment bone mass. Factors that diminish bone mass, such as smoking and alcohol, should be eliminated. Postmenopausal osteoporosis may require the addition of drug therapy (hormone replacement therapy, bisphosphonates, strontium ranelate, raloxifene, and calcitonin). Refer to Chapter 6 for a discussion on management options for a vertebral compression fracture.

Teaching Points

▶ Osteoporosis is the most common metabolic bone disease.
▶ Complications of osteoporosis include vertebral compression fractures.

Further Readings

1. Harvey N, Dennison E, and Cooper C. Epidemiology of osteoporotic fracture. In *Primer on the Metabolic Bone Diseases and Disorders of Metabolism*, 7th ed. (Rosen CJ, Compson JE, and Lian LB, eds.). Washington, DC: American Society for Bone and Mineral Research, 2008, pp.198–203.
2. Cummings SR, Kelsey JL, Nevitt MC, and O'dowd KJ. Epidemiology of osteoporosis and osteoporotic fractures. Epidemiol Rev 1985;7(1):178–208.
3. Deng HW, Chen WM, Recker S, et al. Genetic determination of Colles' fracture and differential bone mass in women with and without Colles' fracture. J Bone Miner Res 2000;15(7):1243–1252.
4. Schousboe J, Taylor B, and Ensurd K. Assessing fracture risk: Who should be screened? In *Primer on the Metabolic Bone Diseases and Disorders of Metabolism*, 7th ed. (Rosen CJ, Compson JE, and Lian LB, eds.). Washington, DC: American Society for Bone and Mineral Research, 2008, pp. 231–237.
5. Harris WH and Heaney RP. Skeletal renewal and metabolic bone disease. N Engl J Med 1969;280:193.
6. Eastell R. Treatment of postmenopausal osteoporosis. N Engl J Med 1998;338(11):736–746.
7. Baba H, Maezawa Y, Kamitani K, et al. Osteoporotic vertebral collapse with late neurological complications. Paraplegia 1995;33(5):281–289.
8. Dawson-Hughes B. Calcium and vitamin D. In *Primer on the Metabolic Bone Diseases and Disorders of Metabolism*, 7th ed. (Rosen CJ, Compson JE, and Lian LB, eds.). Washington, DC: American Society for Bone and Mineral Research, 2008, pp. 276–278.

Chapter 54

Justin Morris Honce

History

▶ A 40-year-old female presented with new onset bilateral upper extremity paresthesias and a reported episode of right-sided blurry vision 3 weeks ago (**Figures 54.1, 54.2, and 54.3**).

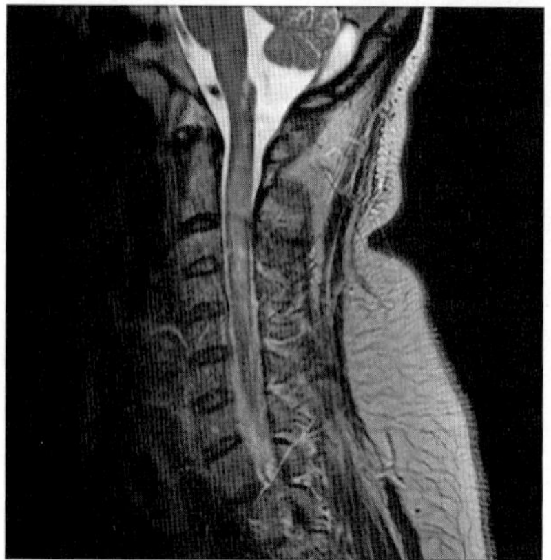

Figure 54.1

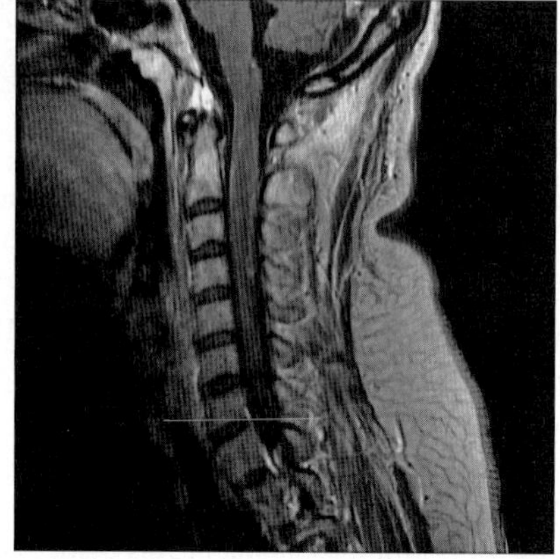

Figure 54.2

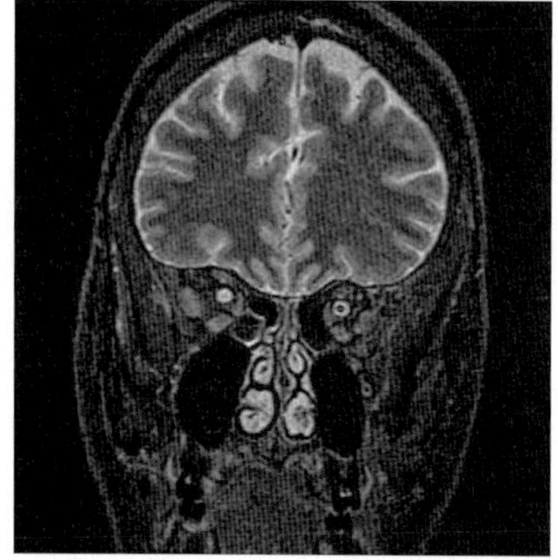

Figure 54.3

Findings

Neuromyelitis optica (Figures 54.1, 54.2, and 54.3). A sagittal T2-weighted image (Figure 54.1) demonstrates a long segment of diffuse T2 hyperintensity within the cervical cord extending from the cervicomedullary junction to about the C5 level. The cord is mildly expanded along the region of signal abnormality. On sagittal postcontrast T1-weighted imaging (Figure 54.2) there is heterogeneous peripheral enhancement along the lesion. A coronal STIR image through the orbits (Figure 54.3) demonstrates abnormal T2 hyperintensity within the right optic nerve. The nerve did not enhance on postcontrast imaging (not shown).

Differential Diagnosis

▶ Multiple sclerosis

▶ Idiopathic transverse myelitis

▶ Acute disseminated encephalomyelitis (ADEM)

Discussion

Neuromyelitis optica (NMO), previously referred to as Devic's syndrome, is a rare disorder characterized by episodes of optic neuritis and transverse myelopathy. While originally considered to be a severe variant of multiple sclerosis (MS), the recent discovery of IgG antibodies targeting aquaporin 4 channels in NMO patients, not seen in MS, has helped solidify the consensus that NMO is a separate and distinct disorder from MS. Aquaporin 4 is found throughout the brain, but is most concentrated in the optic nerves and spinal cord, explaining the predilection of the disease for these two structures. NMO is much rarer than multiple sclerosis, with an estimated prevalence of about 4 per 100,000, occurring more frequently in patients of West Indies or Asian descent. The peak incidence of the disease occurs later than in MS at the end of the fifth decade of life (40 years). There is an even stronger predilection for females than is seen in MS.

Patients with NMO typically present with symptoms of optic neuritis, including orbital pain, blurry vision, or blindness. The onset of symptoms is usually rapid and while usually temporary, residual deficits are not infrequent. With the development of spinal cord involvement patients will develop weakness and paresthesias in the extremities, muscular spasms, and bladder dysfunction. While symptoms related to the optic neuritis and transverse myelitis frequently occur concurrently, it is not uncommon for either to precede the other by days, weeks, months, or in some cases years. As such, the course of the disease may be either monophasic or multiphasic.

The differential diagnoses of NMO by imaging is primarily that of other demyelinating diseases of the central nervous system (CNS) and most commonly include multiple sclerosis, ADEM, and idiopathic transverse myelitis. Spinal cord involvement in multiple sclerosis is typically less extensive than in NMO, with MS cord lesions typically no more than one to two vertebral bodies in length (versus the three or more vertebral body lengths in NMO). Typically cord involvement in MS is more peripheral, rather than the more typical holocord involvement in NMO. The brain is also much more commonly affected in MS than in NMO and typically demonstrates periventricular lesions perpendicular to the plane of the ventricles (so-called "Dawson's fingers") and juxtacortical lesions. A definitive diagnosis of NMO can be made when patients present with optic neuritis, myelitis, and two of the following: contiguous spinal cord involvement of more than three segments, brain MRI not diagnostic of MS, and positive anti-aquaporin 4 antibody. ADEM typically presents with confluent/patchy lesions in the brain and occasionally the spinal cord. A clinical history is usually helpful as there is typically an antecedent viral illness in patients with ADEM. The optic nerves are not affected in patients with ADEM or idiopathic transverse myelitis.

Radiological Evaluation

As is true for all demyelinating diseases of the CNS, MR is the imaging modality of choice to delineate the full extent and severity of the disease. Orbital MR with T2/STIR and postcontrast T1-weighted fat-saturated sequences will demonstrate areas of T2 hyperintensity within the involved portions of the optic nerves. In the acute setting the optic nerves will be swollen and demonstrate patchy or diffuse enhancement, while in later stages enhancement and swelling will resolve and thinning of the optic nerve may develop. The classic appearance of NMO in the spine is extensive areas of a T2 hyperintense signal within the cord typically extending over three or more vertebral bodies in length. In the acute phase there is usually associated cord swelling and enhancement. Enhancement may be homogeneous, patchy, or peripheral. The lesions are hypointense on precontrast T1-weighted imaging. After treatment enhancement resolves and depending on the severity of the initial injury, cord atrophy may develop.

While traditionally it has been thought that the brain is not involved in NMO, more recent studies have demonstrated that T2 hyperintense lesions do occur within the brain in some patients with NMO, more frequently in the relapsing than monophasic type. Most commonly T2 hyperintense lesions have a nonspecific distribution, scattered in the deep white matter of the cerebral hemispheres or cerebellum. In some cases the lesions may have a distribution suggestive of multiple sclerosis. Most intriguingly, however, is the reported predilection in patients for T2 hyperintense lesions to occur in brain regions known to be rich in aquaporin 4 channels, specifically around the third and fourth ventricles and cerebral aqueduct, thalamus, and hypothalamus. These lesions typically do not enhance.

Management

Acute NMO is typically treated with intravenous corticosteroids, as is typical for most acute demyelinating diseases. In resistant cases, plasmapheresis has been used. Most maintenance treatments used are those that produce general immunosuppression and can include azothiprine, rituximab, and cyclophosphamide among others. Of these treatments, rituximab appears to be the most effective; however, as the disease is rare and no large-scale randomized drug trials have been performed, there is no standardized treatment regimens, and practices vary widely. Importantly, treatment of NMO with MS specific therapies such as interferons and natalizumab may lead to worsening of the disease, making correct diagnosis of the disease exceedingly important. With the recent discovery of the anti-aquaporin 4 antibody, emerging treatments are focusing on prevention of binding of the antibody to its receptor in hopes of targeting the underlying pathophysiological mechanism of the disease.

Teaching Points

► Neuromyelitis optica is a severe demyelinating disease characterized by severe attacks of optic neuritis and transverse myelitis.
► In NMO spinal cord involvement is typically more extensive than in multiple sclerosis, with NMO lesions typically greater than three vertebral bodies in length (versus MS win which lesions are one to two vertebral bodies in length).
► Brain lesions do occur in NMO, and have a predilection for brain regions rich in aquaporin 4 channels (specifically around the third and fourth ventricles, cerebral aqueduct, hypothalamus, and thalamus).

Further Reading

1. Filippi M and Rocca MA. MR imaging of Devic's neuromyelitis optica. Neurol Sci 2004;25:S371–S373.
2. Ghezzi A, Bergamaschi R, Martinelli V, et al. Clinical characteristics, course and prognosis of relapsing Devic's neuromyelitis optica. J Neurol 2004;251:47–52.
3. Papadopoulos MC and Verkman A. Aquaporin 4 and neuromyelitis optica. Lancet Neurol 2012;11(6):535–544.
4. Wang F, Liu Y, Duan Y, and Li K. Brain MRI abnormalities in neuromyelitis optica. Eur J Radiol 2011;80(2):445–449.
5. Wingerchuk DM, Lennon VA, Pittock SJ, et al. Revised diagnostic criteria for neuromyelitis optica. Neurology 2006;66(10):1485–1489.

Section 6   **Congenital and Genetic Conditions**

Daniel Varon and Mauricio Castillo

History

► A 15-month-old patient presents with a history of an anorectal malformation (**Figures 55.1 and 55.2**).

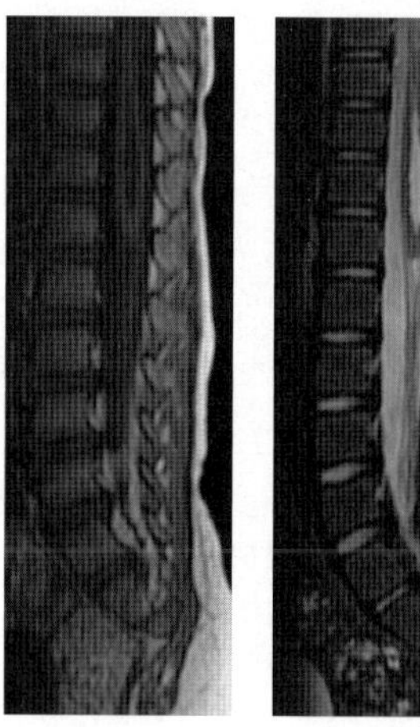

Figure 55.1   Figure 55.2

Chapter 55 **Caudal Regression Syndrome**

Findings

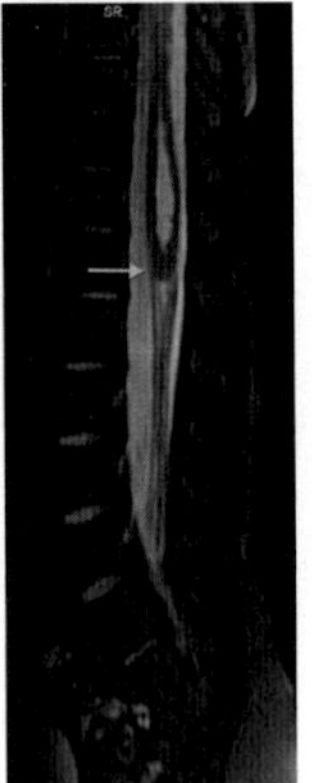

Figure 55.3

Caudal regression syndrome (type 1). Sagittal T1- and T2-weighted images (**Figures 55.1 and 55.3**) show subtotal sacrococcygeal agenesis, with a rudimentary S1 as the last vertebra. The cord terminus is blunt and lies at the level of T12 (arrow), which is too high. The cauda equina has a sparse appearance. The distal cord contains a cyst that may be remnant of the terminal ventricle versus a syrinx.

Discussion

Caudal regression syndrome (CRS) or caudal agenesis is a spectrum of disorders of caudal vertebral agenesis or dysgenesis, often with spinal cord malformations, that is associated with other congenital anomalies especially of the genitourinary and gastrointestinal systems. Over 30% of patients who have CRS are offspring of diabetic mothers. CRS is hypothesized to arise from an early abnormality of gastrulation. Segmental maldevelopment of the caudal notochord and axial–paraxial mesoderm results in an abnormality that interferes with either secondary neurulation alone, or both primary and secondary neurulation, depending on the longitudinal extent of the original notochordal damage.

The congenital spectrum of vertebral abnormalities may range from agenesis of the coccyx to the absence of the sacral, lumbar, and lower thoracic vertebrae, but the majority of these anomalies involve only the sacrum and coccyx.

Traditionally, caudal agenesis has been categorized into two types depending on the location and shape of the conus medullaris: either high and with an abrupt ending (type 1) or low and tethered at the level of the agenesis (type 2; Figure 55.4). Teratomas are known to occur in CRS, particularly with those classified as Type 2. Clinically, these patients often have genitourinary and anorectal malformations as well as malformations of the lower extremities.

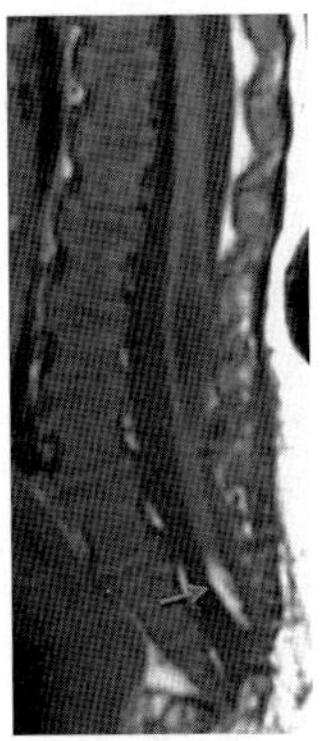

Figure 55.4

Caudal agenesis Type 2 (**Figure 55.4**). Sagittal T1-weighted images show partial sacral agenesis and the spinal cord tethered to a sacral lipoma (arrow). The cord terminus lies at the level of S1. The cord contains a syrinx.

Radiological Evaluation

Radiographs show hypoplasia or agenesis of the distal spine but MR is the mainstay of imaging evaluation showing the following types of lesions:

Caudal Agenesis Type 1

Depending on the severity of the original damage, the eventual degree of vertebral aplasia will vary; however, the last vertebrae are L5, S1, or S2 in the majority of patients. In the sagittal plane, there is often a characteristic abrupt termination of the cord seen as wedge-shaped cord terminus, which is at times slightly longer on its dorsal aspect. The cord terminus in these cases is typically above the L1 level due to the aplasia of the caudal metameres of the spinal cord .The cauda equina has a sparse appearance due to the lack of development of all of its nerve roots (Figure 55.1).

Caudal Agenesis Type 2

In this type, there is a minor degree of distal vertebral dysgenesis compared to Type 1. The spine may be present down to S4 as the last vertebra, and only the most caudal portion of the conus medullaris is absent (its tip). Partial agenesis of the conus can be difficult to recognize, because the conus itself is stretched caudally and tethered to a tight/enlarged filum terminale, lipoma, terminal myelocystocele, lipomyelomeningocele, or teratoma.

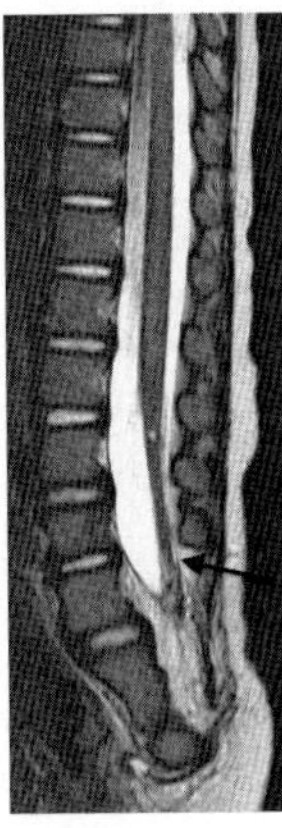

Figure 55.5

Caudal agenesis Type 2 (**Figure 55.5**). A sagittal T2-weighted image shows partial sacral agenesis and a tethered dysplastic cord that lies at the level of L5.

Teaching Points

▶ MRI screening should be performed in patients with characteristic clinical features (shallow and short intergluteal cleft), anorectal and genitourinary anomalies, or X-ray evidence of sacral agenesis.

▶ Vertebral agenesis may begin in the thoracic spine or as caudally as S4.

▶ The cord terminus in CRS Type 1 is typically above the L1 level, but in the Type 2 malformation, the spinal cord is tethered, and may terminate as low as S2.

Management

There is no specific treatment for patients with Type 1 CRS due to their "fixed" spinal cord dysplasia. The prognosis for children with CRS depends on the severity of the lesion (the higher the worse) and the presence of associated anomalies. Surgical untethering may be necessary to improve neurological function in patients with Type 2 CRS.

Further Reading

1. Grimme J and Castillo M. Congenital anomalies of the spine. Neuroimag Clin N Am 2007;17:1–16.
2. Rossi A, Biancheri R, Cama A, et al. Imaging in spine and spinal cord malformations. Eur J Radiol 2004;50:177–200.
3. Nievelstein RAJ, Valk J, Smit LME, et al. MR of the caudal regression syndrome: Embryologic implications. AJNR Am J Neuroradiol 1994;15:1021–1029.

Nima Jadidi and Sylvie Destian

History

▶ A 25-year-old female presents with a headache (**Figures 56.1 and 56.2**).

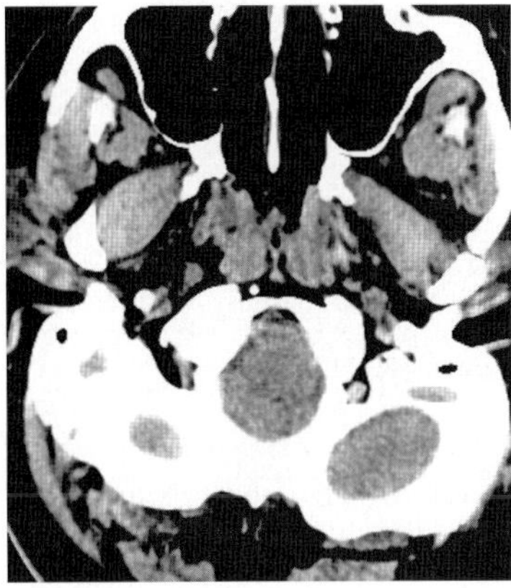

Figure 56.1

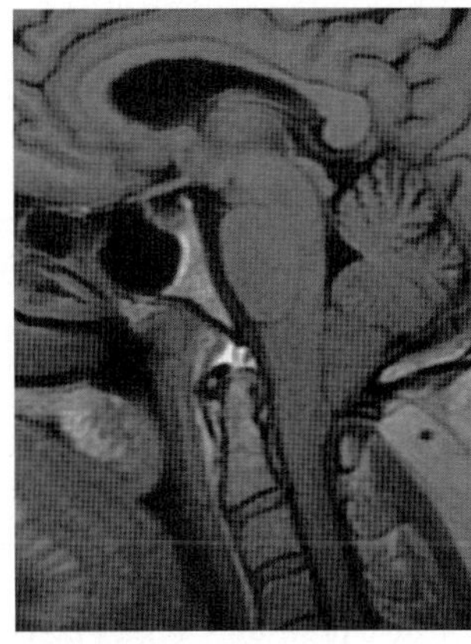

Figure 56.2

Chapter 56 Chiari I Malformation

Findings

Chiari I malformation (Figures 56.1 and 56.2). An axial CT (Figure 56.1) depicts soft tissue crowding at the foramen magnum with lack of cerebrospinal fluid (CSF) around the medulla. This can be seen in the setting of cerebellar tonsillar ectopia and requires further evaluation with an MRI. A sagittal T1-weighted MRI (Figure 56.2) depicts a peg-like configuration of the cerebellar tonsils that extend to the C1–C2 level. This is consistent with a Chiari I malformation.

Differential Diagnosis

► Cerebellar tonsillar ectopia
► Chiari II malformation
► Hydromyelia
► Ependymal cysts
► Myelomalacia
► Cystic tumors

Discussion

With the advent and evolution of imaging modalities, Chiari malformations are diagnosed more frequently as an incidental finding. A Chiari I malformation is displacement of the cerebellar tonsils inferior to the foramen magnum with an otherwise normal brainstem position. Chiari I malformation is believed to arise from a congenital malformation of the posterior fossa. There is a female predominance.

A Chiari I malformation is usually asymptomatic until early adulthood and may be acquired. A common presentation described is nondermatomal upper cervical and occipital pain. A detailed physical examination can yield abnormalities in cervical nerve sensory and motor distributions, hyperreflexia, ataxia, and a positive Babinski response. The latter three symptoms are common findings in the setting of myelopathy.

Tonsils extending more than 5 mm below the foramen magnum and with a pointed configuration is compatible with a Chiari I malformation (Figure 56.3). In 30% of patients with 5–10 mm downward extension of the tonsils, there are no symptoms. Almost all patients with a >12 mm downward extension of tonsils are symptomatic. Associated findings include brainstem compression, hydrocephalus (seen in less than 30% of cases), skeletal anomalies (seen in in 23-45% of cases), and a syrinx (seen in 20–56% of cases). A syrinx is the accumulation of CSF within the spinal cord that dissects through the ependyma creating cavitations.

Syringomyelia is an associated finding of Chiari malformations, and 40–75% of the time occurs in the region of the cervical spine concomitantly with the Chiari I malformation. A syrinx is characterized by a fluid-filled cavity that extends cephalocaudally along one or multiple spinal cord segments due to obstruction of CSF flow at the foramen magnum. While they may be asymptomatic, patients with a cervical syrinx may present with loss of pain and temperature at the level of the lesion due to disruption of the spinothalamic tract fibers crossing to the contralateral side, dysesthesias in the sensory distribution of the nerve roots involved, and atrophy of the intrinsic hand muscles.

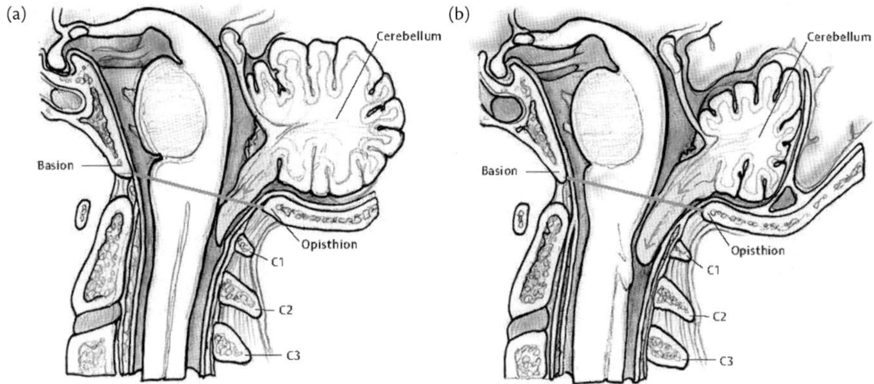

Figure 56.3

Schematic depiction of a Chiari I malformation (**Figure 56.3**). A Chiari I malformation refers to herniation of the cerebellar tonsils greater than 5 mm inferior to an imaginary plane from the tip of the clivus to the posterior margin of the foramen magnum (basion to ophistion).

Radiological Evaluation

On routine noncontrast CT of the brain, the lack of CSF at the foramen and soft tissue around the upper cervical cord suggests at least cerebellar tonsillar ectopia (Figure 56.1). On MR imaging the tonsils are pointed or peg-like and descend below the foramen magnum, most commonly to the C1–C2 level (Figure 56.2). An appropriate evaluation of patients with Chiari I malformations includes an MRI of the cervical spine to determine the presence of a syrinx that may be focal (Figure 56.4), involve the entire cervical cord (Figure 56.5), and in some cases involve the entire cord (Figures 56.6, 56.7, and 56.8).

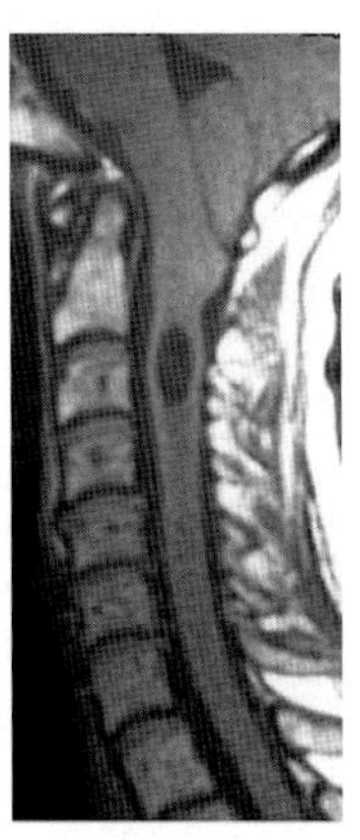

Figure 56.4

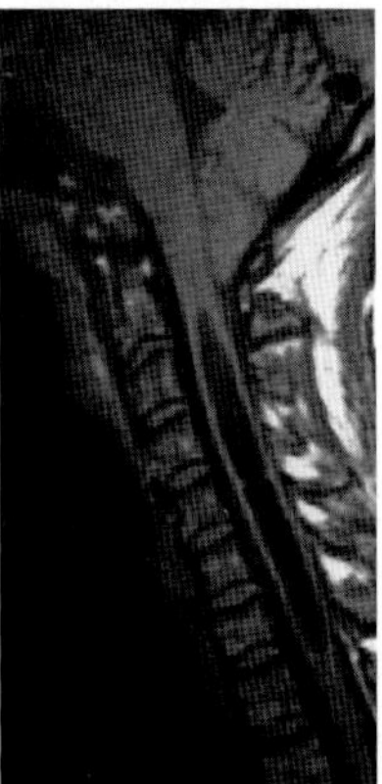

Figure 56.5

Syrinx in a Chiari malformation (**Figures 56.4 and 56.5**). A sagittal MR T1WI (Figure 56.4) depicts an accompanying focal syrinx at the C2–C3 level. A sagittal MR T1WI in a different patient (Figure 56.5) depicts an accompanying syrinx spanning the entire length of the cervical cord.

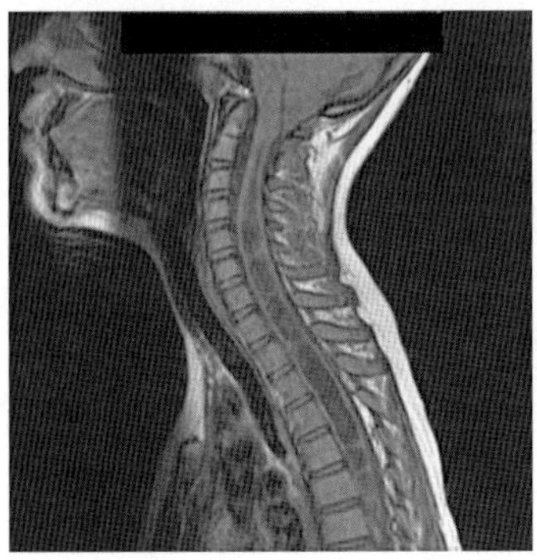

Figure 56.6

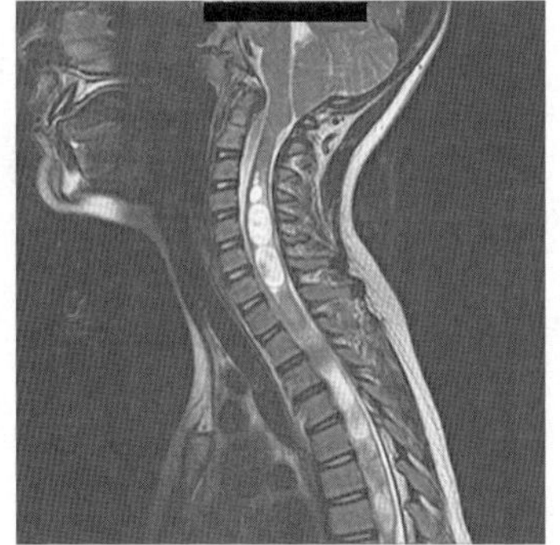

Figure 56.7

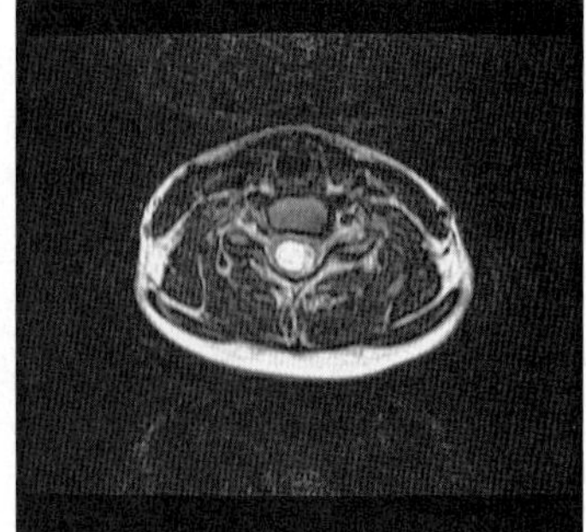

Figure 56.8

Chiari I malformation in a 10-year-old patient (**Figures 56.6, 56.7, and 56.8**). Sagittal T1 (Figure 56.6), sagittal T2 (Figure 56.7), and axial T2 (Figure 56.8) MR images again depict class findings of a Chiari I malformation. The typical peg-like appearance of the cerebellar tonsils is seen on sagittal views. There is a large associated syrinx with involvement of the entire cord (distal thoracic images are not shown).

Management

For Chiari I malformations, observation can be an appropriate initial management in an asymptomatic patient without an associated syrinx. If a syrinx is present, surgical intervention is warranted even in the absence of neurological deficits to prevent further spinal cord damage.

The primary objective of surgery is foramen magnum decompression and thorough decompression of the posterior surface of the cerebellar tonsils. The most common approach is bony decompression through resection of the posterior arch of C1, and occasionally a portion of C2 lamina, and duraplasty. First, a suboccipital craniectomy is performed and the foramen magnum is decompressed with Leksell rongeurs and Kerrison punches. After removal of the C1 posterior arch, and C2 superior lamina as needed, ultrasound can be used to visualize the movement of the cerebellar tonsils and the presence of fibrous bands within the cisterna magna that may need to be released. For duraplasty, the suboccipital dura is opened at the C1 midline in standard Y-shaped fashion and a watertight dural graft is sutured to the margins of the durotomy. The graft has the dual function of providing protection for the neural tissues and optimizing the decompression by enhancing the volume of the posterior fossa.

Teaching Points

▶ Patients with a Chiari I malformation in the absence of syringomyelia and neurological symptoms can be observed for a period of time; the presence of a syrinx is an indication for operative intervention.

▶ The goal of surgical intervention is to restore the normal flow of CSF from the fourth ventricle through the foramen magnum.

Further Reading

1. Grossman RI and Yousem DM. *Neuroradiology, The Requisites*. St. Louis, MO: Mosby, 2003, p. 819.
2. Fernández AA, Guerrero AI, Martínez MI, et al. Malformations of the craniocervical junction (Chiari type I and syringomyelia: classification, diagnosis and treatment). BMC Musculoskelet Disord 2009; 10 Suppl 1:S1.
3. Batzdorf U, McArthur DL, and Bentson JR. Surgical treatment of Chiari malformation with and without syringomyelia. J Neurosurg 2013;118(2):232–242.
4. Winn RH, Tubb RS, Pugh JA, and Oakes JW. In *Youmans Neurological Surgery*, 6th ed. (Winn RH, ed.). Philadelphia, PA: Saunders, 2011, pp. 1918–1927.
5. Khanna, AJ. *MRI Essentials for the Spine Specialist*. New York, NY: Thieme, 2014, pp. 87–110.
6. Elster AD, Chen MY. Chiari I malformations: clinical and radiologic reappraisal. Radiology. 1992;183 (2): 347-53.

History

▶ A newborn of a mother with folic acid deficiency presents with a lower back "bump" (**Figure 57.1**).

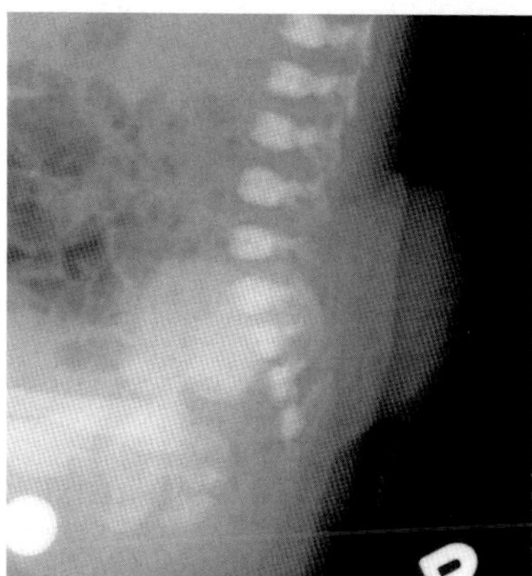

Figure 57.1

Chapter 57 **Myelomeningocele**

Findings

Myelomeningocele (Figure 57.1). A lateral view of the lumbosacral spine in the newborn of a mother with folic acid deficiency demonstrates a mass in the posterior paraspinal soft tissue of the lower back.

Differential Diagnosis

► Lipoma
► Myelocele
► Meningocele
► Syringomeningocele
► Lipomyelocele

Discussion

Myelomeningocele (MMC) is a spinal disraphysm characterized by the presence of a bulging neural tissue on the skin surface at birth. It is an embryological anomaly of neurulation resulting from the lack of closure of the neural tube around day 17 of gestation. The resulting placode is functionally destroyed in the third trimester. However, its anatomical presence will keep the posterior elements of the affected vertebrae open and be visible on the surface of the skin. Multivitamin/folic acid supplementation in early pregnancy reduces the prevalence of MMC.

Radiological Evaluation

No detailed radiological evaluation is required during the newborn period. The clinical presentation suffices to diagnose and warrant surgical intervention. Imaging plays a role in fetal MMC closure and elucidates the causes of neurological deterioration after repair.

While plain radiographs and CT scan help identify the bony anomalies associated with MMC, MRI helps to evaluate for associated malformations of the spinal cord and paraspinal soft tissue. An Arnold–Chiari II malformation is almost always present. Other less common associated malformations are diastematomyelia (35%), dorsal dermal sinus (35%), and hydromyelia (29%). Scoliosis, arachnoid cyst, dermoid, and epidermoid may also be present.

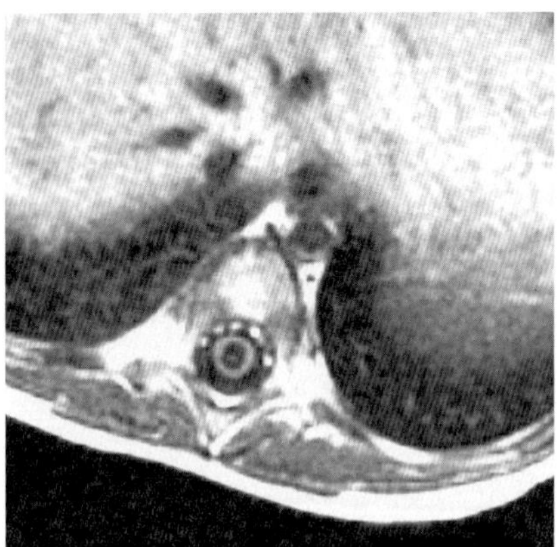

Figure 57.2

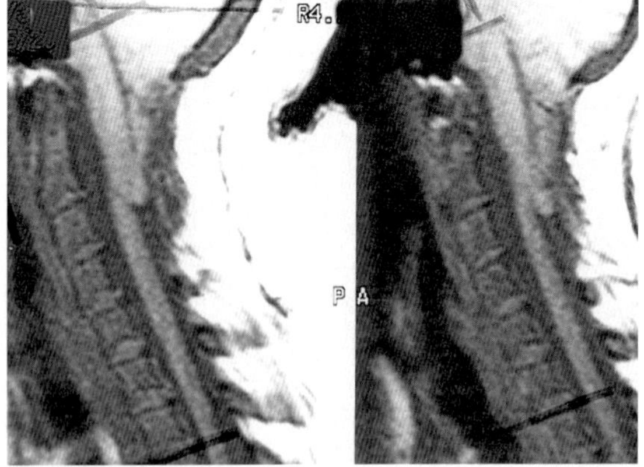

Figure 57.3

Myelomeningocele in a patient with a Chiari II malformation (**Figures 57.2 and 57.3**). An axial T1-weighted image (Figure 57.2) of the thoracic spine in a patient who is deteriorating after surgical repair of a lumbar MMC demonstrates a central cavity of hypointense T1 signal in the thoracic cord consistent with hydromyelia. A sagittal T1-weighted image (Figure 57.3) acquired in the cervical region demonstrates an inferior displacement of the tip of the cerebellar tonsils below the foramen magnum down to the level of C2, compatible with a Arnold-Chiari II malformation.

After surgical repair of a lumbar MMC, the most commonly observed complications are retethering of the cord, inclusion epidermoid, inclusion lipoma, hydromyelia, arachnoid cyst, devascularization of the placode, local wound lesions, and scoliosis. MRI is useful to narrow the differential diagnosis because of its ability to characterize the tissues (Figures 57.4 and 57.5).

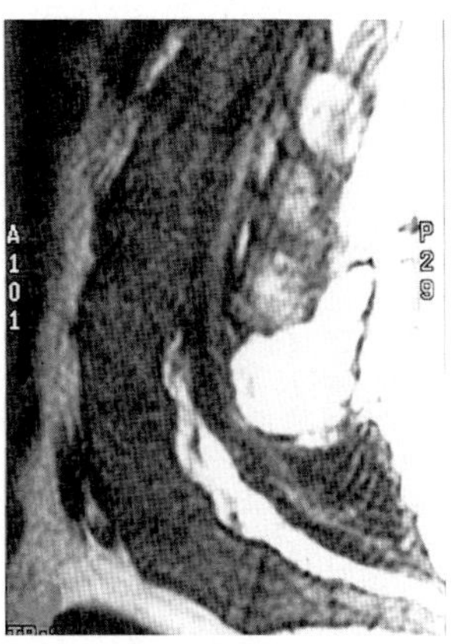

Figure 57.4

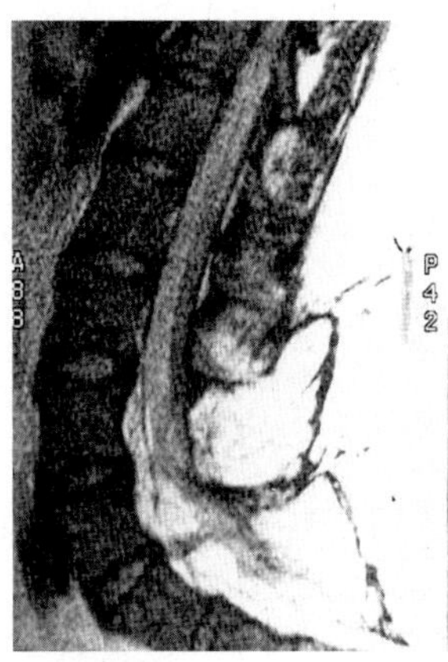

Figure 57.5

MRI evaluation of a different newborn with a soft tissue mass in the back (**Figures 57.4 and 57.5**). Sagittal T1-weighted (Figure 57.4) and T2-weighted (Figure 57.5) images of the lumbosacral spine demonstrate a soft tissue mass with two distinct components. The superior portion (*) is hyperintense on both T1- and T2-weighted sequences indicating fat. The inferior portion (#) is hypointense on T1- and hyperintense on T2-weighted sequences consistent with cerebrospinal fluid (CSF). The MRI clearly identifies a mass with fat and fluid consistent with a lipomyelocele.

Management

Closure during the fetal period can often be performed safely. This is more beneficial to the child instead of postnatal exploration and surgical repair, which is typically reserved for cases in which fetal management is not possible.

Teaching Points

▶ Neurological deteriorations after surgical repair of MMC should prompt an MRI investigation to look for associated malformations, especially Chiari II.

▶ Closing of the skin defect during fetal life is more beneficial than postnatal repair.

Further Reading

1. Milunsky A, Jick H, Jick SS, et al. Multivitamin/folic acid supplementation in early pregnancy reduces the prevalence of neural tube defects. JAMA 1989;262(20):2847–2852.
2. Meuli M and Moehrlen U. Fetal surgery for myelomeningocele is effective: A critical look at the whys. Pediatr Surg Int 2014;30(7):689-697.

Chapter 58

Freddie R. Swain

History

▶ A child presents with gross motor developmental delay (**Figures 58.1 and 58.2**).

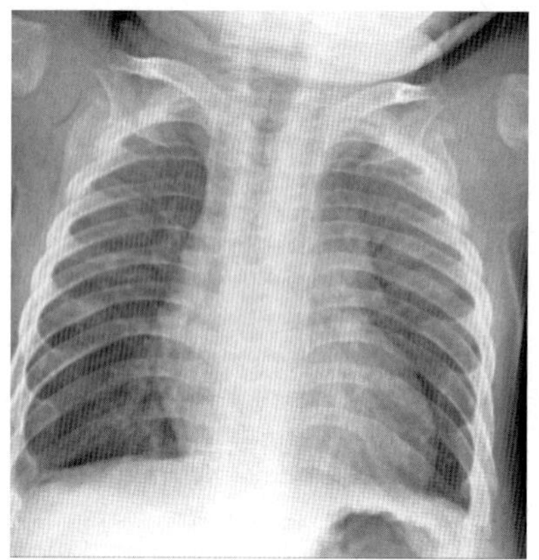

Figure 58.1

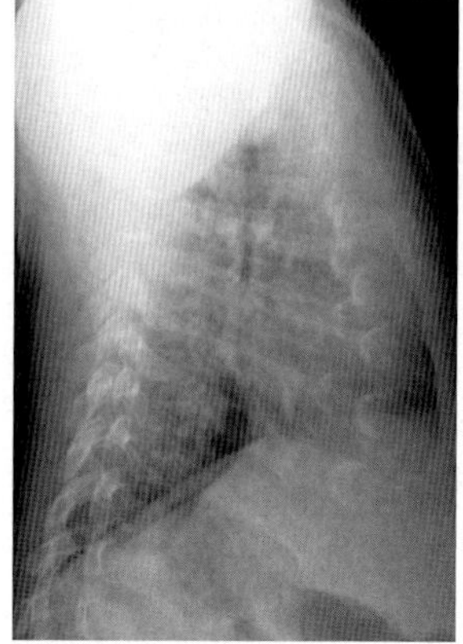

Figure 58.2

Findings

Achondroplasia. A lateral chest radiograph (Figure 58.2) demonstrates shortened pedicles, raising concern for spinal canal stenosis. Anterior rib flaring is also noted on the frontal view (Figure 58.1).

Discussion

Achondroplasia is the most common form of skeletal dysplasia, resulting in a disproportionate short stature along with shortened limbs. It is transmitted as an autosomal dominant trait and is caused by a mutation in the gene that codes for fibroblast growth factor receptor 3 (FGFR3) on the short arm of chromosome 4, which affects the maturation of chondrocytes in the growth plate. Patients with achondroplasia demonstrate spinal cord levels higher than nonachondroplasia patients but no statistical difference is found between symptomatic and asymptomatic achondroplasia patients. Interestingly, cord occupancy is not statistically different among symptomatic versus asymptomatic achondroplasia patients. The incidence of kyphosis, however, has been demonstrated to increase from nonachondroplasia, asymptomatic, and symptomatic patient groups.

Disproportionate growth between endochondral bone and the underlying organs leads to a number of orthopedic, neurological, respiratory, ear, nose, and throat, and dental issues for individuals with achondroplasia. Neurological problems are present in 35-47% of patients with achondroplasia.

Thoracolumbar (TL) kyphosis is a major secondary musculoskeletal impairment thought to arise from the combined impact of other common primary musculoskeletal impairments, such as macrocephaly, hypotonia, and joint hypermobility. TL kyphosis tends to appear around 6 months of age with the majority of patients improving. Nevertheless, approximately 10% of patients progress in kyphosis. Gradual disruption of the vertebral epiphyseal ring that begins during childhood, combined with decreased growth in the anterior vertebral sections, can create a progressive TL kyphosis in adolescents, which is further exacerbated by age-related degenerative changes in the facet joints during adulthood. Wedge-shaped deformities of one or more vertebral bodies, particularly between T10 and L2, can exert a mass effect on the nervous structures, specifically the conus and nerve roots.

Cervical cord compression at the cervicomedullary junction is commonly identified radiographically in children but is less often symptomatic. Significant compression at the foramen magnum can lead to severe neurological complications, including sleep apnea, disordered respiration, myelopathy, hydrocephalus, and sudden infant death.

Radiological Evaluation

Radiographs are the mainstay for initial diagnosis, often depicting several features seen in achondroplasia (**Figure 58.3** and **Table 58.1**). However, some clinicians advocate for routine screening for cervicomedullary compression by MRI or CT in infants because a proportion of these children may require cervicomedullary decompression (CMD).

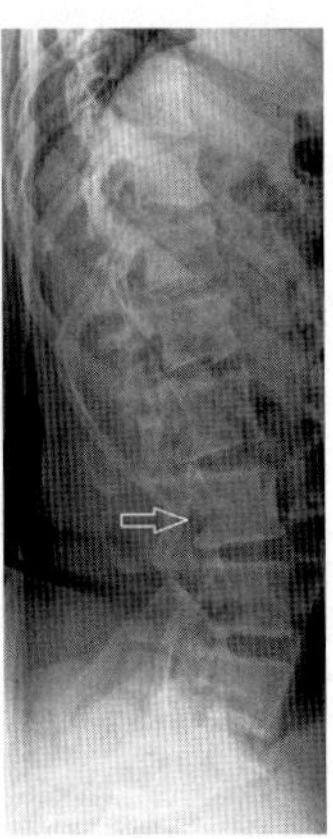

Figure 58.3

Radiographic features of achondroplasia. A lateral lumbar spine radiograph demonstrates posterior vertebral scalloping (Figure 58.3).

Table 58.1. Findings Associated with Achondroplasia

Region	Findings
Spine	▶ Posteriovertebral scalloping
	▶ Decreased interpedicular distance in the lumbar spine
	▶ Gibbus deformity
	▶ Short pedicles
	▶ Increased angle between the lumbar spine and sacrum
Chest	▶ Anterior rib flaring
	▶ Narrowing of ribs in the anteroposterior (AP) direction
Limbs	▶ Metaphyseal flaring
	▶ Trident hand
	▶ Short femori/humeri
Pelvis/hips	▶ Decreased acetabular angle
	▶ "Tombstone" iliac wings
	▶ Trident pelvis
	▶ "Champagne glass" appearance of pelvic inlet
Cranial	▶ Narrowed foramen magnum
	▶ Communicating hydrocephalus
	▶ Cervicomedullary kinking
	▶ Prominent forehead
	▶ Small skull base

Management

In adolescents and adults, the time from symptom onset to surgery is an important predictor of long-term functional outcome. Worsening stenosis of the spinal canal and foramen eventually can lead to spinal cord or root compression, resulting in sensory dysfunction, radicular pain, neurogenic claudication, bladder dysfunction, and in severe cases, fecal incontinence. For these patients, laminectomy is one option to relieve the symptoms of spinal stenosis and prevent permanent neurological deficit. However, postoperative instability can occur and thoracolumbar kyphosis has been cited as the main reason for developing paraparesis. Decompression techniques may need to be combined with instrumented fixation or spinal reconstructions in certain circumstances.

Further Reading

1. Engberts AC, Jacobs WC, Castelijns SJ, Castelein RM, Vleggeert-Lankamp CL. The prevalence of thoracolumbar kyphosis in achondroplasia: a systematic review. J Child Orthop. 2012 Mar;6(1):69–73. doi: 10.1007/s11832-011-0378-7. Epub 2011 Dec 3.
2. Modi HN, Suh SW, Hong JY, Yang JH. Magnetic resonance imaging study determining cord level and occupancy at thoracolumbar junction in achondroplasia – A prospective study. Indian J Orthop. 2011 Jan;45(1):63–8. doi: 10.4103/0019-5413.73661.
3. Penny J Ireland, Verity Pacey, Andreas Zankl, Priya Edwards, Leanne M Johnston, and Ravi Savarirayan Optimal management of complications associated with achondroplasia. Appl Clin Genet. 2014; 7: 117–125.
4. Carlisle ES, Ting BL, Abdullah MA, Skolasky RL, Schkrohowsky JG, Yost MT, Rigamonti D, Ain MC. Laminectomy in patients with achondroplasia: the impact of time to surgery on long-term function. Spine (Phila Pa 1976). 2011 May 15;36(11):886–92. doi: 10.1097/BRS.0b013e3181e7cb2a.

Chapter 59

Freddie R. Swain and Gary Shapiro

History

▶ An adolescent girl presents with worsening deformity (**Figure 59.1**).

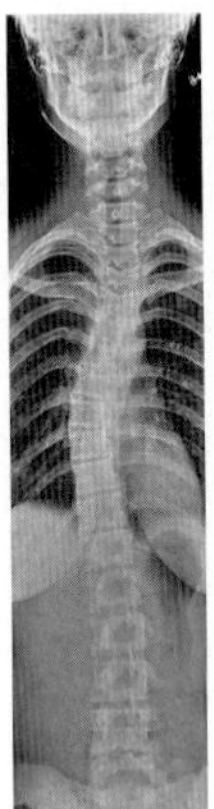

Figure 59.1

Findings

Scoliosis (Figure 59.1). A standing posteroanterior (PA) radiograph demonstrates a scoliotic (Cobb) angle of 29 degrees measured from the superior endplate of T2 to the inferior endplate of T12.

Discussion

Scoliosis is defined as a spinal deformity with a Cobb angle of over 10 degrees. It is the most common spinal disorder in children and adolescents, divided into cohorts of idiopathic and nonidiopathic scoliosis. Adolescent idiopathic scoliosis affects 2–3% of the population with 0.1% of patients requiring surgery.

Idiopathic scoliosis is categorized by age:

▶ Infantile scoliosis: 0–3 years of age
▶ Juvenile scoliosis: 4–10 years of age
▶ Adolescent scoliosis: 11–18 years of age
▶ Adult scoliosis: >18 years of age

Nonidiopathic scoliosis can be further divided into the following groups:

▶ Congenital scoliosis: secondary to a malformation of vertebrae such as hemivertebra, unilateral bar, or block vertebra.
▶ Neuromuscular scoliosis: secondary to insufficiency of active (muscular) stabilizers of the spine; i.e., cerebral palsy, spinal muscular atrophy, spina bifida, muscular dystrophies, or spinal cord injuries.

Adult scoliosis patients consist of two groups: idiopathic and degenerative. Idiopathic begins during adolescence and continues throughout adulthood while degenerative scoliosis begins around 50 years of age.

While the main symptom of adolescent scoliosis is deformity (**Figure 59.2**), the symptoms of adult scoliosis often include back pain and radiating pain to the legs. Adult scoliosis is more often accompanied by sagittal and coronal imbalance when compared to adolescent scoliosis. Medical comorbidity such as cardiopulmonary disease may increase perioperative complications, and osteoporosis may result in lack of firm fixation.

Curve Types

Thoracic curves are the most common (48%), followed by thoracolumbar/lumbar curves (40%). Double curves (9%) and double thoracic curves (3%) are less common.

Radiological Evaluation

The most common measurement of spinal curvature is the Cobb angle on a full spine radiograph. The standing anteroposterior (AP) or PA radiograph of the full spine is the basic tool for radiographic characterization and quantification of the deformity. The Cobb angle is the measurement between two end vertebrae of a curve, defined as the most tilted vertebrae at the top and bottom of a curve.

MRI of the spine is indicated in nonidiopathic curves, atypical curve patterns, or when there are abnormal reflexes on physical examination. An MRI of the brain and entire spine is obtained in such cases to evaluate for tethered cord or syrinx.

CT scans can be obtained to better define bony abnormalities and, on occasion, as a preoperative planning tool. The benefits of a CT scan must be weighed with the risk of radiation exposure to the patient.

Management

To select the therapeutic regime for patients with idiopathic scoliosis, it is necessary to analyze the extent of curvature (Cobb angle) in both the sagittal and coronal planes and the remaining growth potential of the patient.

Treatment consists of observation in curves less than 25 degrees in skeletally immature patients or in curves up to 45 degrees at skeletal maturity. In skeletally immature patients, surveillance is performed at regular intervals to assess curve progression. Physical therapy can be used for core strengthening, but has not been shown to affect the magnitude of the curve or the likelihood of progression.

Bracing is indicated in skeletally immature patients with curves of 25–40 degrees. Bracing has been shown to be most effective when worn for 20–22 hours/day. Bracing is not indicated in skeletally mature patients.

Surgery is indicated when curves are 45 degrees or greater in skeletally immature patients or in adults who have documented curve progression over time, worsening back or radicular pain, or a progressive neurological deficit.

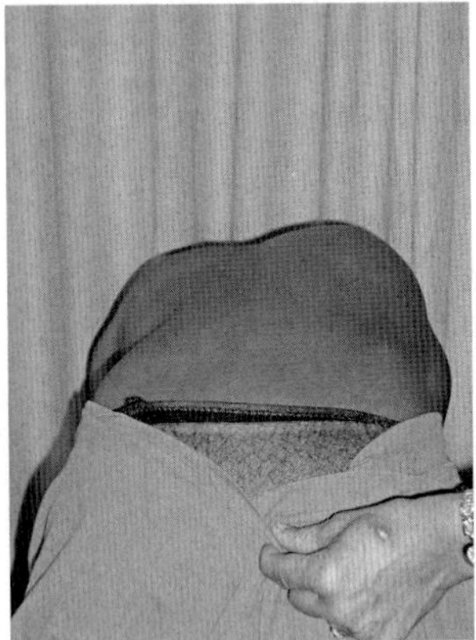

Figure 59.2

Figure 59.2 is a clinical photograph of a patient with a forward bend.

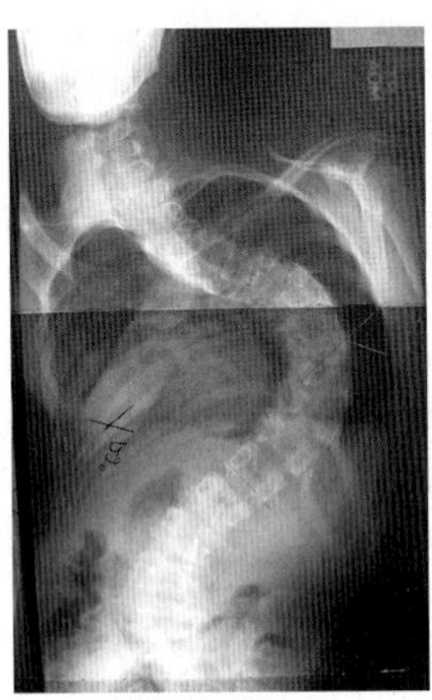

Figure 59.3

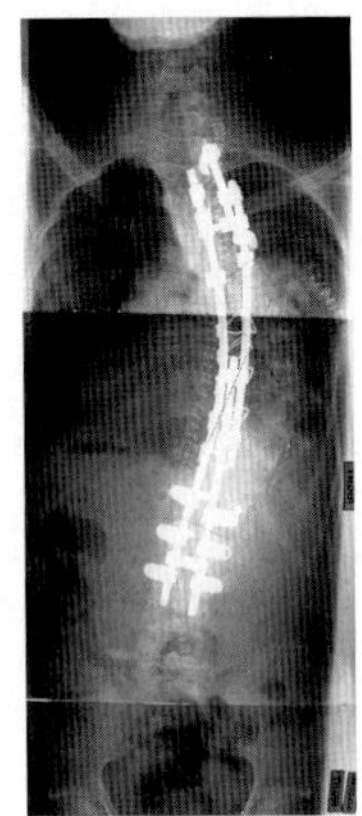

Figure 59.4

Preoperative and postoperative imaging appearance (**Figures 59.3 and 59.4**). Preoperative (Figure 59.3) and postoperative (Figure 59.4) AP radiographs of a different patient demonstrate surgical correction of a scoliosis.

Most surgeries are performed from a posterior approach with pedicle screw fixation (Figures 59.3 and 59.4). Other options include anterior only and combined approaches for severe deformity. Research is being conducted on spinal growth modulation in children to achieve curve correction without fusion.

Teaching Points

▶ Scoliosis affects both children and adults.
▶ Treatment varies based on age, curve magnitude, and clinical findings.

Further Reading

1. Jin-Hyok Kim, Sung-Soo Kim, and Se-Il Suk Incidence of Proximal Adjacent Failure in Adult Lumbar Deformity Correction Based on Proximal Fusion Level. Asian Spine J. 2007 Jun; 1(1): 19–26.
2. Konieczny MR,Senyurt H, Krauspe R. Epidemiology of adolescent idiopathic scoliosis. J Child Orthop. 2013 Feb;7(1):3–9. doi: 10.1007/s11832-012-0457-4. Epub 2012 Dec 11.
3. Montgomery F, Willner S. The natural history of idiopathic scoliosis. Incidence of treatment in 15 cohorts of children born between 1963 and 1977. Spine (Phila Pa 1976). 1997 Apr 1;22(7):772–4.
4. Smith JS, Shaffrey CI, Glassman SD, Carreon LY, Schwab FJ, Lafage V, Arlet V, Fu KM, Bridwell KH; Spinal Deformity Study Group. Clinical and radiographic parameters that distinguish between the best and worst outcomes of scoliosis surgery for adults. Eur Spine J. 2013 Feb;22(2):402–10. doi: 10.1007/s00586-012-2547-x. Epub 2012 Oct 18.
5. Waldt, Gersing, and Brugel Seminars in musculoskeletal radiology (Impact Factor: 0.95). 07/2014; 18(3):219–227. DOI: 10.1055/s-0034-1375565
6. Dalal A, Upasani VV, Bastrom TP, Yaszay B, Shah SA, Shufflebarger HL, Newton PO. Apical vertebral rotation in adolescent idiopathic scoliosis: comparison of uniplanar and polyaxial pedicle screws. J Spinal Disord Tech. 2011 Jun;24(4):251–7. doi: 10.1097/BSD.0b013e3181edebc4.

Chapter 60

Justin Morris Honce

History

▶ A 51-year-old female presents with worsening low back pain and radiation of discomfort, numbness, and tingling into the bilateral lower extremities (**Figures 60.1, 60.2, 60.3, and 60.4**).

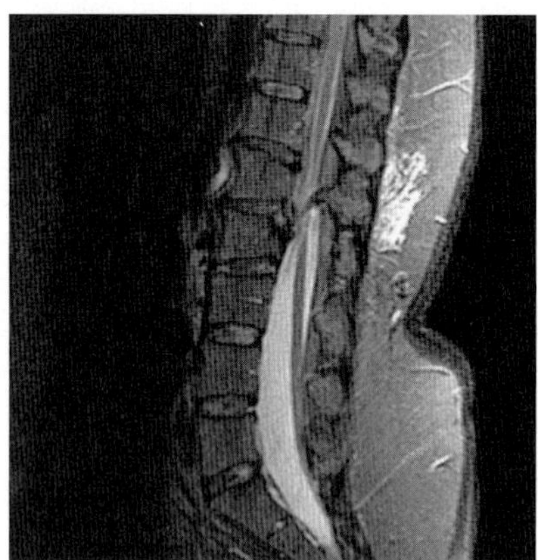

Figure 60.1

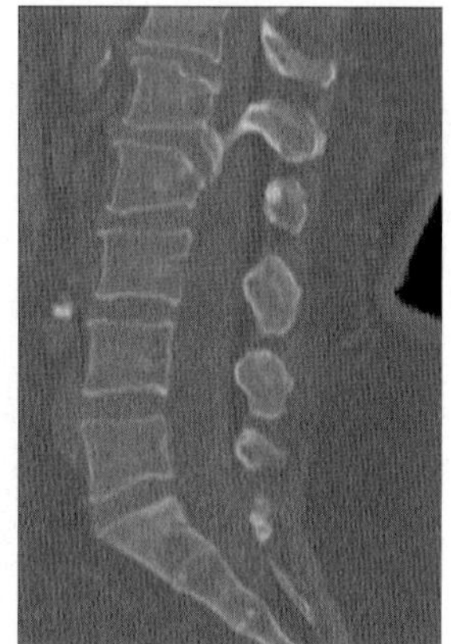

Figure 60.2

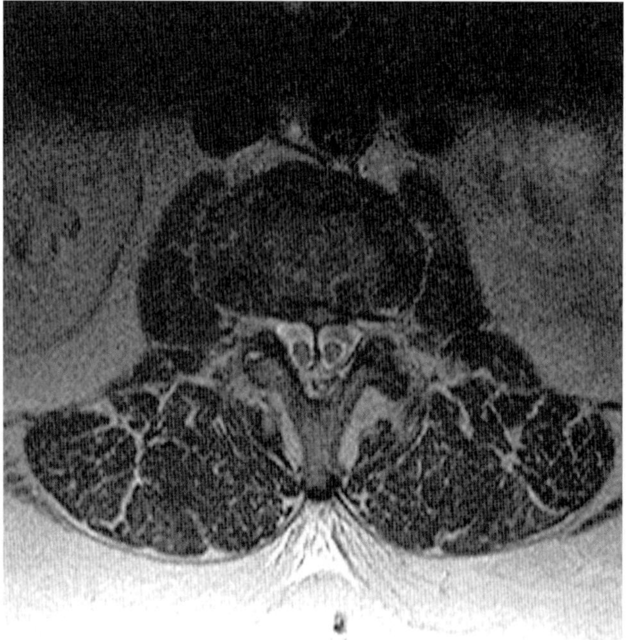

Figure 60.3

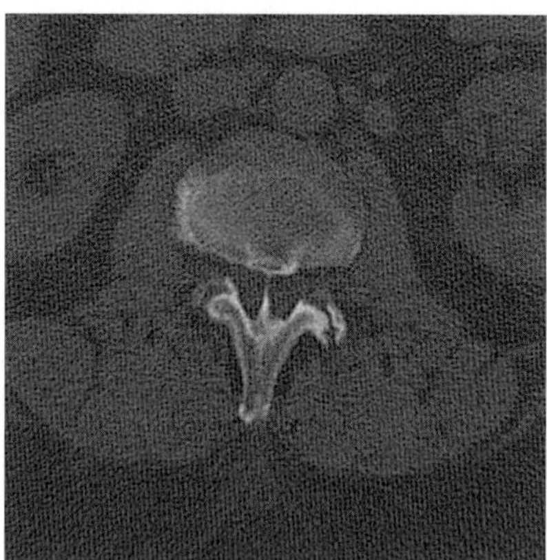

Figure 60.4

Findings

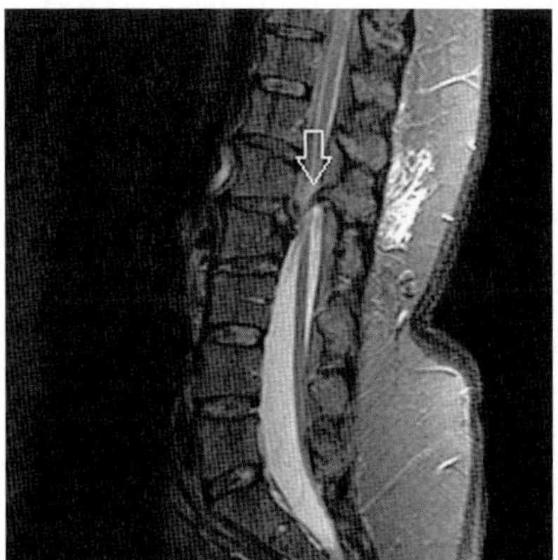

Figure 60.5

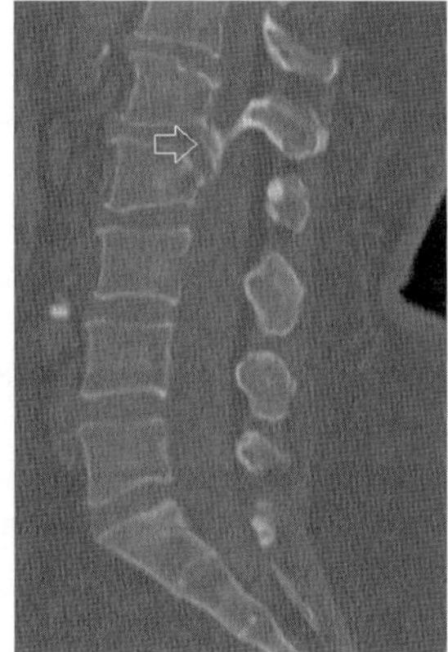

Figure 60.6

Diastematomyelia. A sagittal STIR image (Figure 60.5) demonstrates a linear, low-signal structure traversing obliquely inferiorly across the spinal canal from the posterior elements of L1 to the posterior edge of L2 (Arrow). The sagittal CT reconstruction image (Figure 60.6) shows that this structure is ossified. Note also on the sagittal STIR image that the cord is low lying, ending in the upper sacral region (arrow).

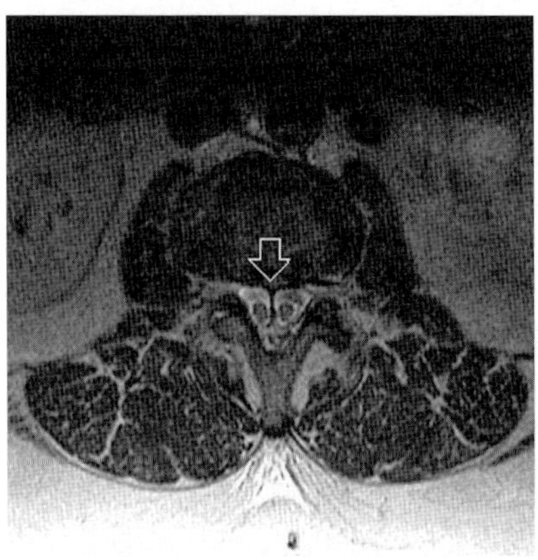

Figure 60.7

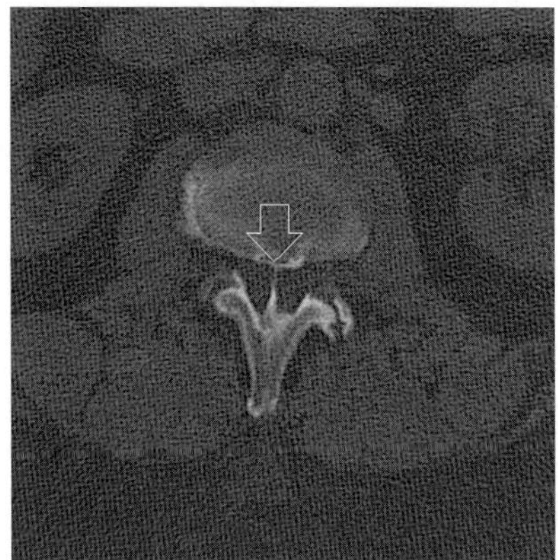

Figure 60.8

Axial T2-weighted imaging (Figure 60.7) demonstrates a thin cleft that divides the thecal sac and spinal cord into two symmetric halves (Arrow). The axial CT image (Figure 60.8) again shows that this septum/cleft is ossified (Arrow).

Differential Diagnosis

Diplomyelia.

Discussion

Diastematomyelia (or split cord malformation) is a congenital malformation in which there is a longitudinal division of the spinal cord into two separate hemicords as the result of separation by a midline septum. Each of the hemicords contains a dorsal and ventral horn and a central canal. From each dorsal or ventral horn a unilateral dorsal and ventral nerve root arises. There are two types of diastematomyelia. In Type I, both the cord as well as the arachnoid and dura are split, resulting in two separate dural sacs; each hemicord has a separate arachnoid and pial covering. In Type II, while the cord is split into two halves, both hemicords are contained within an intact pial and arachnoid layering and a single dural sac. The intervening septum may be osseous, cartilaginous, or fibrous and in cases of Type II malformations this band may not be visible.

The level of the cleft/septum and associated longitudinal division of the cord is variable. Most commonly these malformations occur in the lumbar spine (~60%); however, they can also be found in the thoracic spine (typically lower thoracic) and, very rarely, in the cervical region. Most typically the cleft/septum is located at midline and results in the division of the cord into relatively symmetric hemicords. They are not always midline, however, and in rare cases may traverse the spinal canal in an oblique fashion, resulting in asymmetry in the size of the hemicords and their dural sacs. This is especially true in patients with concomitant scoliosis.

The spinal column is abnormal in nearly all patients with diastematomyelia. The most common abnormalities are thickening and fusion of the lamina at adjacent levels, spina bifida, and vertebral body segmentation anomalies. In addition to the split cord malformation, numerous other spinal cord malformations can be seen. A low-lying, tethered cord is identified in up to 80% of patients, myleomeningoceles and syringohydromelia are present in up to 20% of patients, and intraspinal lipomas, dermoids, and neuroenteric cysts occur more rarely. Chiari malformation can be seen in patients as well.

Radiological Evaluation

Diastematomyelia is best evaluated with both MRI and CT imaging. CT imaging is best able to visualize the osseous/cartilaginous spur and provides excellent visualization of the associated vertebral body/posterior element anomalies; however, MRI is far superior in evaluating the morphology of the splitting of the cord/dura/arachnoid. T1-weighted images are well suited to visualize the splitting of the cord, whereas T2-weighted images allow the dorsal and ventral nerve roots and the separation of the dural sacs to be delineated. The midline cleft/septum is typically hypointense on T1 and T2 imaging, but if the osseous spur has internal marrow, it can appear T1 hyperintense. MR imaging is also ideal for the evaluation of associated congenital anomalies (low lying/tethered cord, thickening of nerve roots, and intraspinal masses/cysts, etc.).

The imaging appearance is pathognomonic; however, in cases in which the midline septum/spur cannot be identified, diplomyelia is the major differential diagnosis. Diplomyelia is an extremely rare malformation in which the cord is duplicated, without a midline septum. In contradistinction to diastematomyelia each hemicord in diplomyelia has paired dorsal and ventral horns from which bilateral dorsal and ventral nerve roots arise.

Management

In the absence of progressive neurological deficit, no surgical intervention is indicated. In cases of progressive deficits, surgical intervention with resection of the midline cleft and repair of associated tethering or other abnormalities may be performed. Typically there may be partial improvement in deficits over time but no dramatic reversal.

Teaching Points

▶ Diastematomyelia is a longitudinal splitting of the cord (and frequents the dural sac, arachnoid, and pia) by an osseous, cartilaginous or fibrous band, typically midline in location.

▶ In contradistinction to diplomyelia (cord duplication), each hemicord has a signal dorsal and ventral horn that gives rise to unilateral nerve roots.

▶ Diastematomyelia in nearly all cases is associated with other congenital spinal column and spinal cord malformations, including vertebral body segmentation anomalies, spina bifida, tethered cord, myelomeningocele, and hydromyelia, among others. Careful examination of all images is crucial to evaluate for these other abnormalities.

Further Reading

1. Basak M, Ozel A, and Erturk M. An unusual case of diastematomyelia: Presence of one dural sheath associated with a bony spur. Neurology 2003;60(3):491.

2. Breningstall GN, Marker SM, and Tubman DE. Hydrosyringomyelia and diastematomyelia detected by MRI in myelomeningocele. Pediatr Neurol 1992;8:267–271.

3. Han JS, Benson JE, Kaufman B, et al. Demonstration of diastematomyelia and associated abnormalities with MR imaging. AJNR Am J Neuroradiol 1985;6:215–219.

4. Miller AW, Guille JT, and Bowen JR. Evaluation and treatment of diastematomyelia. J Bone Joint Surg Am 1993;75A:1308–1317.

5. Naidich TP and Harwood-Nash DC. Diastematomyelia: Hemicord and meningeal sheath; single and double arachnoid and dural tubes. AJNR Am J Neuroradiol 1983;4:633–636.

Chapter 61

Ernst Garcon

History

▶ A full-term infant of a diabetic mother is unable to move her legs (**Figures 61.1 and 61.2**).

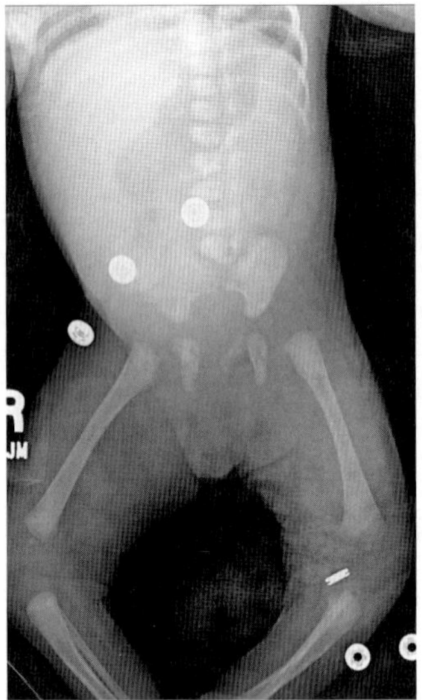

Figure 61.1

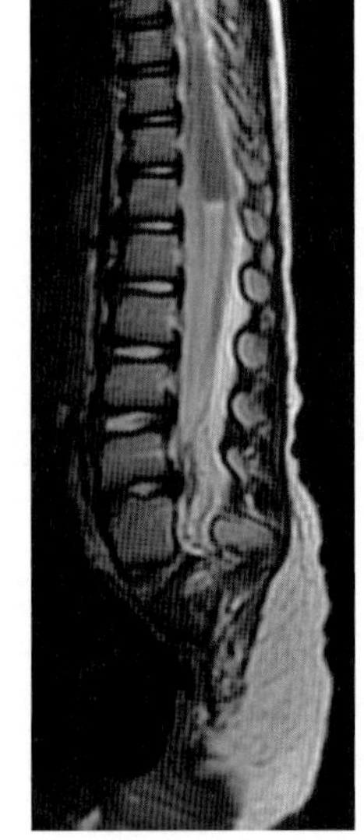

Figure 61.2

Findings

Sacral agenesis with caudal regression syndrome. An anteroposterior (AP) view of the pelvis (**Figure 61.1**) demonstrates the absence of the sacrum. The iliac wings are hyperplastic and in close proximity to one another. A sagittal T2-weighted MRI of the lower spine (**Figure 61.2**) shows partial agenesis of the sacrum. The spinal cord is club-shaped and abruptly ends at T12.

Discussion

Sacral agenesis (SA) is a skeletal malformation that can be seen in infants with Caudal Regression Syndrome (CRS) and sirenomyelia (a congenital deformity in which the legs are fused together, resulting in a mermaid appearance). CRS includes partial agenesis of the thoracic, lumbar, and sacral spine, imperforated anus, malformed genitalia, bilateral renal dysplasia or aplasia, and pulmonary hypoplasia. It is an embryological anomaly of the caudal cell mass that fails to properly involute around day 38 of gestation. Its incidence is approximately 1/7500 births and equally affects boys and girls. Many associations have been reported with a diabetic mother being the most consistent.

Radiological Evaluation

The radiological evaluation of an infant with SA begins with a plain radiograph of the spine to assess the integrity of the axial skeleton. Spine malformations may also be incidental findings on chest X-rays (**Figure 61.3**).

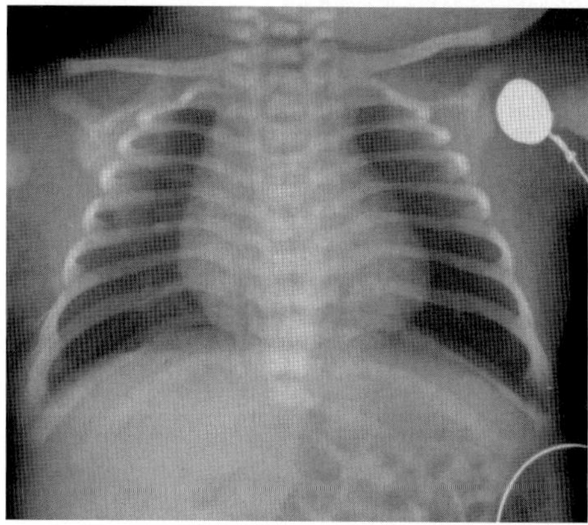

Figure 61.3

A chest radiograph (**Figure 61.3**) shows an abrupt cut off of the spinal column below T11 despite a normal cardiopulmonary shadow. This is a finding that can easily be overlooked if a systematic approach is not applied during film interpretation.

Recent advances in musculoskeletal ultrasound allow it to be used in the investigation of the spine of infants with CRS. The lack of ionizing radiation makes ultrasound very attractive in pediatric imaging (**Figures 61.4 and 61.5**).

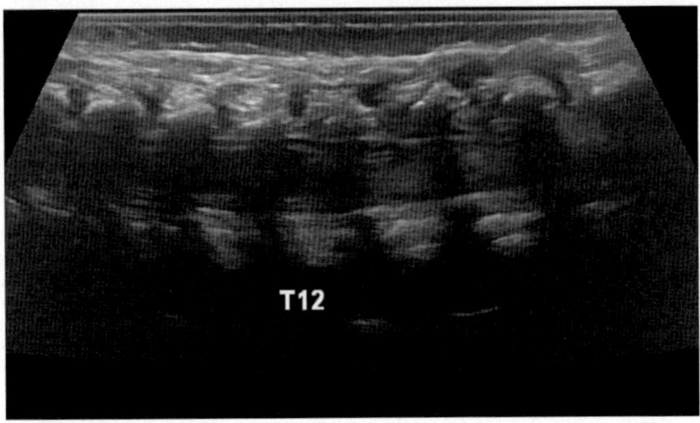

Figure 61.4

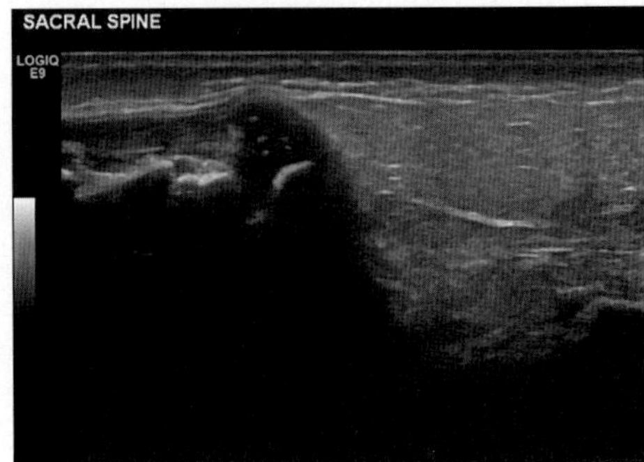

Figure 61.5

Gray scale sagittal ultrasound evaluation of the lower spine in a CRS infant shows a hyperechoic cord that terminates normally at L2 (**Figure 61.4**) within the hypoechoic spinal canal. Note the absence of a fully developed sacrum when the transducer is moved below L3 (**Figure 61.5**).

A CT scan is an important tool in the surgical planning. It provides information about the spinal column and its content when iodinated contrast media is administered intrathecally through a spinal tap. The resulting CT myelogram is more sensitive for the detection of spinal canal and cord anomalies (**Figures 61.6 and 61.7**).

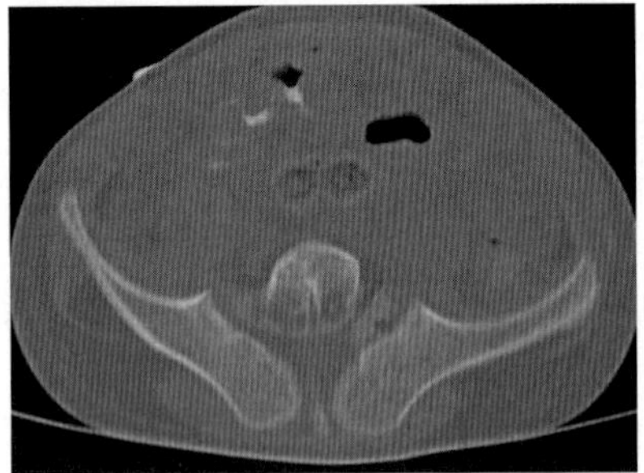

Figure 61.6

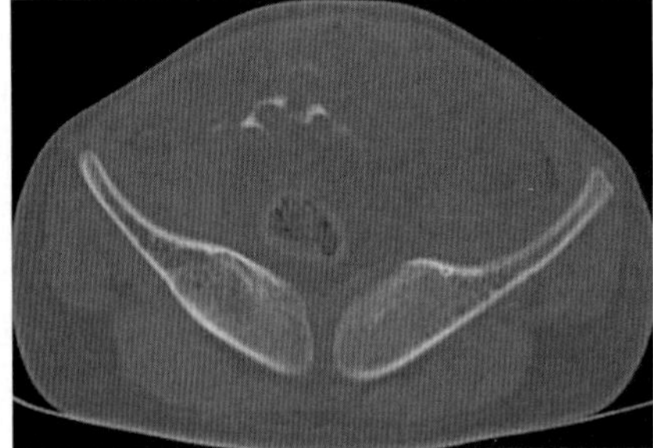

Figure 61.7

A CT scan of the pelvis done without intravenous or intrathecal contrast demonstrates a hypoplastic S1 segment of the sacrum (**Figure 61.6**). The distal sacrum is completely absent and the iliac wings are in close proximity (**Figure 61.7**).

MRI is considered today the gold standard to evaluate patients with SA. A prenatal MRI plays a critical role in assessing the extension and severity of CRS, especially in the decision of terminating the pregnancy. A postnatal MRI is better than a CT scan to evaluate the spinal cord, conus medullaris, and cauda equina. The position of the conus is very important in predicting neurological deteriorations when it ends below L1.

Management

Management involves a multidisciplinary approach aimed at addressing specific problems with various organ systems.

Teaching Points

▶ SA is a skeletal feature of CRS and sirenomyelia.

▶ Hyperglycemia is the most commonly recognized teratogen involved in SA associated with CRS.

Further Reading

1. Stroustrup Smith A, Grable I, and Levine D. Case 66: Caudal regression syndrome in the fetus of a diabetic mother. Radiology 2004;230:229–233.

Chapter 62

Gustavo A. Tedesqui and Mauricio Castillo

History

▶ A 17-year-old female presents with hearing loss and weakness in the legs (**Figures 62.1, 62.2, and 62.3**).

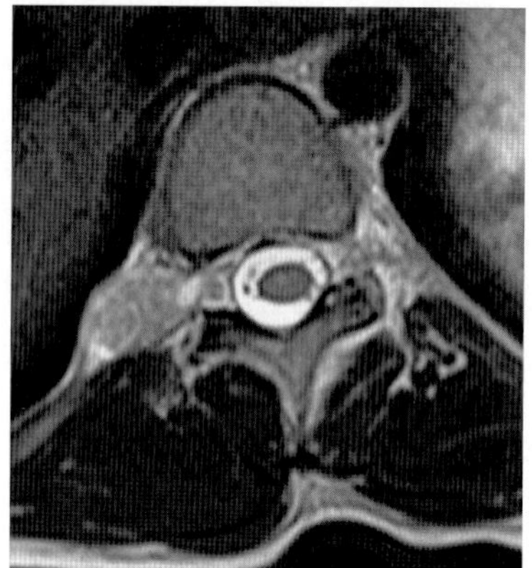

Figure 62.1

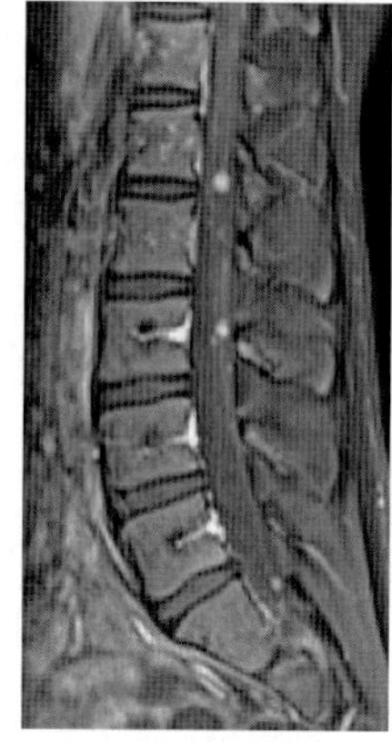

Figure 62.2

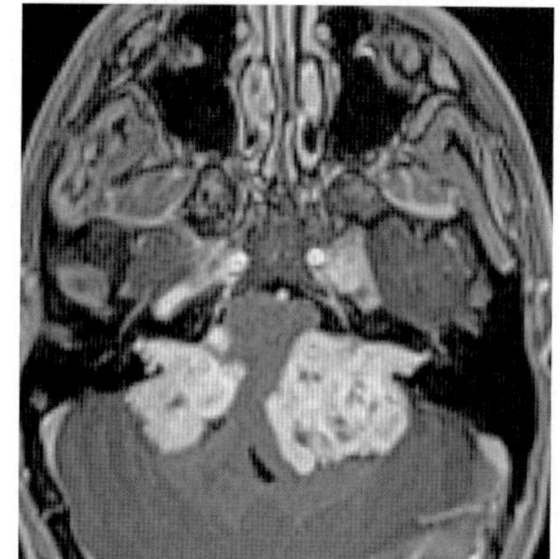

Figure 62.3

Findings

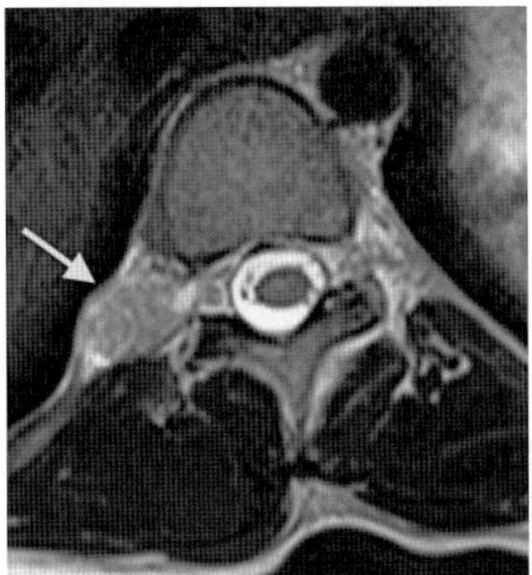
Figure 62.4

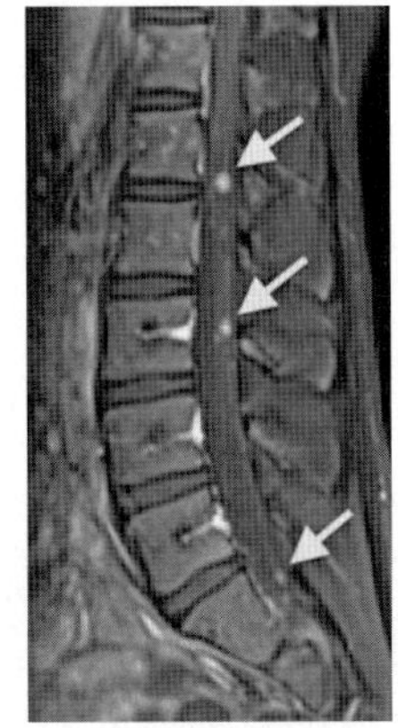
Figure 62.5

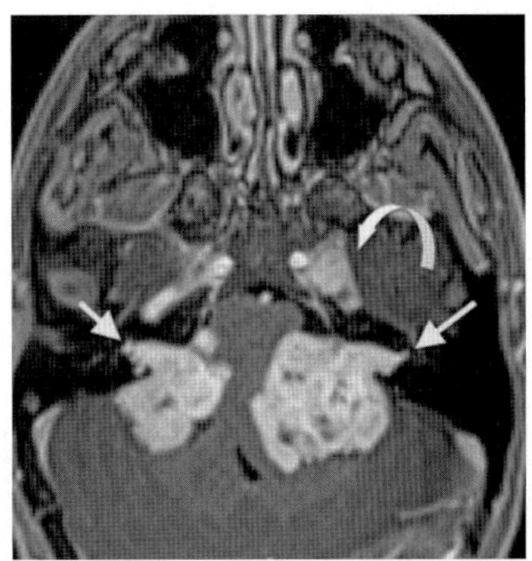
Figure 62.6

Neurofibromatosis type 2 (**Figures 62.4, 62.5, and 62.6**). A spinal axial T2-weighted MR image (Figure 62.4) demonstrates a hyperintense thoracic, well-defined, ovoid mass (arrow) following a nerve root as it exits the medullary canal through an enlarged neuroforamen. A lumbar midsagittal T1 contrast-enhanced MR image (Figure 62.5) shows multiple lesions enhancing after intravenous gadolinium administration (arrows) typical of neural sheath tumors. An axial T1 contrast-enhanced MR image (Figure 62.6) in the same patient demonstrates bilateral cerebellopontine angle masses (straight arrows) arising from the internal auditory canals compatible with vestibular schwannomas. Note also a schwannoma within the left Meckel's cave (curved arrow).

Differential Diagnosis

► Neurofibromas
► Hemangioblastoma
► Metastases
► Chronic inflammatory demyelinating polyneuropathy (CIDP)
► Lymphoma

Discussion

Neurofibromatosis (NF) is an autosomal dominant disorder that primarily affects cell growth of neural tissues causing a high risk of tumor formation. Two distinctive forms are recognized, but variant forms may exist.

The most common type, NF type 1 (NF1) or peripheral neurofibromatosis, has presentations that can vary widely from patient to patient and that include neurofibromas, optic gliomas, osseous lesion café-au-lait macules, freckles in axillary or inguinal regions, and Lisch nodules.

NF type 2 (NF2) or central neurofibromatosis is characterized by the development of various tumors. Unlike NF1, it is not associated with neurofibromas. Instead, patients with this disease have schwannomas, meningiomas, and ependymomas. A useful mnemonic commonly used to remind the components of the disease is MISME (multiple inherited schwannomas, meningiomas, and ependymomas).

Radiological Evaluation

The spinal manifestations of NF1 have been well documented with CT and MR and include kyphoscoliosis, dural ectasia, and neurofibromas. Spinal manifestations of NF2 include schwannomas, meningiomas, and ependymomas.

Schwannomas and neurofibromas are both benign, slowly growing tumors that present as sharply marginated, spherical, and lobulated masses in the paraspinal region most commonly in the cervical region. CT provides information related to the consequences of the tumor on the adjacent bones. As they are slow growing, they remodel the adjacent bones often resulting in foraminal enlargement with erosion of the pedicles, thin laminae, and posterior vertebral scalloping due the presence of a dumbbell-shaped mass (**Figure 62.7**). MRI provides excellent delineation of nerve sheath tumors that appear as solid, circumscribed masses, isointense to slightly hypointense on T1W images and hyperintense on T2W images (Figures 62.1 and 62.2). Schwannomas often demonstrate a heterogeneous signal on T2W images. Schwannomas and neurofibromas are often indistinguishable by imaging. Although the "target sign" (hyperintense rim and central area of low signal) on T2W images has been described classically with neurofibromas, it can still be seen in a schwannoma. Plexiform neurofibromas are the hallmark of NF1 and may resemble a larger, lobulated "bags of worms" infiltrating neural elements (**Figure 62.8**). On postcontrast images, plexiform tumors show intense contrast enhancement (Figures 62.2 and 62.3).

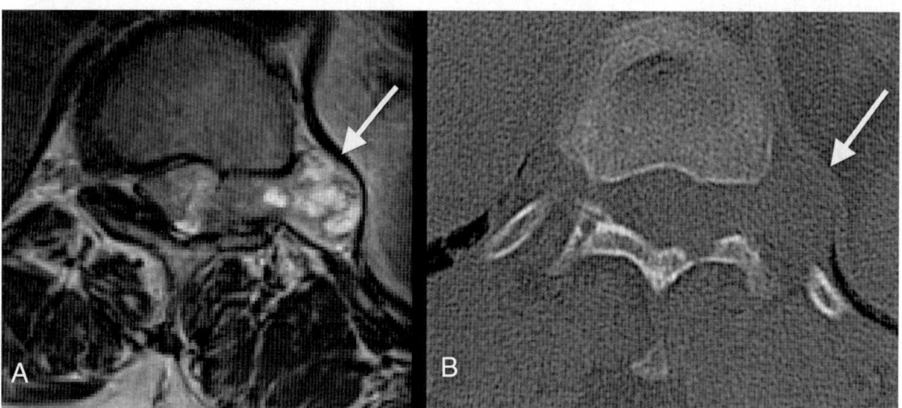

Figure 62.7

Schwannoma in a patient with NF. An axial T2-weighted MR image (**Figure 62.7A**) and CT (**Figure 62.7B**) show a dumbbell-shaped mass (arrows) with expansion and remodeling of the left T11–T12 neural foramen consistent with slow growth as seen in nerve sheath tumors. This was a pathology-proven schwannoma.

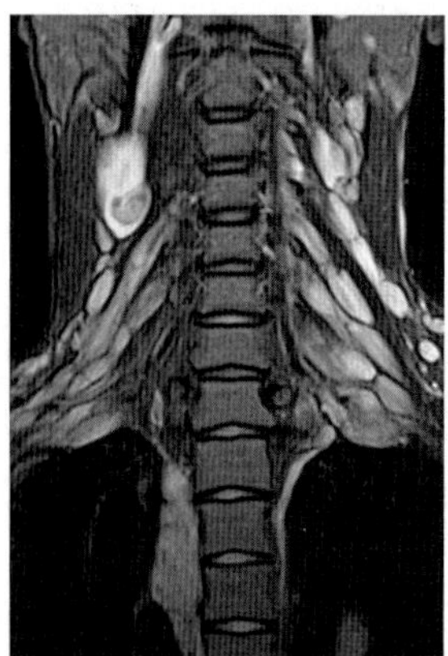

Figure 62.8

Plexiform neurofibromas in NF1 (**Figure 62.8**). Coronal STIR MR demonstrates extensive bilateral plexiform neurofibromas arising from both brachial plexi and paraspinal regions. Findings are compatible with the patient's history of NF1.

Management

There is no cure for neurofibromatosis. Patients should be routinely monitored for complications. Surgery may be used to remove tumors that cause pain, a loss of function, and/or compression of the spinal cord, neural structures, and brain.

Teaching Points

- ► A tumor associated with the nerve roots suggests either a schwannoma or neurofibroma. Schwannomas and neurofibromas are often indistinguishable by imaging.
- ► Spinal neurofibromas are very rare outside NF1 and multiple schwannomas are typical of NF2.
- ► In case of tumors involving multiple nerve roots, the presence of bilateral vestibular schwannomas suggests NF2, whereas the presence of subcutaneous neurofibromas suggests NF1.

Further Reading

1. Rossi SE, Erasmus JJ, McAdams HP, and Donnelly LF. Thoracic manifestations of neurofibromatosis-I. AJR Am J Roentgenol 1999;173(6):1631–1638.
2. Ruggieri M, et al. Earliest clinical manifestations and natural history of neurofibromatosis type 2 (NF2) in childhood: A study of 24 patients. Neuropediatrics 2005;36(1):21–34.
3. Khong PL, Goh WHS, Wong VCN, and Fung CW. MR imaging of spinal tumors in children with neurofibromatosis 1. AJR Am J Roentgenol 2003;180:413–417.

Chapter 63

Shamir Rai, Ismail Tawakol Ali, and Savvas Nicolaou

History

► A 33-year old male, with a prenatal diagnosis of tuberous sclerosis (TSC) with lesions involving the brain and kidney, presents to the emergency department with renal flank pain and hematuria (**Figures 63.1, 63.2, 63.3, and 63.4**).

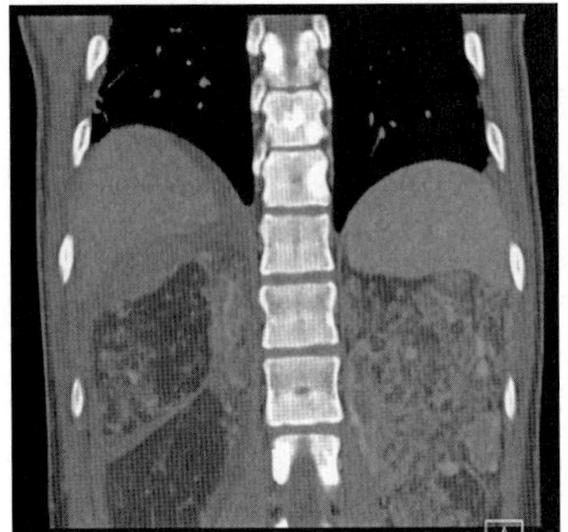

Figure 63.1

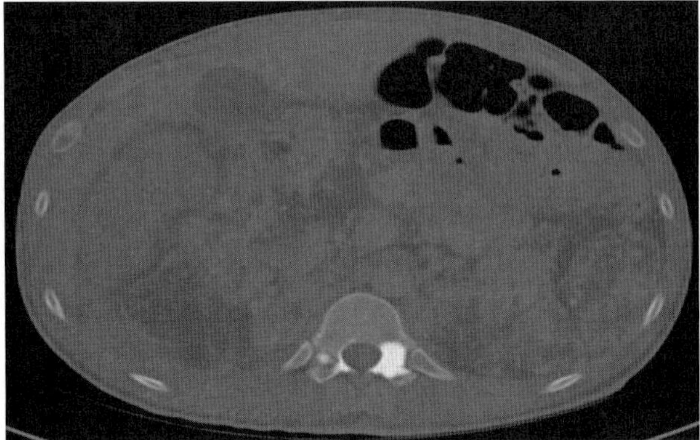

Figure 63.2

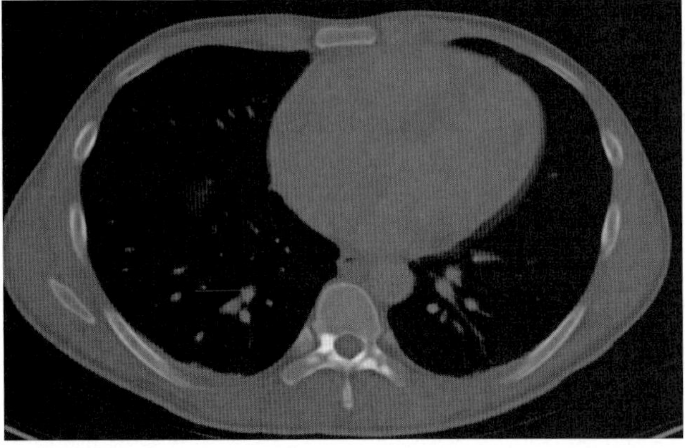

Figure 63.3

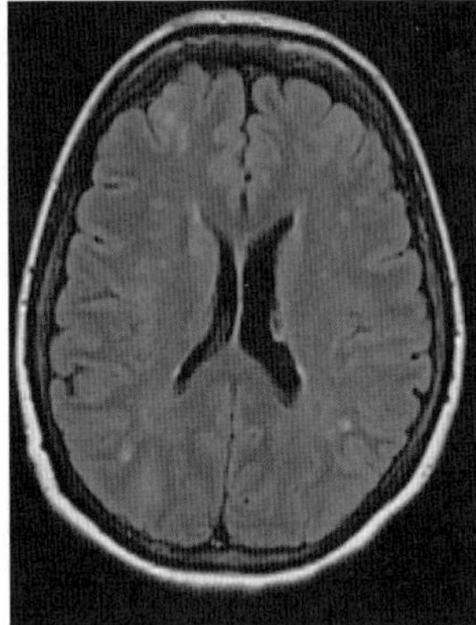

Figure 63.4

Chapter 63 Spinal Involvement in Tuberous Sclerosis

Findings

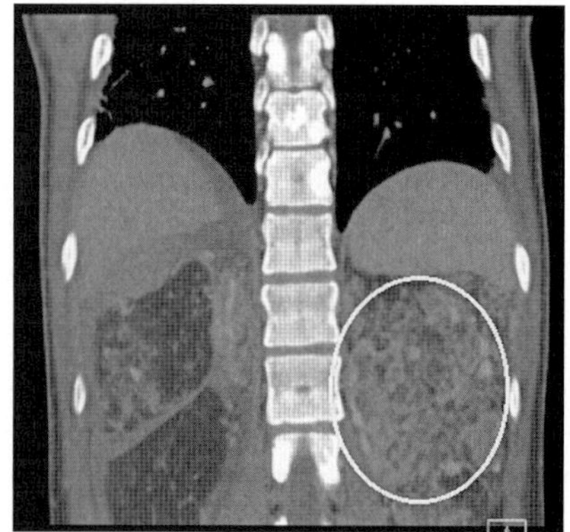

Figure 63.5

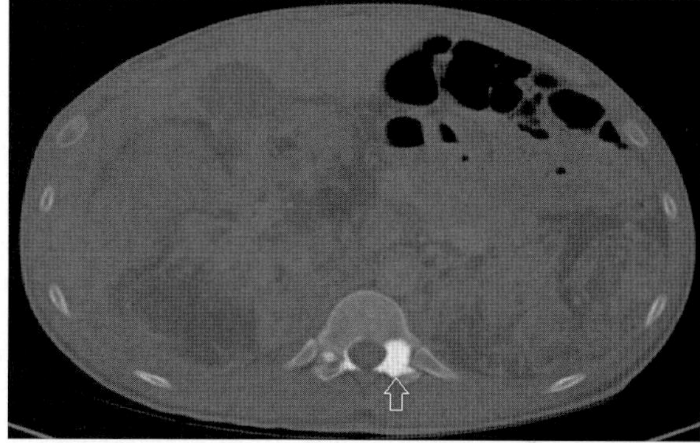

Figure 63.6

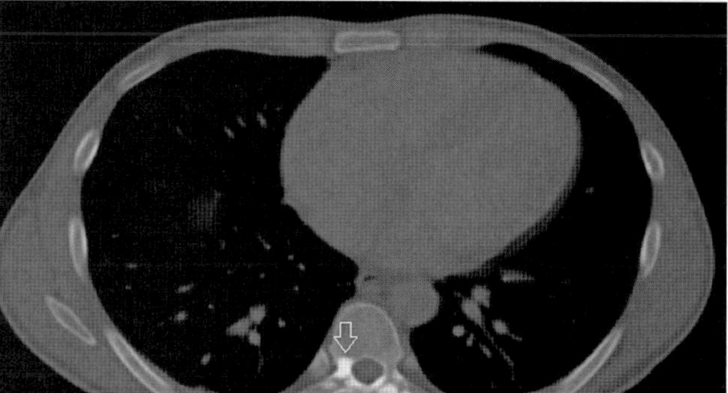

Figure 63.7

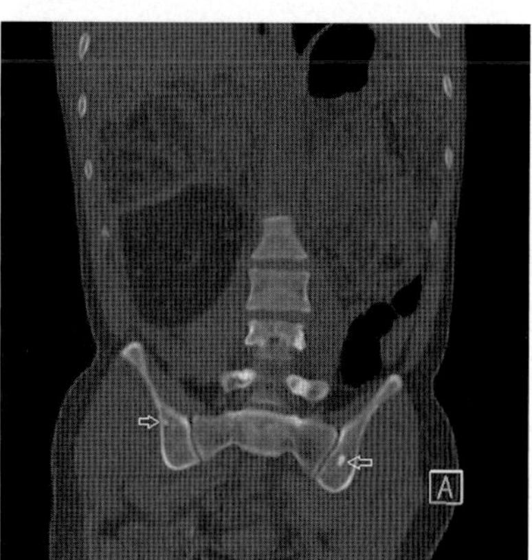

Figure 63.8

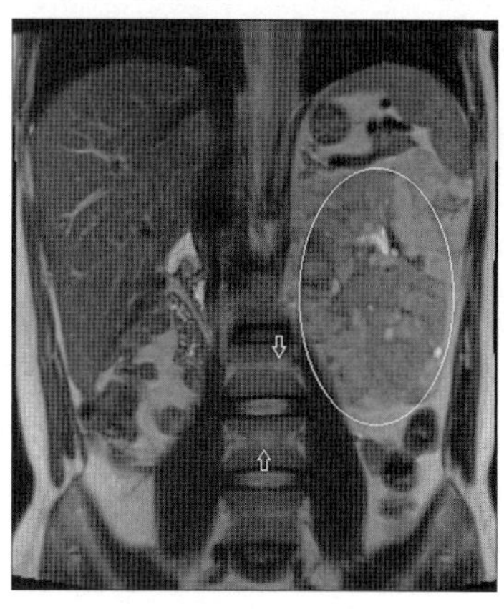

Figure 63.9

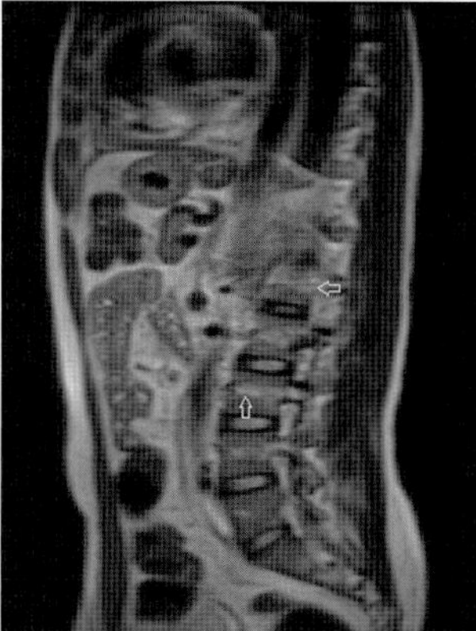

Figure 63.10

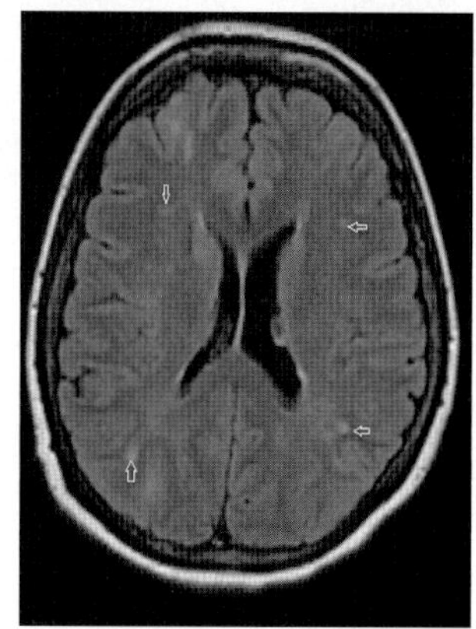

Figure 63.11

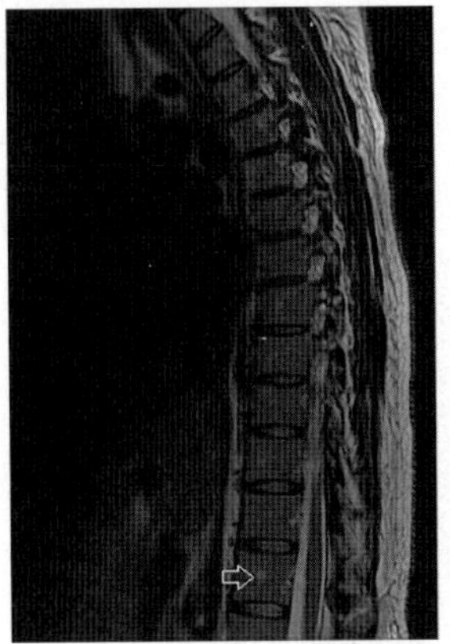
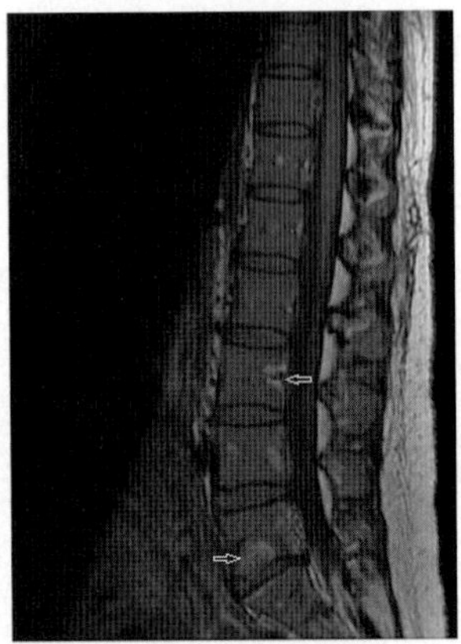

Figure 63.12   Figure 63.13

TSC (**Figures 63.5, 63.6, 63.7, 63.8, 63.9, 63.10, 63.11, 63.12, and 63.13**). A postcontrast portal venous phase coronal image (Figure 63.5) and axial images (Figures 63.6 and 63.7) demonstrate multiple sclerotic bony lesions within the thoracic vertebral bodies. The characteristic appearance of sclerotic ovoid or round lesions with poorly defined margins is evident (arrows). A prominent large left-sided renal angiomyolipoma is present (circle) and can be seen on the coronal image. CT KUB (kidneys, ureters, and bladder) (Figure 63.8) demonstrates characteristic ill-defined sclerotic lesions along the iliac sides of the sacroiliac joints. Coronal (Figure 63.9) and sagittal (Figure 63.10) T2 HASTE MR images demonstrate multiple sclerotic bony lesions (arrows) within the lumbar vertebral bodies. A prominent large left-sided renal angiomyolipoma (circle) is visualized on the coronal image. An axial T2 FLAIR MR head image (Figure 63.11) demonstrates multiple subependymal nodules. There are multiple areas of mild cortical expansion and hyperintensity in keeping with cortical tubers. Multiple vertebral hyperintense ovoid foci with ill-defined margins are present on T2-weighted (Figure 63.12) and T1-weighted (Figure 63.13) MR sagittal images of the mid and lower spines, respectively. These findings are in keeping with bone islands in TSC. The findings are all consistent with a diagnosis of TSC.

Differential Diagnosis

The differential diagnosis of focal or multifocal sclerotic bone lesions includes the following:

Congenital:
- ▸ TSC
- ▸ Bone islands (enostoses)
- ▸ Osteopoikilosis (rare inherited benign bone islands that develop during childhood and persist through life)

Trauma:
- ▸ Stress fracture
- ▸ Previous instrumentation

Vascular:
- ▸ Infarct
- ▸ Hemangiomas

Infection:
- ▸ Chronic osteomyelitis

Neoplasm:
- ▸ Primary:
- ▸ Osteoma
- ▸ Osteosarcoma

Metastatic:
- Prostate
- Breast
- Lymphoma
- Other

Endocrine/Metabolic:
- Paget's disease
- Calcium and phosphate metabolism abnormalities

Other:
- Erdheim–Chester disease (rare, non-Langerhan's cell, nonfamilial granulomatosis)

Discussion

TSC is a rare autosomal dominant neurocutaneous syndrome characterized by the presence of multiple benign congenital tumors in multiple organs. It is the second most common neurocutaneous syndrome after neurofibromatosis Type 1. Classically, a triad of clinical features was described consisting of epilepsy, mental retardation, and adenoma sebaceum, known as the Vogt triad, although not commonly seen in patients with TSC. The prevalence of TSC ranges from 1 in 6000 to 1 in 12,000 and affects both genders and all ethnicities equally. Obvious signs may be visible at birth, while in others it may not be diagnosed for years. TSC is considered to be caused by mutations in the tumor suppressor genes TCS1 (long arm chromosome 9) and TCS2 (short arm chromosome 16). If these genes are altered by mutation, unregulated growth of tumors results throughout the body.

The diagnosis of TSC is made through characteristic dermatological findings in TSC (facial angiofibroma, periungual fibromas), a family history of TSC, and imaging findings on CT and MRI. Common imaging findings of the head and body include cortical tubers, subependymal nodules, giant cell astrocytomas, white matter abnormalities, cardiac rhabdomyomas, lung cysts and renal angiomyolipomas.

Sclerotic bone lesions are the third most common imaging finding in patients with TSC after brain tubers and renal angiomyolipomas. Spinal tumors have been reported very rarely and they are mainly represented by sacrococcygeal and cervical chordomas (see chordoma case for further details). Only one case report of a giant cell tumor of the bone in the spine has been reported in the setting of TSC.

Radiological Evaluation

Because the classical Vogt triad is uncommonly seen at clinical examination, radiological examinations play an important role in the diagnosis of TSC and in treatment (**Figures 63.14, 63.15, 63.16, and 63.17**). From the perspective of the spine, the sclerotic bone lesions in TSC closely resemble bone islands, which are foci of dense, compact bone within the medullary cavity of bones. The bone lesions of TSC are commonly seen in the ribs, vertebral bodies, and along the iliac side of the sacroiliac joints. They appear as sclerotic ovoid or round lesions with poorly defined margins. These sclerotic lesions are typically asymptomatic and are most commonly found in vertebral bodes on CT images obtained to evaluate renal or lung disease, as seen in this case.

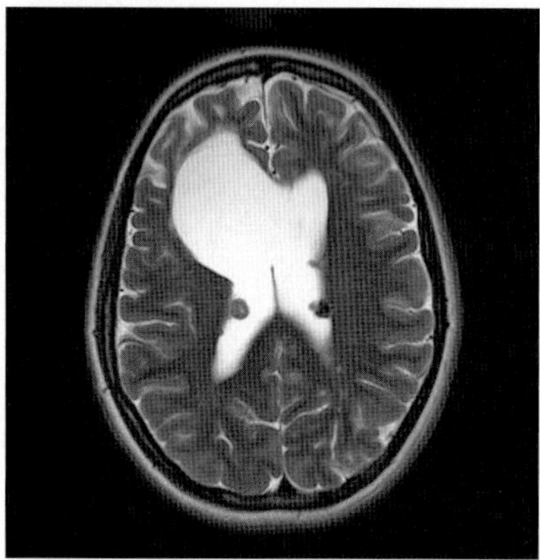

Figure 63.14

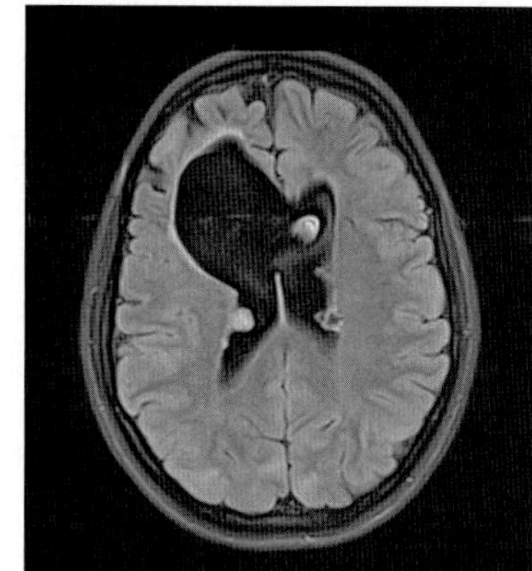

Figure 63.15

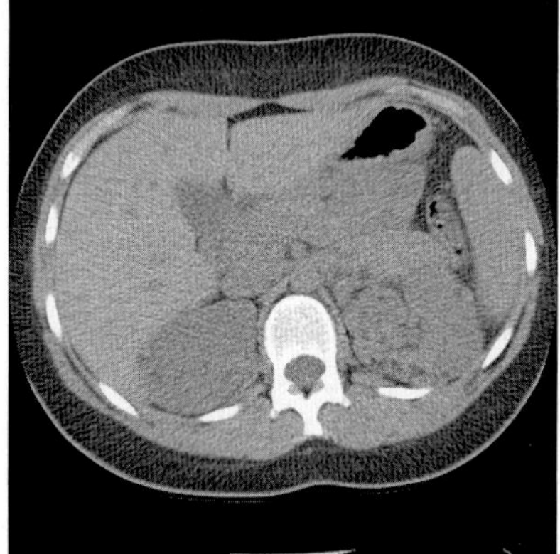

Figure 63.16

Figure 63.17

A constellation of findings is seen in a 19-year-old patient with TSC (**Figures 63.14, 63.15, 63.16, and 63.17**). Axial T2 (Figure 63.14) and FLAIR (Figure 63.15) images through the brain demonstrate subependymal nodules in both lateral ventricles. Focal dilatation of the frontal horn of the right lateral ventricle is also seen. A noncontrast axial CT image (Figure 63.16) shows fat-attenuation lesions mainly in the left kidney, but are seen bilaterally on a coronal postcontrast MR image (Figure 63.17) consistent with angiomyolipomas.

Management

The sclerotic lesions are of unclear etiology but are probably hamartomas based on the histological appearance. Hamartomas are composed of tissues normally found in the location of origin but in abnormal quantity, mixture, or arrangement. These lesions are benign in nature and if the patient is asymptomatic from the lesions no treatment is required. Follow-up specifically for these asymptomatic sclerotic lesions is not recommended in the setting of TSC.

Teaching Points

- ► TSC is a rare autosomal-dominant neurocutaneous syndrome associated with mutation in the tumor suppressor genes TCS1 and TCS2.
- ► Sclerotic bone lesions are the third most common imaging finding in patients with TSC after brain tubers and renal angiomyolipomas.
- ► Lesions are commonly seen in the ribs, vertebral bodies, and along the iliac side of the sacroiliac joints and appear as sclerotic ovoid or round lesions with poorly defined margins.

► The sclerotic bone lesions seen in TSC are thought to be hamartomas, which are benign in nature and do not require specific follow-up if the patient is asymptomatic.

► Spinal tumors, mainly consisting of sacrococcygeal and cervical chordomas, have been rarely reported in the setting of TSC.

Further Reading

1. Avila N, Dwyer A, Rabel A, et al. CT of sclerotic bone lesions: Imaging features differentiating tuberous sclerosis complex with lymphangioleiomyomatosis from sporadic lymphangioleiomyomatosis. Radiology 2010;254(3):851–857.
2. Baskin HJ. The pathogenesis and imaging of the tuberous sclerosis complex. Pediatr Radiol 2008;38:936–952.
3. Benli IT, Akalin S, Boysan E, et al. Epidemiological, clinical and radiological aspects of osteopoikilosis. J Bone Joint Surg Br 1992;74(4):504–506.
4. Francesco M, Lecce M, Fraioli M, et al. Case report: Spinal giant cell tumor in tuberous sclerosis: Case report and review of the literature. J Spinal Cord Med 2013;36(2):157–159.
5. Green GJ. The radiology of tuberose sclerosis. Clin Radiol 1968;19:135–147.
6. Lee-Jones L, Aligianis I, Davies PA, et al. Sarcoccygeal chordomas in patients with tuberous sclerosis complex show somatic loss of TSC1 or TSC2. Cancer 2004;41(1):80–85.
7. Storm PB, Magge SN, Kazahaya K, et al. Cervical chordoma in a patient with tuberous sclerosis presenting with shoulder pain. Pediatr Neurosurg 2007;43(2):167–169.
8. Umeoka S, Koyama T, Miki Y, et al. Pictorial review of tuberous sclerosis in various organs. RadioGraphics 2008;28(7):e32.

Chapter 64

Bita Ameri and Shivani Gupta

History

▶ A 20-year-old male presents with back pain and a history of frequent fractures (**Figures 64.1 and 64.2**).

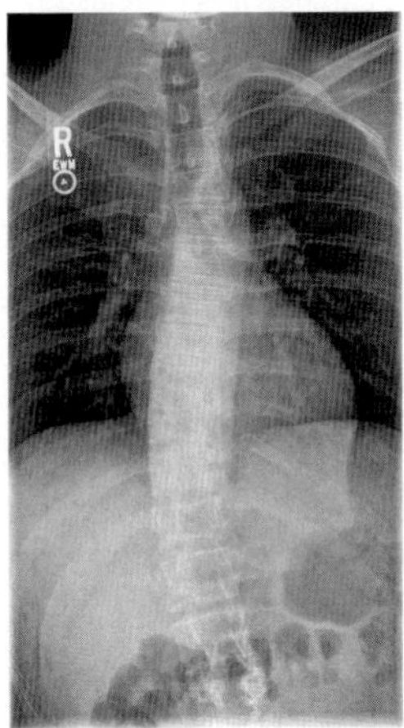

Figure 64.1

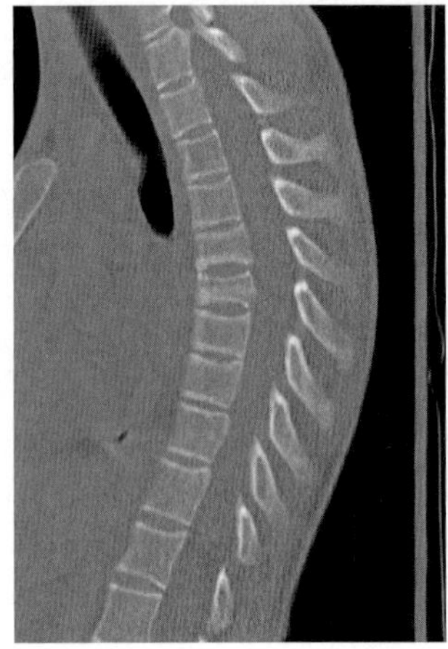

Figure 64.2

Findings

Osteogenesis imperfecta (OI). A frontal radiograph (**Figure 64.1**) shows gracile osteopenic bones. Sagittal nonenhanced computed tomography (NECT) (**Figure 64.2**) shows diffuse osteopenia, thoracic vertebral body compression fractures, and a slightly exaggerated thoracic kyphosis.

Differential Diagnosis

▶ Idiopathic juvenile osteoporosis
▶ Osteoporosis–pseudoglioma syndrome
▶ Bruck syndrome
▶ Chronic steroid use
▶ Hypophosphatasia
▶ Rickets
▶ Skeletal dysplasias

Discussion

OI is a group of rare collagen mutation disorders with the common feature of bone fragility. It is classified into eight different types based on clinical, genetic, and radiographic criteria. It is often possible to make the diagnosis clinically with a history of frequent fractures due to minor trauma. However, collagen or DNA testing can be used for a definitive diagnosis. OI types I through IV are the classic types, and types V through VIII are newly described and less understood. Clinical features vary, even among patients with the same type of OI. The four main types of OI are as follows:

▶ Type I: the mildest form, bones fracture easily
▶ Type II: the most severe form, severe bone deformity and small stature diagnosed by ultrasound during pregnancy; most die within the first year of life due to respiratory failure or intracerebral hemorrhage
▶ Type III: often severe bone deformity, bones fracture easily often before birth, can sometimes have normal life expectancy
▶ Type IV: between I and III in severity, mild to moderate bone deformity

Osteoporotic compression fractures and kyphoscoliosis are commonly seen among all types of OI. Other characteristic clinical findings include blue sclera, early hearing loss, brittle teeth, thin fragile skin, and joint laxity.

Radiological Evaluation

While ultrasound is the most helpful modality for prenatal diagnosis, conventional radiography becomes the most used modality after birth. On radiography, the most severe forms of OI (Types II and III) demonstrate severe osteopenia, delayed or absent calvarial ossification, and short and bowed bones that are thickened and show exuberant callus formation due to multiple fractures in utero and early childhood. Milder forms of OI (Types I and IV) demonstrate mild osteopenia, wormian bones of the skull, and thin gracile bones that are nearly normal in length. Radiography and CT imaging can be used to evaluate osteoporotic vertebral fractures, which commonly occur among all types of OI due to osteopenia (Figure 64.4). More severe forms of OI are associated with platyspondyly (Figure 64.3). Basilar invagination is a potentially fatal but rare complication of OI (usually Type IV), which is best evaluated with CT imaging.

The differential diagnosis for OI in an adolescent or young adult would include diseases associated with diffuse osteopenia, increased risk of fracture, or bone deformities, such as idiopathic juvenile osteoporosis, Bruck syndrome, osteoporosis-pseudoglioma syndrome, chronic steroid use, metabolic bone disease (i.e., hypophosphatasia, rickets), and skeletal dysplasias. Idiopathic juvenile osteoporosis will show resolution over time but OI will not. Hypophosphatasia is radiographically indistinguishable from milder forms of OI. Rickets is characterized by wide and frayed metaphyses, unlike OI. Bruck syndrome, osteoporosis-pseudoglioma syndrome, and skeletal dysplasias can be distinguished by their extraskeletal findings. Bruck syndrome is associated with congenital joint contractures and osteoporosis-pseudoglioma syndrome is associated with blindness.

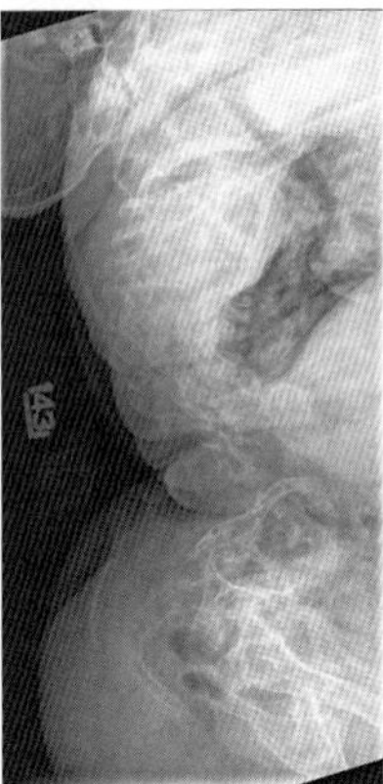

Figure 64.3

Spinal findings in a patient with OI. A lateral radiograph (**Figure 64.3**) of the thoracolumbar spine demonstrates diffuse osteopenia, deformed bones, and platyspondyly with a severely kyphotic spine in a patient with OI.

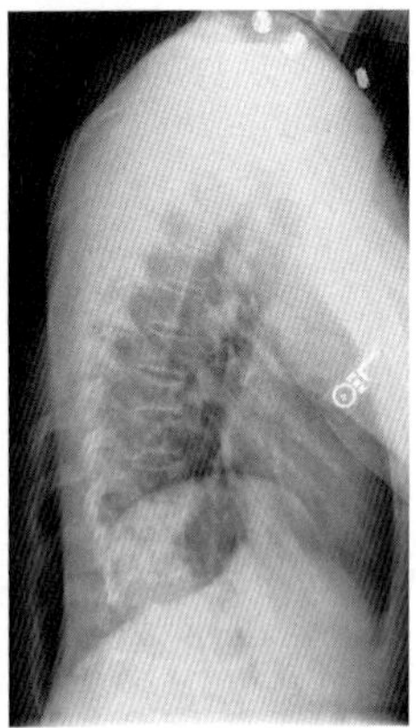

Figure 64.4

Spinal findings in a patient with OI. Lateral radiograph (**Figure 64.4**) of the chest demonstrates several compression deformities in the thoracic spine in this young patient with OI.

Management

Given the spectrum of disease severity in OI, the prognosis and management also vary greatly. Overall, treatment of the disease is chiefly supportive and directed toward improvement of mobility (e.g., braces and walkers) and development of optimal bone mass and muscle strength (e.g., bisphosphonates and physical therapy). In more severe cases, kyphoplasty/vertebroplasty can be performed for symptomatic compression fractures. Intramedullary fixation can be used to correct long bone deformities or fractures, and growth hormone treatments can be administered for short stature.

Teaching Points

► OI is a connective tissue disorder associated with mutations in collagen.

▶ OI is classified into multiple types based on clinical, radiographic, and genetic findings; Type I is the most common and mildest form with a normal life expectancy, whereas Type II is the most severe form and is lethal before 1 year of age.

▶ OI is characterized by generalized osteopenia and bone deformities. Compression fractures, kyphoscoliosis, and rarely basilar invagination are key neuroradiological findings.

Further Reading

1. Renaud A, et al, Radiographic features of osteogenesis imperfecta. Insights Imaging 2013;4(4):417–429.
2. Basel D, et al. Osteogenesis imperfecta: Recent findings shed new light on this once well-understood condition. Genet Med 2009;11(6):375–385.

Chapter 65

Manpreet Bajwa and Shivani Gupta

History

▶ An 8-month-old female presents with failure to thrive (**Figures 65.1 and 65.2**).

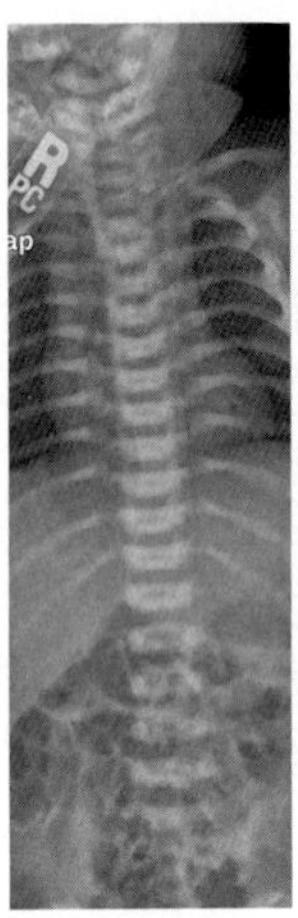
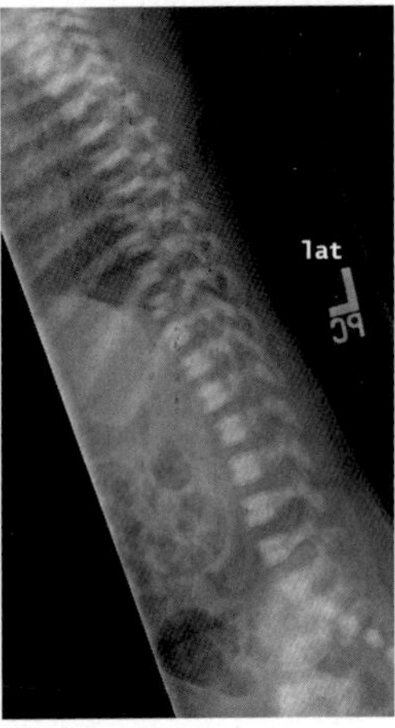

Figure 65.1   Figure 65.2

Findings

Autosomal recessive osteopetrosis in an 8-month-old female (**Figures 65.1 and 65.2**). Anteroposterior (AP) and lateral radiographs of the spine demonstrate diffusely increased density of the vertebral bodies with a "sandwich" appearance created by a radiolucent central area.

Differential Diagnosis

► Heavy metal poisoning
► Melorheostosis
► Hypervitaminosis D
► Pyknodysostosis
► Fibrous dysplasia (facial bones/skull)

Discussion

Osteopetrosis is also known as Albers–Schönberg disease or "marble bone disease." It is a hereditary disorder due to abnormal osteoclastic function, resulting in structurally weak, sclerotic bone. Two forms are described: infantile (autosomal recessive) and adult (autosomal dominant) types. The infantile form has a poor prognosis whereas the adult form can be asymptomatic in up to 50% of patients.

Complications of osteopetrosis include recurrent fractures, extramedullary hematopoiesis, cranial nerve palsies, failure to thrive in children, renal tubular acidosis, and hematological abnormalities (anemia, leukocytopenia, and thrombocytopenia). In children, leukemia is another complication that may require a bone marrow transplant.

Radiological Evaluation

On radiographs, the bones demonstrate a diffuse increase in density. Cortical thickening is seen, which has a smooth appearance and results in a decreased caliber of the medullary cavity. A bone-within-bone appearance is seen. In the spine, sandwich vertebrae are noted (alternating sclerotic and radiolucent transverse lines). The Erlenmeyer flask deformity (lack of tubulization of the long bones, particularly the femur, with flaring of the distal metaphyseal aspects; **Figure 65.3**) can be seen in osteopetrosis, although it is also a feature in several other skeletal dysplasias as well as systemic disorders (Gaucher disease, Niemann–Pick disease, thalassemia). Multiple healed fractures are often seen throughout the skeleton.

MRI demonstrates diffusely decreased signal intensity of the marrow on both T1- and T2-weighted images.

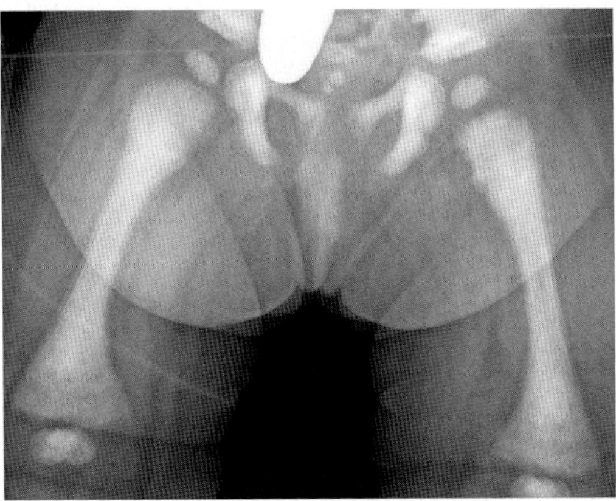

Figure 65.3

Autosomal recessive osteopetrosis in an 8-month-old female (**Figure 65.3**). A frontal radiograph of the femurs demonstrates the Erlenmeyer flask deformity with flaring of the distal femoral metaphyses. This patient also has diffusely increased bone density with a bone-within-bone appearance.

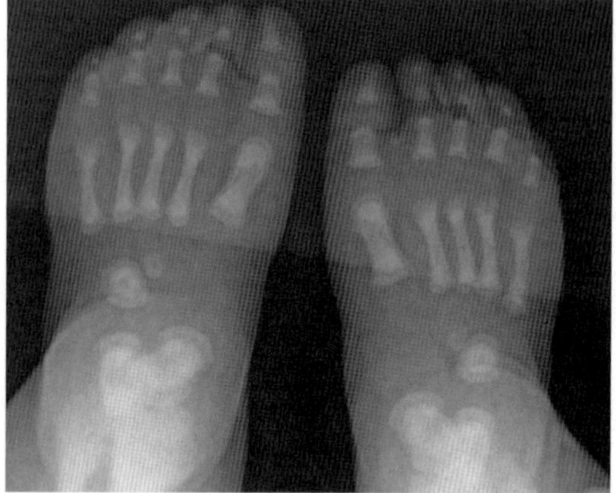

Figure 65.4

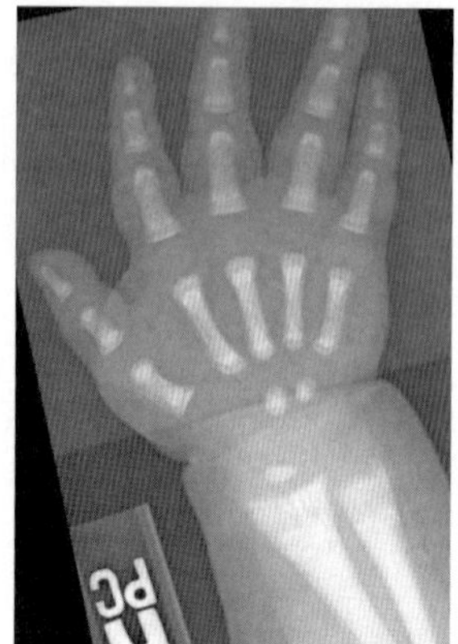

Figure 65.5

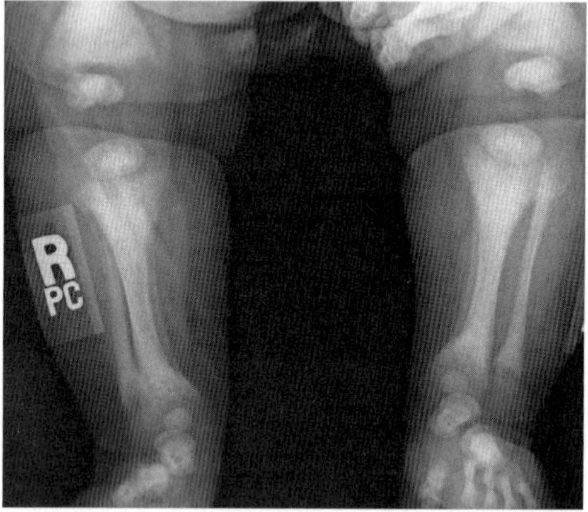

Figure 65.6

Autosomal recessive osteopetrosis in an 8-month-old female (**Figures 65.4, 65.5, and 65.6**). Radiographs of the bilateral feet, right hand, and bilateral lower extremities demonstrate the bone-within-bone appearance, which occurs due to abnormal osteoclast function. This sign can also be seen in other conditions such as sickle cell disease, Caffey's disease, and congenital syphilis, among others.

Management

Treatment is largely centered on a bone marrow transplant. The prognosis for the adult autosomal dominant type is good whereas the prognosis for the infantile autosomal recessive type is poor. Stillbirths or death in infancy are often seen; the remaining patients rarely survive past teenage years due to complications.

Teaching Points

▶ Osteopetrosis results in dense but structurally weak bones.
▶ The autosomal recessive infantile form has a poor prognosis.
▶ Look for the bone-within-bone sign as well as osteosclerosis.

Further Reading

1. Bollerslev J and Mosekilde L. Autosomal dominant osteopetrosis. Clin Orthop Relat Res 1993;294:45–51.
2. Gerritsen EJ, Vossen JM, van Loo IH, et al. Autosomal recessive osteopetrosis: Variability of findings at diagnosis and during the natural course. Pediatrics 1994;93(2):247–253.
3. Bourke E, Delaney VB, Mosawi M, et al. Renal tubular acidosis and osteopetrosis in siblings. Nephron 1981;28:268–272.
4. Elster AD, Theros EG, Key LL, and Chen MY. Cranial imaging in autosomal recessive osteopetrosis. Part I. Facial bones and calvarium. Radiology 1992;183:129–135.
5. Wilson CJ and Vellodi A. Autosomal recessive osteopetrosis: Diagnosis, management, and outcome. Arch Dis Child 2000;83(5):449–452.
6. Srinivasan M, Abinun M, Cant AJ, et al. Malignant infantile osteopetrosis presenting with neonatal hypocalcaemia. Arch Dis Child Fetal Neonatal Ed. 2000;83(1):F21–23.

Section 7   Vascular

Safia Cheeney and Kathleen R. Fink

History

▶ A previously healthy 18-year-old male presents with acute onset bilateral upper extremity weakness, paresthesias, and urinary retention (**Figures 66.1 and 66.2**).

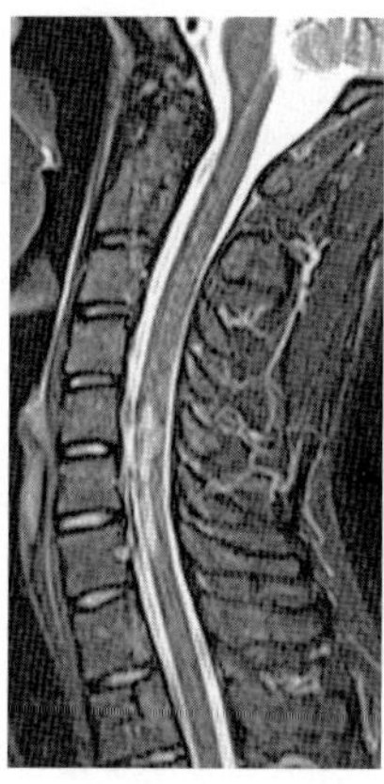

Figure 66.1

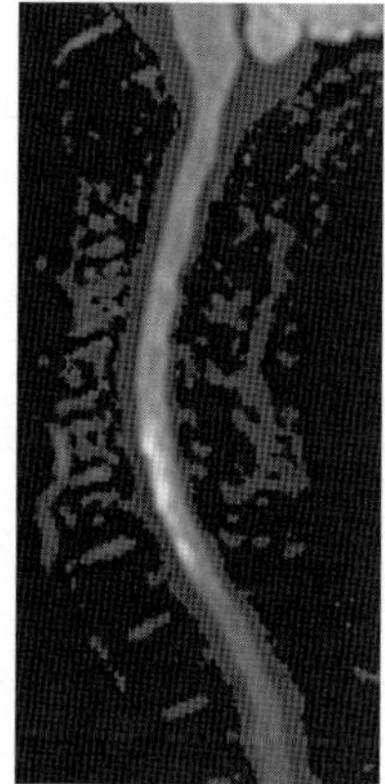

Figure 66.2

Chapter 66 Spinal Cord Infarction

Findings

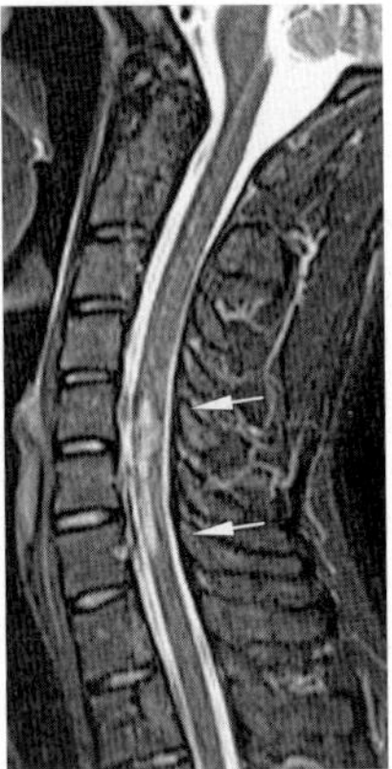

Figure 66.3

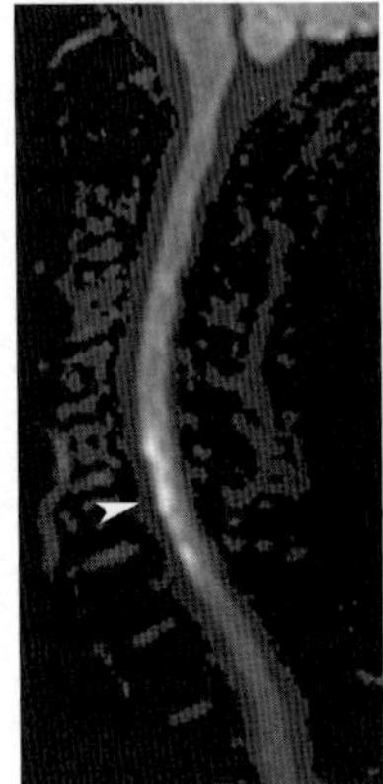

Figure 66.4

Spinal cord infarct. A sagittal T2-weighted MRI (Figure 66.3) shows signal hyperintensity within the cervical spinal cord (arrows), which demonstrates restricted diffusion (Figure 66.4, arrowhead). Axial images demonstrate an "owl eyes" appearance in the anterior horn cells with T2 hyperintensity (**Figure 66.5, arrow**) and restricted diffusion (**Figure 66.6, arrowhead**). ADC map confirms diffusion restriction (**Figure 66.7, arrowhead**).

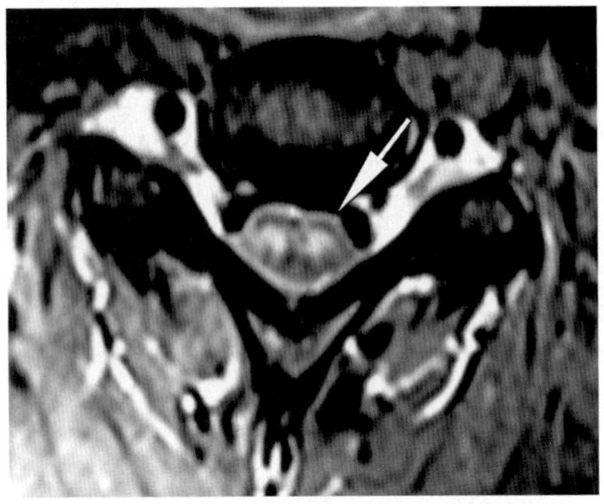

Figure 66.5

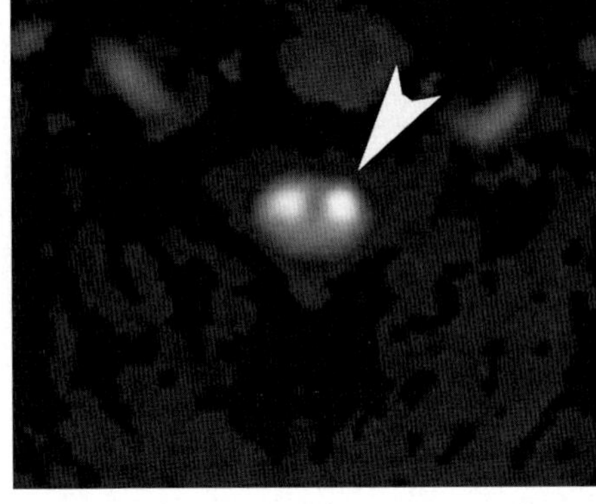

Figure 66.6

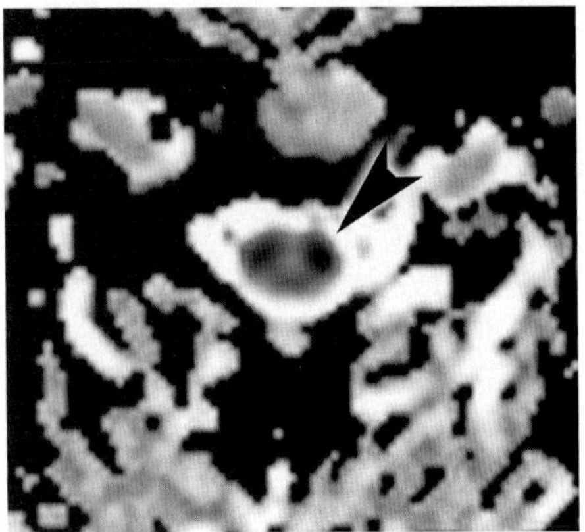

Figure 66.7

Differential Diagnosis

▶ Transverse myelitis
▶ Demyelinating disease

Discussion

T2 signal hyperintensity in the cervical spinal cord may be seen in cord infarction, transverse myelitis, and demyelinating disease. In this case, the signal abnormality corresponds to the vascular distribution of the anterior spinal artery and demonstrates restricted diffusion, suggesting an acute anterior spinal cord infarction.

Radiological Evaluation

Spinal cord infarction is a rare and potentially debilitating condition with symptoms reflecting the level and extent of the spinal cord involved. Risk factors include vascular disease (atherosclerosis, aortic dissection, aortic surgery), hypotension, embolism, and trauma. An identifiable cause is found less than half the time, as in this case.

MRI is the imaging test of choice for suspected spinal cord infarct (**Figures 66.8, 66.9, 66.10, and 66.11**). Sagittal and axial T2-weighted images are the mainstay for diagnosis, although diffusion-weighted sequences can help narrow the differential. The most common location for spinal cord infarction is in the territory of the anterior spinal artery. Infarct involving this vascular territory results in an abnormal T2/FLAIR and DWI signal in the central cord, which can produce an "owl eyes" appearance on axial imaging.

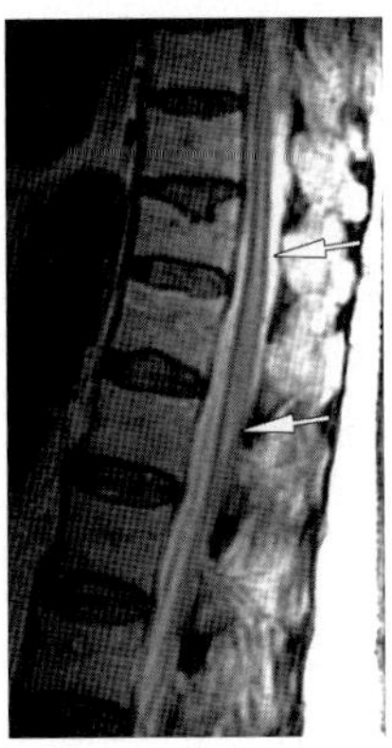

Figure 66.8

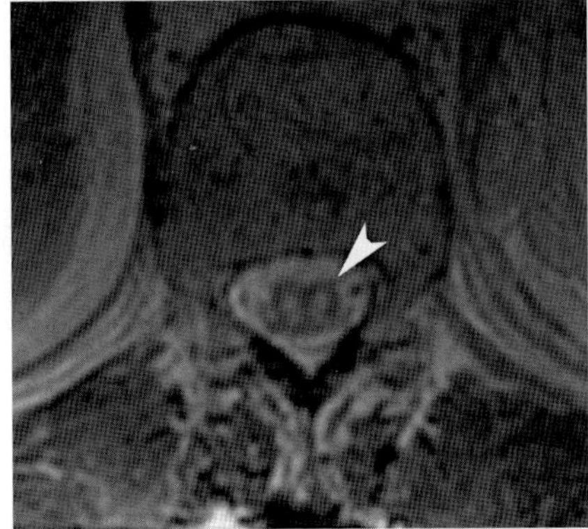

Figure 66.9

Spinal cord infarction after abdominal aortic surgery (**Figures 66.8 and 66.9**). A sagittal and axial T2-weighted MRI image shows expansion of the lower spinal cord and conus medullaris (Figure 66.8, arrows) with involvement of the central gray matter (Figure 66.9, arrowhead). This patient awoke from surgery with T10 paraplegia.

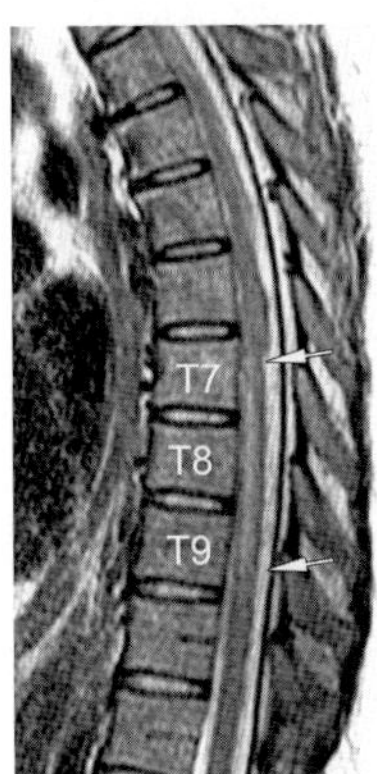

Figure 66.10

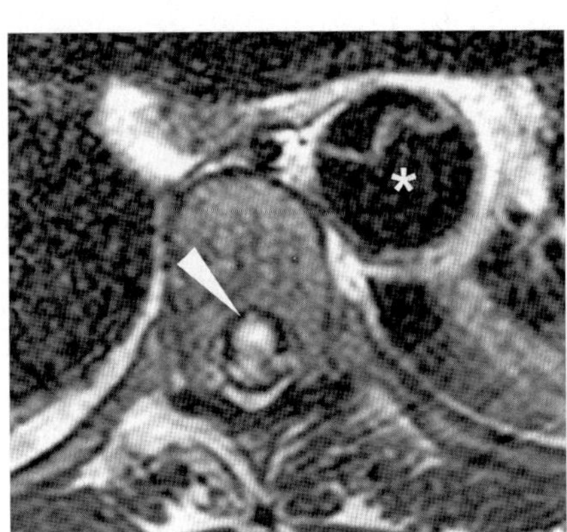

Figure 66.11

Spinal cord infarction complicating acute aortic dissection. A sagittal T2-weighted MRI image shows increased cord signal spanning T7 through T9 (**Figure 66.10, arrows**). Axial T2 redemonstrates the cord signal abnormality (**Figure 66.11, arrowhead**) as well as the aortic dissection (*).

Management

Management of a spinal cord infarct can include steroids, antiplatelet therapy, treatment of the patient's underlying disease, and eventually rehabilitation therapy.

Teaching Points

▶ Spinal cord infarction is a rare condition that is associated with aortic disease and aortic surgery.
▶ MRI imaging with T2 and DWI sequences is the imaging modality of choice for the evaluation of spinal cord infarction.
▶ The most common location for spinal cord infarction is the vascular territory of the anterior spinal artery.

Further Reading

1. Thurnher MM and Bammer R. Diffusion-weighted MR imaging (DWI) in spinal cord ischemia. Neuroradiology 2006;48:795–801.
2. Nedeltchev K, Loher T, Stepper F, et al. Long-term outcome of acute spinal cord ischemia syndrome. Stroke 2004;35:560–565.
3. Masson C, Pruvo JP, Meder JF, et al. Spinal cord infarction; clinical and magnetic resonance imaging findings and short term outcome. J Neurol Neurosurg Psychiat 2004;75:1431–1435.
4. Kuker W, Weller M. Klose U, et al. Diffusion-weighted MRI of spinal cord infarction; high resolution imaging and time course of diffusion abnormality. J Neurol 2004;251:818–824.
5. Lynch K, Oster J, Apetauerova D, and Hreib K. Spinal cord stroke: Acute imaging and intervention. Case Rep Neurol Med 2012;2012:706780.
6. Bracken M, Shepard M, Collins W, et al. Methylprednisolone or naloxone treatment after acute spinal cord injury: 1 year follow up data. J Neurosurg 1992;76:23–31.

Martin Arrigan and Manraj Kanwal Singh Heran

History

▶ A 64-year-old male presented with a history of low back pain and progressive painless spastic paraparesis (**Figures 67.1, 67.2, and 67.3**).

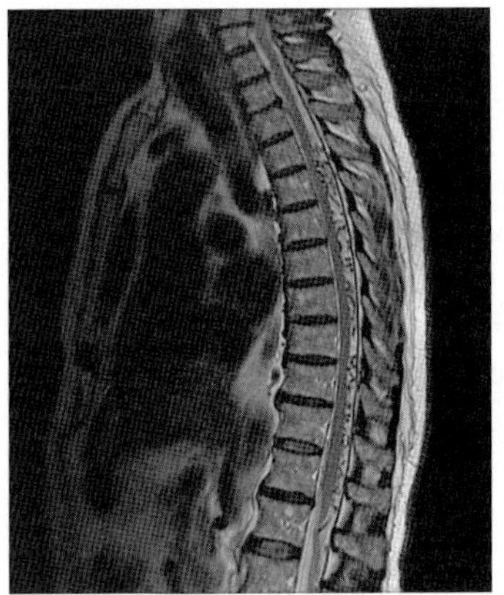

Figure 67.1

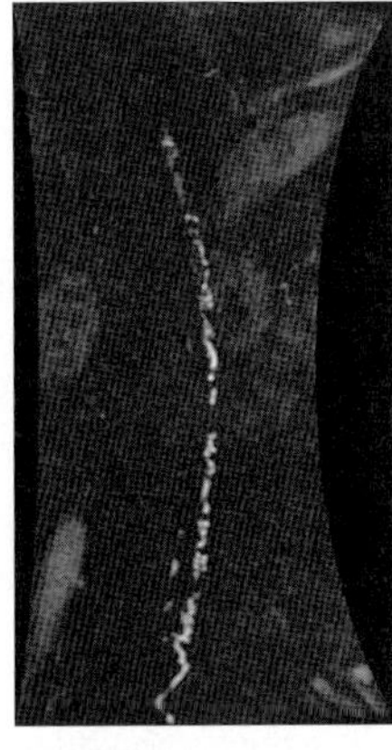

Figure 67.2

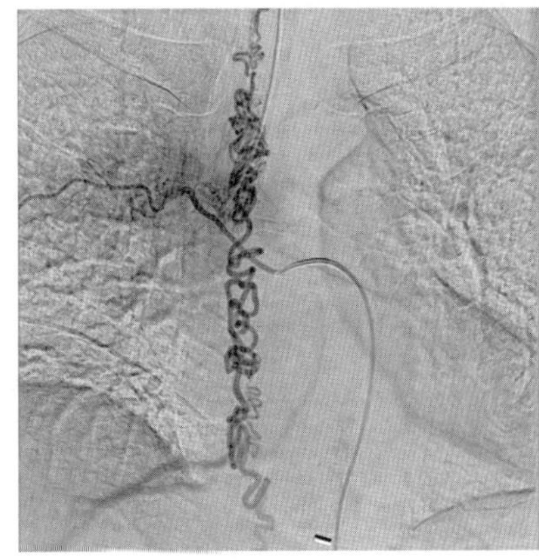

Figure 67.3

Chapter 67 Spinal Dural Arteriovenous Fistula

Findings

Spinal dural arteriovenous fistula (Figures 67.1, 67.2, and 67.3). Thoracolumbar T2-weighted MRI demonstrates an extensive network of flow voids extending from the T4 thoracic cord to the conus at T12 (Figure 67.1). A time-resolved MR angiogram demonstrated arteriovenous shunting centered at the T5 level (Figure 67.2). These findings represented a spinal dural arteriovenous fistula (SDAVF), confirmed on spinal angiography, with arterial supply to the fistula via the right T3 (Figure 67.3), and T4 and T5 intercostal arteries (not shown).

Differential Diagnosis

Arteriovenous malformation (AVM), pial AV fistula, and neoplastic, inflammatory, and ischemic conditions are included in the differential. However, the appearance as seen in this case is often classic for a- SDAVF.

Discussion

SDAVF is the most common vascular malformation of the spine, accounting for approximately 70% of all spinal vascular malformations. The shunt is typically located deep to the dura at the dorsal aspect of the intervertebral foramen. The arterial supply is via one (or more) radiculomeningeal artery that shunts to a radicular vein where the radicular vein passes through the dura of the exiting root.

Clinically, the classical presentation of a spinal dural AVF is painless, progressive paraparesis in the middle-to-older aged Caucasian male. However, symptoms can range widely, from asymptomatic to pain (radicular, polyradicular, nonspecific), with many patients experiencing more focal neurological signs, such as lower extremity weakness and bowel/bladder concerns.

Identification of a radiculomeningeal artery feeding the fistula differentiates the lesion from other spinal cord vascular malformations. SDAVF can be divided into three categories (lateral, ventral, dorsal) according to embryological development. The lateral type is the classic lesion, accounting for almost 90% of SDAVFs, occurring at the lateral epidural space where the radicular veins connect the spinal cord venous drainage to the epidural venous plexus.

Radiological Evaluation

SDAVF results in venous congestion, hypoxia, and eventual myelopathy of the cord. The reduced number of venous channels in the lower thoracic region makes the lower cord more prone to congestion, even in the case of remotely located shunts. Thus, the fistula itself and its supplying vessels may be located away from the level of myelopathy. Blood spinal cord barrier breakdown may occur, leading to enhancement with gadolinium. On conventional MRI, in addition to dilated veins on the surface of the spinal cord, the cord should be assessed for size, signal characteristics, and enhancement. A hypointense rim from deoxygenated blood can be present. Temporally resolved MR angiography increasingly allows for improved characterization of the fistula and level of the shunt. Digital subtraction angiography remains the gold standard for complete characterization of the SDAVF vascular anatomy.

Management

Treatment options include surgical occlusion of the intradural vein draining the shunt, or radiological intervention with liquid embolization, penetrating through the supplying radiculomeningeal arterial branches into the draining vein.

Teaching Points

- ► SDAVF is the most common vascular lesion of the spine, having a wide variety of presentations.
- ► Radiological assessment involves MRI and digital subtraction imaging (DSA), with the goal to identify the vascular anatomy of the fistula, and should involve assessment of the entire cord as myelopathy can occur at levels remote from the actual lesion.

Further Reading

1. Krings TW and Geibprasert SD. Spinal dural arteriovenous fistulas. AJNR. 2009;30:639–648.
2. Geibprasert S, Pereira V, Krings T, et al. Dural arteriovenous shunts: A new classification of craniospinal epidural venous anatomical bases and clinical correlations. Stroke 2008;39:2783–2789.

Richard Silbergleit, Anant Krishnan, and Daniel M. Sciubba

History

▶ A 55-year-old female presents with back pain and fatigue (**Figures 68.1, 68.2, 68.3, and 68.4**).

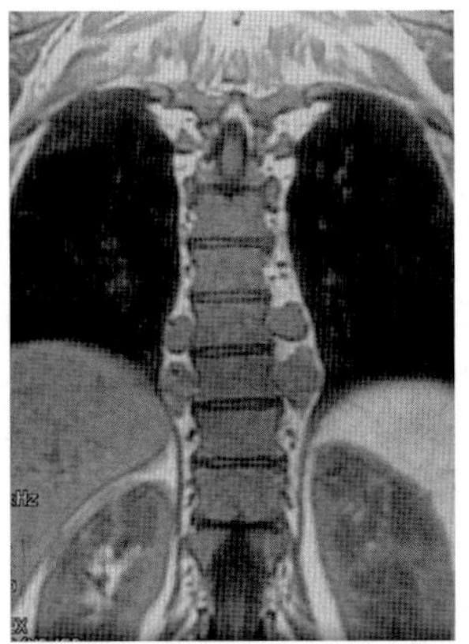

Figure 68.1

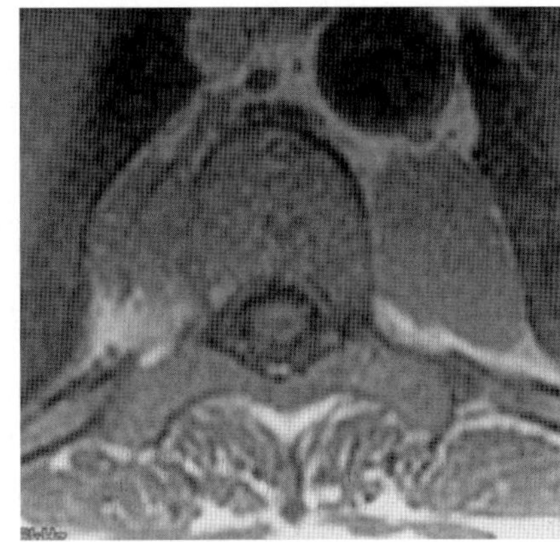

Figure 68.2

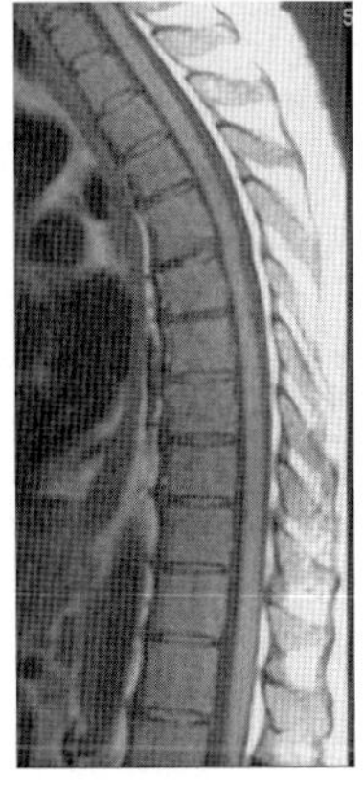

Figure 68.3

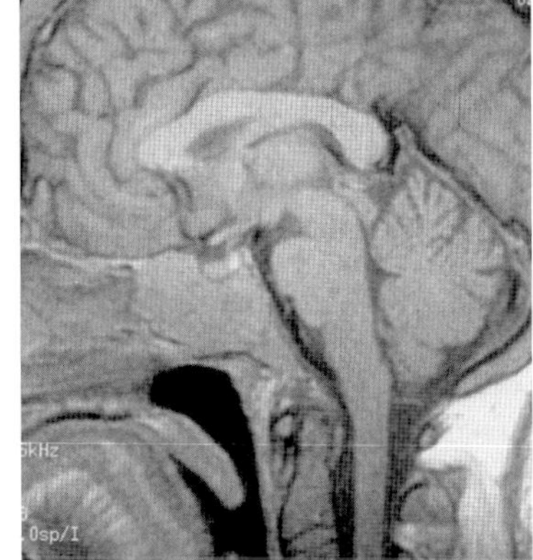

Figure 68.4

Chapter 68 Extramedullary Hematopoiesis

Findings

Extramedullary hematopoiesis. Coronal T1-weighted (**Figure 68.1**) and axial T1-weighted (**Figure 68.2**) images of the thoracic spine demonstrate low signal intensity in the bone marrow and paraspinal soft tissue masses. This patient has a history of thalassemia. A sagittal T1-weighted image (**Figure 68.3**) of the thoracic spine shows diffuse and homogeneous low signal intensity in the marrow. A sagittal T1-weighted image of the brain (**Figure 68.4**) demonstrates expansion and low signal intensity in the clivus.

Differential Diagnosis

Diffuse low signal intensity in the marrow:
► Normal in infants and children (hematopoietic marrow)
► Anemias (thalassemia, sickle cell disease)
► Chronic disease states
► Myelofibrosis
► Chemotherapy
► Metastatic disease
► Leukemia
► Multiple myeloma
► Monoclonal gammopathies
► Sarcoidosis

Paraspinal masses:
► Lymphadenopathy
► Lymphoma
► Extramedullary hematopoiesis
► Nerve sheath tumors (neurofibromatosis I and II)

Discussion

Focal low signal intensity areas in the spine on T1-weighted MRI are often due to metastatic disease, osteomyelitis, or edema from fracture. Diffuse low signal intensity in the marrow suggests a systemic process that may be benign or malignant. The presence of paraspinal soft tissue masses further narrows the differential diagnosis with chronic anemias being the most common when both low signal intensity in the marrow and paraspinal soft tissue masses are present. In chronic anemias, hematopoietic marrow never converts to fatty marrow or fatty marrow may convert back to hematopoietic marrow. Other bones in the axial and appendicular skeleton may be involved as well.

Hereditary anemias that may lead to extramedullary hematopoiesis include alpha-thalassemia, beta-thalassemia, sickle cell anemia, and hereditary spherocytosis. Thalassemia is the most common anemia to cause extramedullary hematopoiesis. Paravertebral lesions are common (**Figure 68.1**). Mediastinal, epidural (**Figure 68.5**), and presacral (**Figure 68.6**) lesions may also occur. Epidural extramedullary hematopoiesis may cause cord compression. Osteoporosis is typically also present. This may lead to compression fractures. The appearance in a given patient is the result of a combination of the primary disease and therapy (transfusion and chelation).

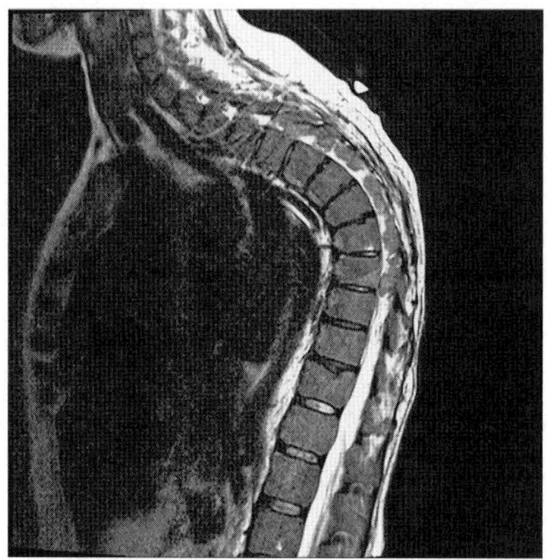
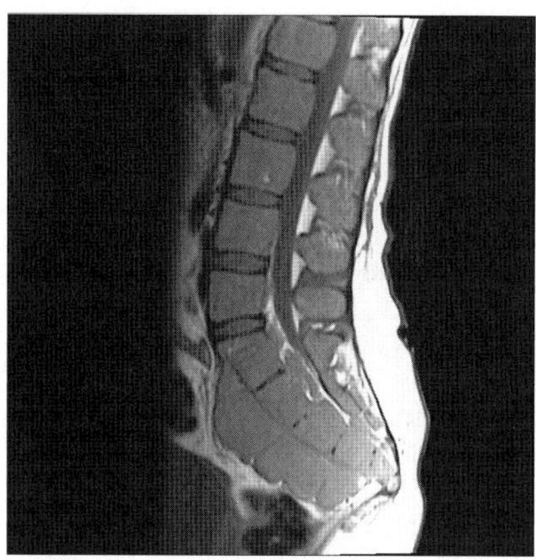

Figure 68.5

Figure 68.6

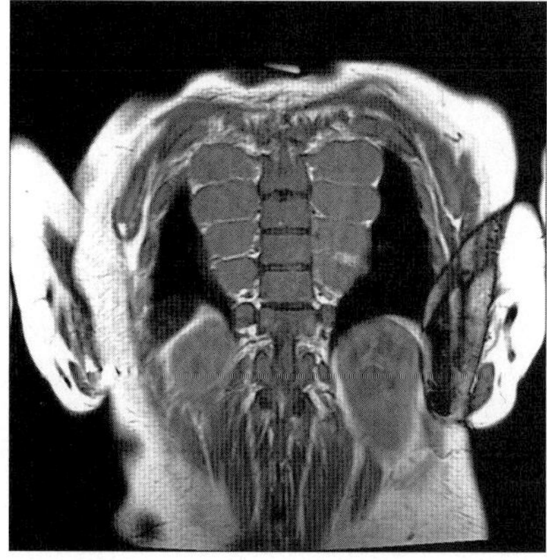

Figure 68.7

Imaging of thalassemia (**Figures 68.5, 68.6, and 68.7**). A sagittal T2-weighted image (**Figure 68.5**) in another patient (40-year-old female) demonstrates multiple epidural masses. This patient has a history of thalassemia. A sagittal T1-weighted image in the same patient (**Figure 68.6**) demonstrates presacral and epidural masses due to extramedullary hematopoiesis. A coronal T1-weighted image (**Figure 68.7**) demonstrates extensive paraspinal extramedullary hematopoiesis.

Radiological Evaluation

MRI typically demonstrates diffuse low signal intensity in the bone marrow on T1-weighted images. The bone marrow may be expanded and there may be compression fractures. Paraspinal and epidural masses are common and are frequently large and multiple.

Management

Clinical suspicion of extramedullary hematopoiesis should be entertained in any patient with a history of a hereditary anemia who presents with a spinal mass. CT-guided biopsy will confirm the diagnosis even if not suspected, and thus biopsy should always be considered in the setting of a spinal mass of unclear etiology. In general, such lesions respond well to conventional radiation combined with treatment of the underlying anemia (e.g., transfusion). In cases of poor response to radiation or presentation with progressive neurological decline, surgical resection or debulking should be considered.

Teaching Points

▶ Chronic anemias may present with low signal intensity marrow on T1-weighted images.

► The presence of extramedullary soft lesions in conjunction with low signal intensity marrow on T1-weighted images is suggestive of a chronic anemia.

► The appearance in a given patient is the result of a combination of the primary disease and therapy.

Further Reading

1. Tunaci M, Tunaci A, Engin G, et al. Imaging features of thalassemia. Eur Radiol 1999;9:1804–1809.
2. Shah LM and Hanrahan CJ. MRI of spinal bone marrow: Part 1. Techniques and normal age-related appearances. AJR 2011;197:1298–1308.
3. Hanrahan CJ and Shah LM. MRI of spinal bone marrow: Part 2. T1-weighted imaging-based differential diagnosis. AJR 2011;197:1309–1321.
4. Levin TL, Sheth SS, Ruzal-Shapiro C, et al. MRI marrow observations in thalessemia: The effects of the primary disease, transfusional therapy, and chelation. Pediatr Radiol 1995;25:607–613.

Section 8   **Miscellaneous**

History

▶ A 23-year-old man presented with a several month history of bilateral hand cramping and atrophy of the left hand musculature (**Figures 69.1, and 69.2**).

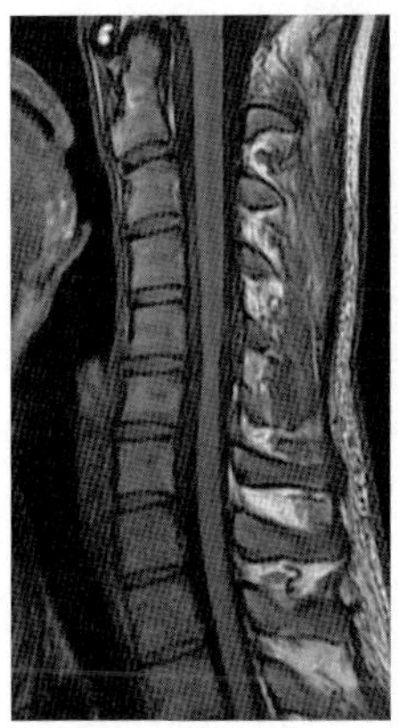

Figure 69.1

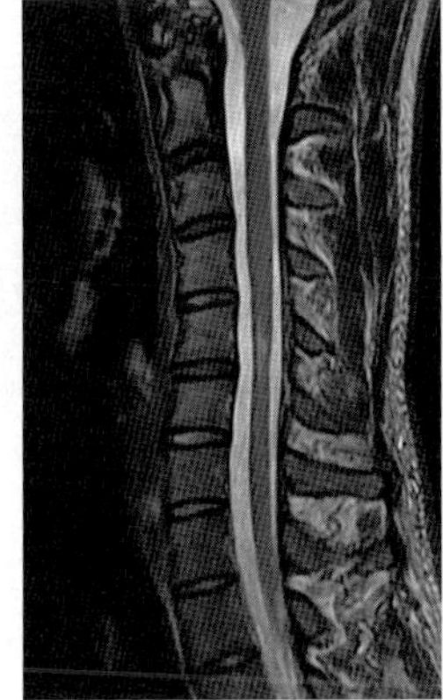

Figure 69.2

Chapter 69 **Hirayama Disease**

Findings

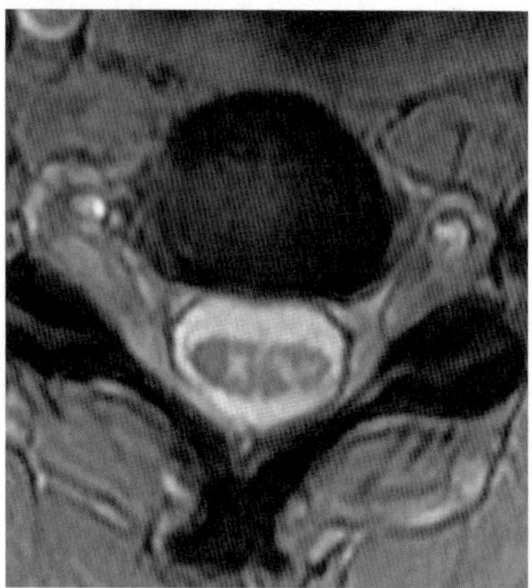

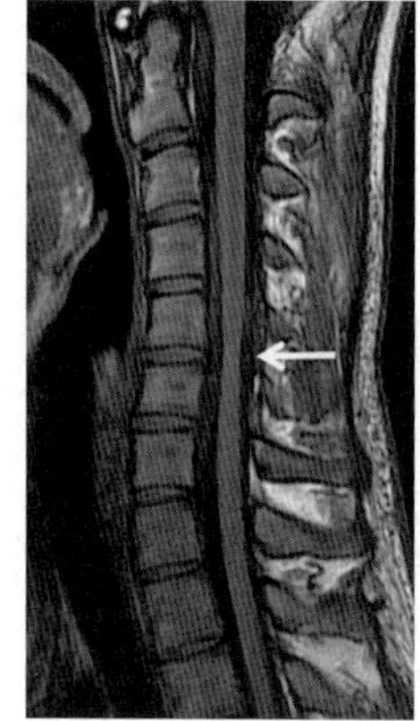

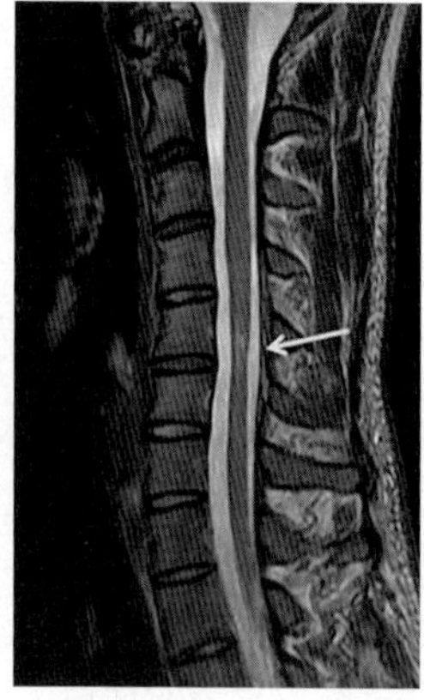

Figure 69.3

Figure 69.4

Figure 69.5

Hirayama disease (**Figures 69.3, 69.4, and 69.5**). Standard MRI imaging was initially performed with the patient in the neutral position. Sagittal T1-weighted (Figure 69.4) and T2-weighted (Figure 69.5) images of the cervical spine demonstrate focal cord atrophy centered at C5–C6 with increased signal intensity in the cord on T2-weighted images in the area of atrophy. An axial T2*-weighted image (Figure 69.3) shows greater atrophy of the left half of the cord and more T2 signal abnormality in the left half of the cord. The findings suggested a condition that typically shows greater abnormality on flexion MR imaging.

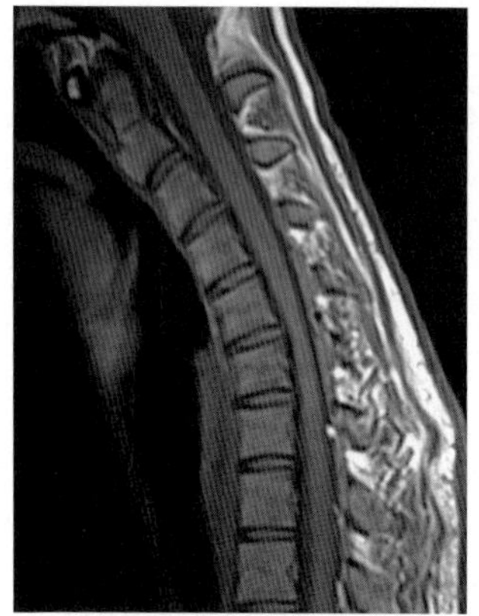

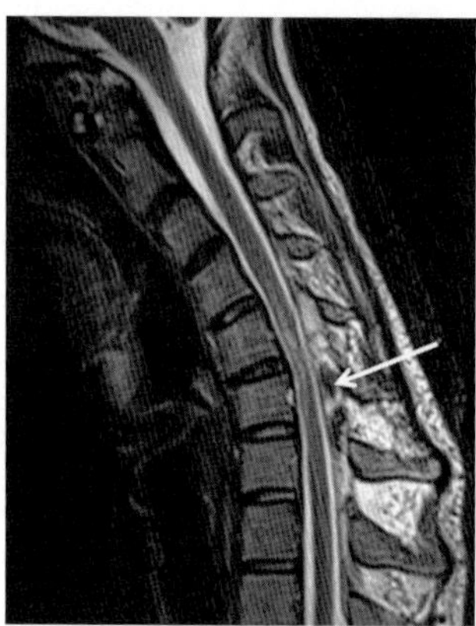

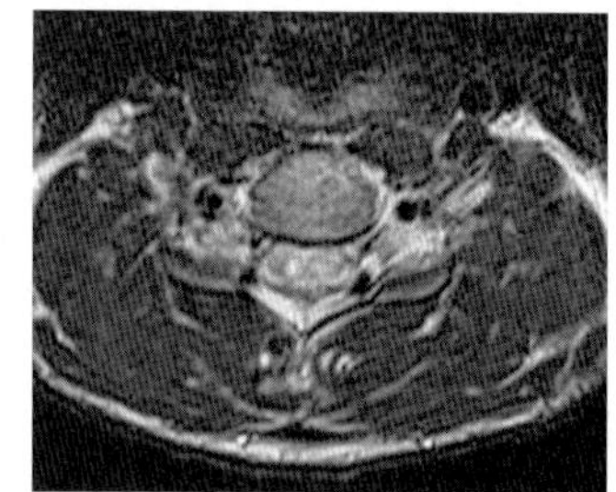

Figure 69.6

Figure 69.7

Figure 69.8

The patient returned and was imaged in flexion. Sagittal T1-weighted (**Figure 69.6**) and T2-weighted (**Figure 69.7**) images show enlargement of the posterior epidural space and anterior displacement of the dorsal dura. Loss of signal in the posterior epidural space suggesting flow voids (arrow) was seen on the sagittal T2-weighted images. An axial T2-weighted image (**Figure 69.8**) confirms the enlargement of the posterior epidural space.

Differential Diagnosis

▶ Hirayama disease
▶ Demyelination/multiple sclerosis
▶ Spinal cord infarct
▶ Spinal cord trauma

Discussion

Hirayama disease (nonprogressive juvenile spinal musculature atrophy of the distal upper limbs) is a myelopathic process that was first described by Hirayama in 1959. This disease typically affects young males between the ages of 15 and 25 years. The symptoms develop over several months to years and there is usually significant weakness at presentation. Asymmetric involvement of the distal upper extremities is common. The underlying cause is a relative shortening of the dura. The dura is relaxed in extension and tightens in flexion. This causes an anterior displacement of the dorsal dura in flexion, which causes cord compression. The anterior spinal artery may be compromised and the anterior horn motor cells can be damaged. This leads to focal cord injury and atrophy. The disease usually progresses for several years and then stabilizes. The reason for the preferential involvement of young males is uncertain.

Radiological Evaluation

MRI in the neutral position demonstrates focal cord atrophy in the lower cervical spinal cord, which is classically asymmetric. There is frequently but not always increased signal intensity in the atrophic segment of the cord on T2-weighted images. The cervical vertebral bodies and discs are usually normal. Recognition of focal atrophy in the lower cervical cord in a young male should suggest the diagnosis and lead to additional imaging in the flexed position. MRI in flexion shows anterior displacement of the posterior dura with cord compression. The posterior epidural space is enlarged. Flow voids are often seen in the enlarged posterior epidural space representing dilated epidural veins. The posterior epidural space enhances consistent with dilated veins. CT myelography in flexion and extension has also been shown to demonstrate the cord atrophy, dural displacement, and enlargement of the posterior epidural space.

Management

When treated nonoperatively, a cervical collar can reduce the ability to flex the neck and regular use can arrest the progression of the cord injury. Surgical treatment with duraplasty or anterior reconstruction is a consideration in select cases.

Teaching Points

▶ Atrophy of the lower cervical cord in a young male should suggest the diagnosis of Hirayama disease.
▶ Involvement of the cord by Hirayama disease is often asymmetric.
▶ The radiologist should suggest MRI in flexion when Hirayama disease is suspected.
▶ Flexion imaging demonstrates anterior displacement of the posterior dura.
▶ The epidural space enlarges in flexion and the epidural veins become prominent.
▶ Wearing a cervical collar can arrest the progression of Hirayama disease.

Further Reading

1. Hirayama K, Toyokura Y, and Tsubaki T. Juvenile muscular atrophy of unilateral upper extremity: A new clinical entity. Psychiat Neurol Jpn 1959;61:2190–2197.
2. Gandhi D, Goyal M, Boutque PR, and Jain R. Case 68: Hirayama disease. Radiology 2004;230:692–696.
3. Chen CJ, Chen CM, Wu CL, et al. Hirayama disease: MR diagnosis. AJNR Am J Neuroradiol 1998;19:365–368.

4. Kikuchi S, Tashiro K, Kitagawa K, et al. A mechanism of juvenile muscular atrophy localized in the hand and forearm (Hirayama's disease): Flexion myelopathy with tight dural canal in flexion. Clin Neurol (Tokyo) 1987;27:412–419.
5. Tokumaru Y and Hirayama K. A cervical collar therapy for nonprogressive juvenile spinal muscular atrophy of the distal upper limb (Hirayama's disease). Clin Neurol (Tokyo) 1992;32:1102–1106.
6. Hassan KM, Sahni H, and Jha A. Clinical and radiological profile of Hirayama disease: A flexion myelopathy due to tight cervical dural canal amenable to collar therapy. Ann Indian Acad Neurol 2012;15:106–112.

Anant Krishnan and Richard Silbergleit

History

▶ A 49-year-old female presented with progressive ataxia, diplopia, and lower extremity weakness over 18 months. Lumbar punctures demonstrated elevated protein and lymphocyte predominance with negative cultures and cytology. MRI images of the thoracic and cervical spine are displayed (**Figures 70.1, 70.2, 70.3, 70.4, and 70.5**).

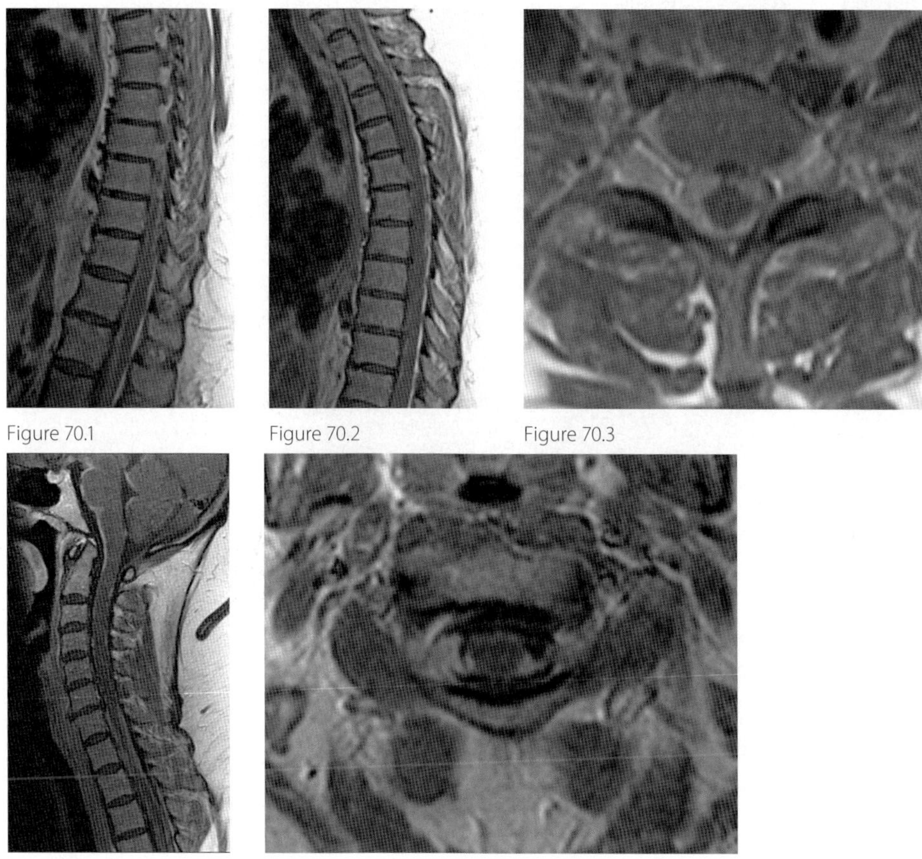

Figure 70.1

Figure 70.2

Figure 70.3

Figure 70.4

Figure 70.5

Chapter 70 **Neurosarcoidosis of the Spine**

Findings

Neurosarcoidosis of the spine. Sagittal and axial postcontrast T1-weighted images (**Figures 70.6, 70.7, and 70.8**) demonstrate significant leptomeningeal enhancement (arrows) coating the conus and thoracic spinal cord. Sagittal (**Figure 70.9**) and axial (**Figure 70.10**) postcontrast T1-weighted images of the cervical spine demonstrate leptomeningeal enhancement along the spinal cord (arrows). Intracranially, enhancement along the basilar meninges (interrupted arrows) and hypothalamus (circle) is also seen.

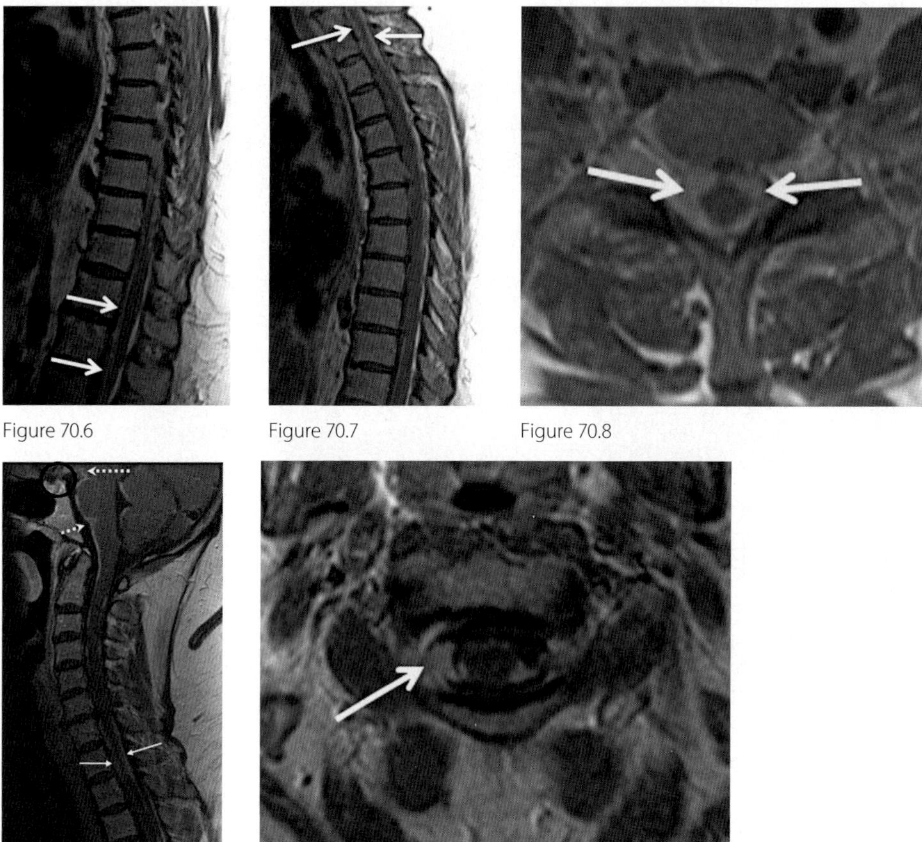

Figure 70.6   Figure 70.7   Figure 70.8

Figure 70.9   Figure 70.10

Differential Diagnoses

Sarcoidosis, the great mimicker, is often a diagnosis of exclusion, and the differential is dependent on its appearance.

Leptomeningeal manifestation (as in above case):
- Leptomeningeal carcinomatosis (breast and lung particularly) and drop metastases
- Other granulomatous infections such as tuberculosis and fungal infections
- Leukemia and lymphoma
- Inflammatory disease (when spinal nerve involvement and enhancement are seen) including Guillain–Barré and cytomegalovirus radiculitis

Intramedullary mass:
- ▶ Primary spinal cord tumors including astrocytoma and ependymoma
- ▶ Hemangioblastoma
- ▶ Demyelination, spinal cord inflammation

Dural-based and osseous lesions:
- ▶ Meningiomatosis
- ▶ Metastases

Discussion

Sarcoidosis was probably first described around the late nineteenth century with various names applied to it such as "Mortimer's malady" and "lupus pernio." It was histologically first best described by the Norwegian dermatologist Caesar Boeck, who coined the term sarcoidosis for the benign sarcoma-like lesions of the skin.

A multisystem disorder, characterized by noncaseating granulomas, sarcoidosis affects the central nervous system in approximately 10% of patients (based on imaging findings) and probably as much as 25% of all patients based on autopsy series. Isolated neurosarcoidosis is believed to be less than 1%.

Radiological Evaluation

The spectrum of involvement of the spine by sarcoidosis ranges from (inside to out) involvement of the spinal cord and nerve roots, leptomeninges and dura, extradural space, and even the vertebrae and discs. Leptomeningeal involvement constitutes a common finding and occurs in approximately 40% of cases. Leptomeningeal disease presents as a thin, smooth enhancement with a few associated nodules. Intracranial involvement, especially of the basilar meninges and hypothalamus–pituitary, is a helpful feature to assess for on cervical spine imaging. This combination of findings is most commonly seen in granulomatous processes including neurosarcoidosis and tuberculous and fungal infections.

Intramedullary involvement by neurosarcoidosis is a rare manifestation and mimics primary spinal cord tumors. The spinal cord is enlarged, with an elevated T2 signal and patchy enhancement (Figures 70.11 and 70.12). Leptomeningeal enhancement can be seen concurrently in approximately 60% of patients. Junger et al. described a progression of disease from the leptomeninges to the cord including the following:
- ▶ Phase 1: Normal spinal cord size with linear leptomeningeal enhancement.
- ▶ Phase 2: Presumed spread of leptomeningeal inflammation through Virchow-Robin spaces results in diffuse spinal cord enlargement with early faint enhancement.
- ▶ Phase 3: Decrease in cord swelling and the presence of focal/multifocal enhancement.
- ▶ Phase 4: Resolution of enhancement and the cord can become normal in size or atrophic.

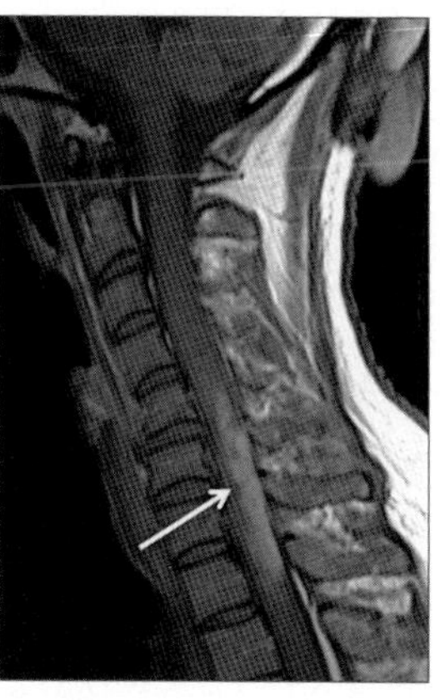

Figure 70.11

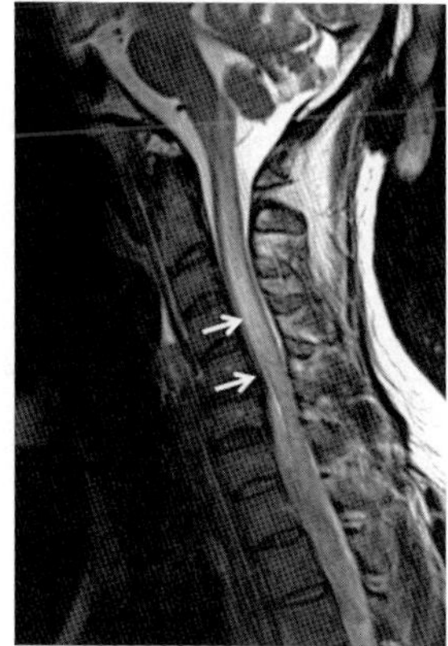

Figure 70.12

Neurosarcoidosis in the spine (Figures 70.11 and 70.12). A sagittal T1-weighted postcontrast image (Figure 70.11) demonstrates patchy but intense enhancement (arrow) within the cervical spinal cord in a patient with pathologically proven intramedullary neurosarcoidosis. A sagittal T2-weighted image (Figure 70.12) in the same patient demonstrates cord edema (short arrows) and expansion.

Dural involvement is also described in sarcoidosis and presents as bulky, peripheral masses with homogeneous enhancement and a low T2 signal though some authors report a higher than typical T2 signal. Mass effect on the spinal cord can be present. Lastly, osseous lesions are uncommon. In the spine they are most commonly seen in the lower thoracic and upper lumbar spine but are nonspecific by imaging, mimicking many other lesions such as metastases.

Management and Prognosis

▶ A definitive diagnosis requires pathological evaluation of samples, which can be difficult to obtain in isolated neurosarcoidosis. A surgical biopsy can typically be attempted for dural/leptomeningeal masses near the C1–C2 level and intradural extramedullary masses in the lumbar spine.

▶ Cerebrospinal fluid (CSF) testing is primarily performed to exclude other conditions. Elevated CSF protein and lymphocyte predominance may be seen in neurosarcoidosis. CSF angiotensin-converting enzyme (ACE) levels have been described as an option and are insensitive (24–55%) but specific (94–95%) for neurosarcoidosis.

▶ Treatment includes early medical treatment primarily with steroids, but also in some cases with steroid-sparing immunosuppressive agents such as methotrexate, cyclophosphamide, and infliximab among others. Radiation treatment has also been tried in patients with drug-resistant central nervous system (CNS) sarcoidosis.

Teaching Points

▶ Neurosarcoidosis has a broad spectrum of presentation ranging from involvement of the cord, spinal nerves, and leptomeninges through dural and osseous lesions.

▶ Consider sarcoidosis when extensive leptomeningeal enhancement is present along the spinal cord in a patient with long standing symptoms and "negative" LP for infection or malignancy. A lymphocyte predominance in CSF is typical. Assessment of the basilar meninges for similar findings is a helpful feature.

▶ Intramedullary sarcoidosis can mimic a spinal cord tumor. Identifying concurrent leptomeningeal enhancement may assist in distinguishing the two.

Further Reading

1. Danbolt N. The historical aspects of sarcoidosis. Postgrad Med J 1958;34(391):245–267.
2. Lury K, Smith K, Matheus M, and Castillo M. Neurosarcoidosis—Review of imaging findings. Semin Roentgenol 2004;39(4):495–504.
3. Vargas DL and Stern BJ. Neurosarcoidosis: Diagnosis and management. Semin Respir Crit Care Med 2010;31(4):419–427.
4. Junger SS, Stern BJ, Levine SR, et al. Intramedullary spinal sarcoidosis: Clinical and magnetic resonance imaging characteristics. Neurology 1993;43:333–337.
5. Khoury J, Wellik, K, Demaerschalk, B, and Wingerchuk, D. Cerebrospinal fluid angiotensin-converting enzyme for diagnosis of central nervous system sarcoidosis. Neurologist 2009;15(2):108–111.

Jaysson T. Brooks, Brian Neuman, Cornelia Wenokor, and A. Jay Khanna

History

► A 34-year-old male presents to the emergency department with complaints of persistent neck pain, bilateral arm weakness, and an unsteady gait since he was involved in a minor car accident 3 weeks ago (**Figures 71.1 and 71.2**).

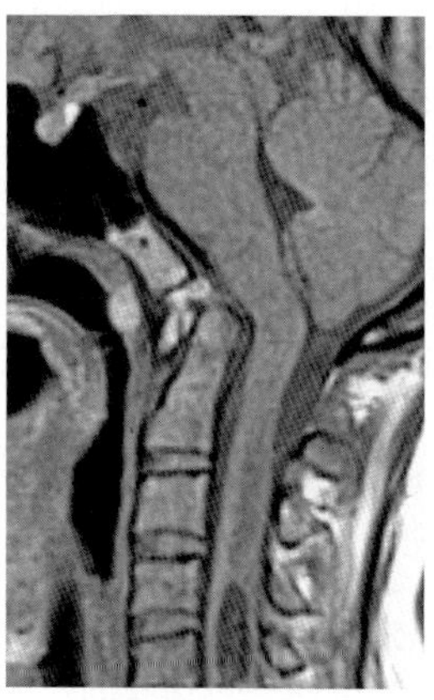

Figure 71.1

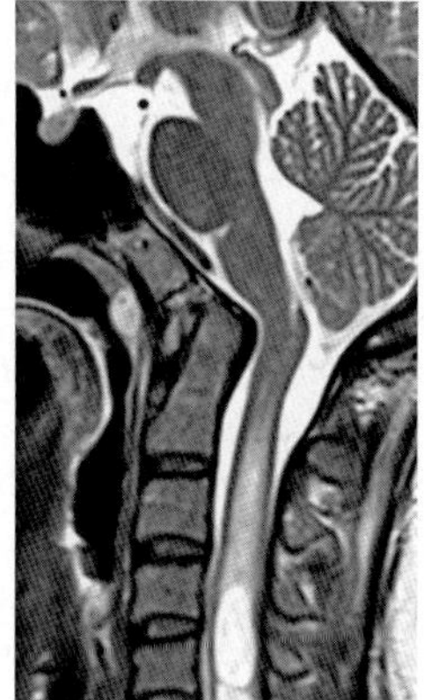

Figure 71.2

Chapter 71 **Basilar Invagination**

Findings

Basilar invagination (**Figures 71.1 and 71.2**). A T1-weighted image of the cervical spine (Figure 71.1) shows compression of the brainstem by the odontoid, also known as basilar invagination (BI). A T2-weighted image (Figure 71.2) of the cervical spine shows an intraspinal syrinx and a concomitant BI.

Differential Diagnosis

► Basilar impression
► Congenital basilar invagination
► Cranial settling
► Atlantooccipital assimilation

Discussion

This patient has BI, which is defined as a congenital abnormality at the craniovertebral junction (CVJ) resulting in the protrusion of the odontoid process of C2 into the foramen magnum. In patients without an associated Chiari malformation, trauma is often the most frequent precipitating factor.

While often used interchangeably, true BI is distinct from the conditions in the differential diagnosis. Platybasia is a flattening of the skull base that often occurs in conjunction with BI; basilar impression refers to superior migration of the odontoid process in the setting of softening of the skull base seen in conditions such as Paget's disease and osteomalacia, and cranial settling is a vertical subluxation of the odontoid caused by a loss of supporting ligamentous structures typically seen in rheumatoid arthritis (**Figures 71.3 and 71.4**). Atlantooccipital assimilation is characterized by the incorporation of C1 into the occiput, with a resultant dens extending into the foramen magnum.

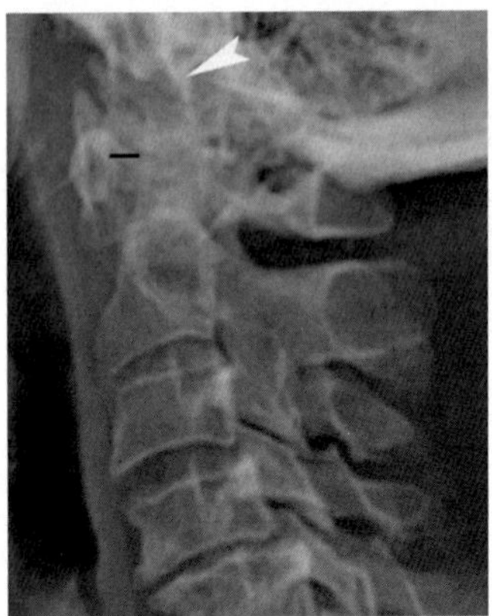

Figure 71.3

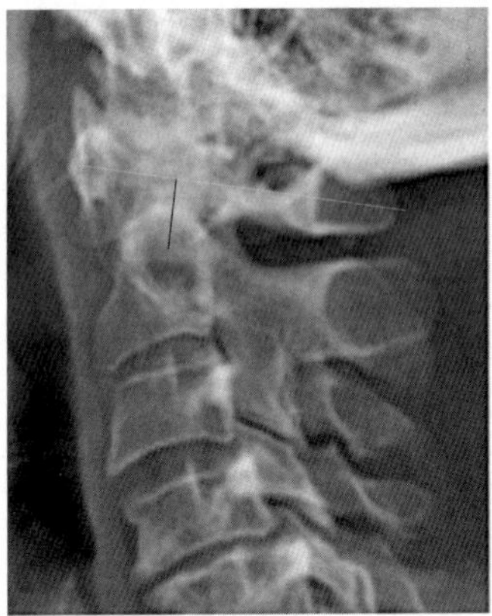

Figure 71.4

Rheumatoid arthritis (Figures 71.3 and 71.4). There is atlantoaxial settling, with the dens (white arrowhead) extending too far cephalad, essentially contacting the clivus. An easy way to assess this is using Ranawat's line, a line drawn through the axis of C1 (white line) and measuring the distance from the center of the C2 pedicle (black line). A distance of less than 13 mm is consistent with impaction. Also seen is widening of the atlantodental interval (horizontal black line in Figure 71.3).

Radiological Evaluation

Normal relationships at the CVJ are illustrated below (**Figure 71.5**). BI can be positively diagnosed when the dens is above Wackenheim's and McRae's line, >3 mm above Chamberlain's line, and >4.5 mm above McGregor's line.

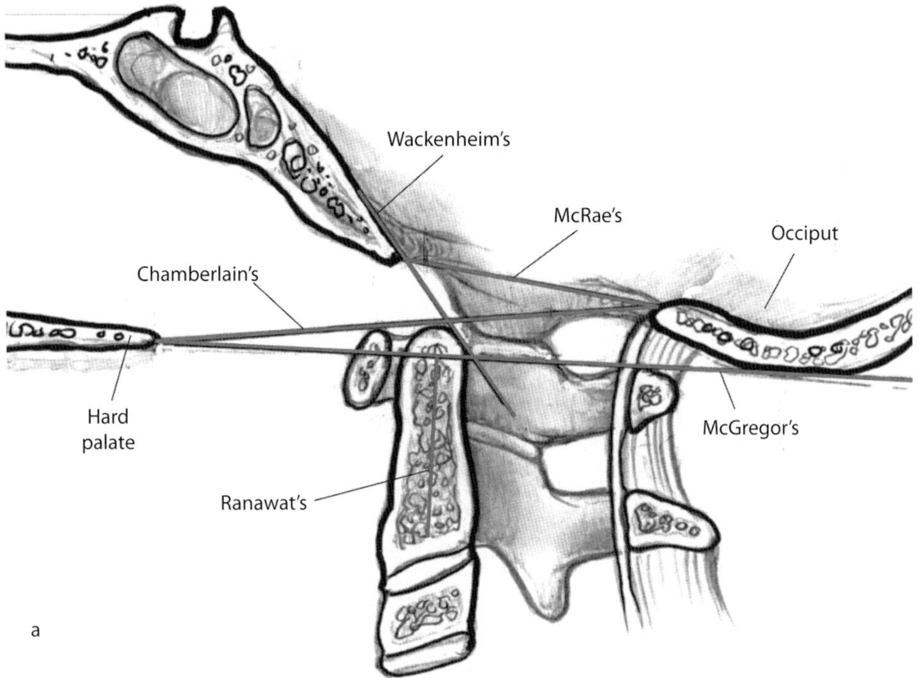

Figure 71.5

Normal craniocervical junction anatomical landmarks (**Figure 71.5**). Wackenheim's clivus baseline is drawn along the superior surface of the clivus; McRae's line is drawn from the basion to the opisthion; Chamberlain's line is drawn from the hard palate to the opisthion; Chamberlain's line is drawn from the hard palate to the most caudal point on the midline occipital curve.

Management

Although still controversial, neurologically intact, asymptomatic patients with mild basilar invagination and compression of neural structures can be monitored closely. For all other patients surgery is indicated. It is important to obtain CT and MRI scans of the CVJ as well as angiography of the vertebral arteries preoperatively to define the regional anatomy before surgical treatment is undertaken.

A trial of axial cervical traction is routinely performed to assess the degree to which reduction of the odontoid can be achieved. If reduction of the odontoid is achievable with traction then only posterior decompression and fusion are indicated. If the odontoid is not reducible, then additional ventral decompression may be considered through a transoral approach. The presence of a Chiari malformation is important as previous studies have shown that 82% of patients without an associated Chiari malformation improved clinically after traction, while only 5% of patients with a Chiari malformation improved with traction.

Teaching Points

▶ Adequate advanced imaging and vascular studies should be performed preoperatively.
▶ Reduction of the odontoid with axial cervical traction allows treatment with posterior decompression and fusion alone.
▶ Severe ventral compression or an associated Chiari malformation often leads to combined anterior and posterior decompressions with fusion.

Further Reading

1. Daniel RT, Muzumdar A, Ingalhalikar A, et al. Biomechanical stability of a posterior-alone fixation technique after craniovertebral junction realignment. World Neurosurg 2012;77(2):357–361.

2. Goel A, Bhatjiwale M, and Desai K. Basilar invagination: A study based on 190 surgically treated patients. J Neurosurg 1998;88(6):962–968.
3. Khanna AJ. *MRI for Spine Surgeons and Specialists*. Retrieved from Google Books, 2014.
4. Klekamp J. (2014). Treatment of basilar invagination. Eur Spine J 2014;23(8):1656–1665.
5. Menezes AH. (2008). Craniocervical developmental anatomy and its implications. Child's Nervous Syst: ChNS 2008;24(10):1109–1122.
6. Smith JS, Shaffrey CI, Abel MF, and Menezes AH. (2010). Basilar invagination. Neurosurgery 2010;66(3 Suppl):39–47.

Freddie R. Swain

History

▶ An 18-year-old female presents to the emergency room with right arm and hand tingling, especially after gymnastic practice (**Figures 72.1 and 72.2**).

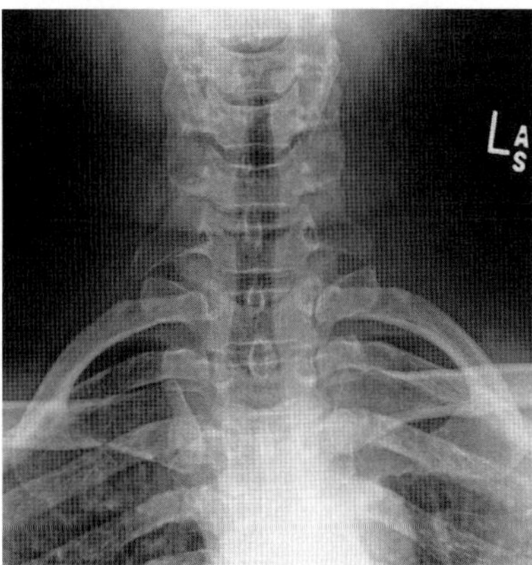

Figure 72.1

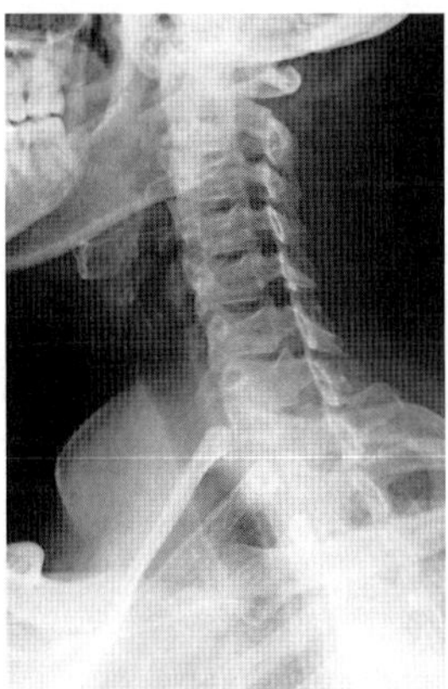

Figure 72.2

Chapter 72 Cervical Rib

Findings

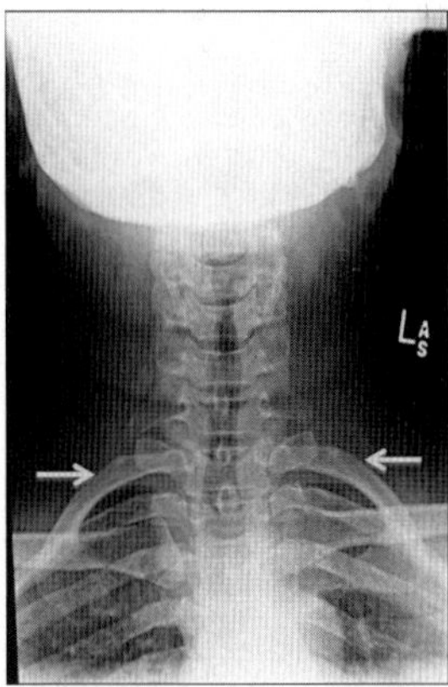

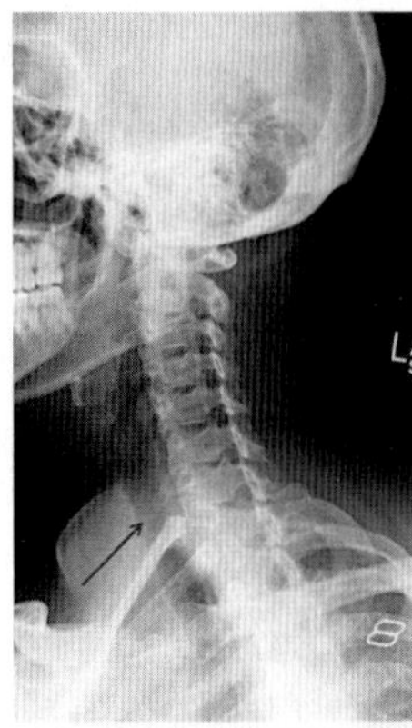

Figure 72.3

Figure 72.4

Bilateral cervical ribs (**Figures 72.3 and 72.4**). Anteroposterior and right oblique radiographs demonstrate bilateral cervical ribs, with the right greater in size than the left.

Discussion

Cervical ribs (supernumerary or accessory ribs arising from the seventh cervical vertebra) are a common incidental finding on chest radiographs and CTs. They are seen in up to 0.5% of the population, and are more common in females than males. While the majority of patients are asymptomatic, cervical ribs can lead to vascular and neurological compromise (thoracic outlet syndrome or brachial plexopathy). Studies have shown that of patients requiring an operative procedure for thoracic outlet syndrome (TOS), cervical ribs accounted for 69%.

Radiological Evaluation

In 1869, Gruber described four types of cervical ribs: (1) cervical ribs extending just beyond the transverse process, (2) cervical ribs extending beyond the transverse process with a free tip almost touching the first rib, (3) cervical ribs extending beyond the transverse process with fibrous bands or cartilage attaching to the first rib, and (4) cervical ribs completely fused to the first rib. Patients with Gruber class 1 tend to be asympomatic, while Gruber classes 2–4 make up the majority of patients who become symptomatic.

Vascular compromise can be arterial or venous. A subset of these patients can have an associated subclavian artery aneurysm. Duplex ultrasound with the affected arm in abduction and adduction is an important tool to make the diagnosis. CT imaging can also be performed with arms in abduction and adduction. Neurogenic compromise can present with symptoms of pain, paresthesias, and/or weakness in the affected arm.

Management

Current treatment options include Transaxillary first rib resection and scalenectomy (FRRS) with cervical rib resection for patients not requiring vascular reconstruction. Supraclavicular FRRS with cervical rib resection should be considered for patients requiring arterial bypass. Due to the risk of compression and subsequent thrombosis, subclavian artery stents should not be placed before rib resection.

Teaching Points

► Cervical ribs are classified into four types based on an anatomical system.
► Cervical ribs can result in thoracic outlet syndrome or a brachial plexopathy.
► The presence of a cervical rib is often underreported.

Further Reading

1. Chang KZ1, Likes K, Davis K, Demos J, Freischlag JA. The significance of cervical ribs in thoracic outlet syndrome. J Vasc Surg. 2013 Mar;57(3):771–5. doi: 10.1016/j.jvs.2012.08.110.
2. Weber AE, Criado E. Relevance of bone anomalies in patients with thoracic outlet syndrome. Ann Vasc Surg. 2014 May;28(4):924–32. doi: 10.1016/j.avsg.2013.08.014. Epub 2013 Dec 6.

Chapter 73

David Rodriguez, Tao Ouyang, and Vikas Agarwal

History

▶ A 35-year-old male with a history of neurofibromatosis type 1 presents with chronic low back pain (**Figures 73.1 and 73.2**).

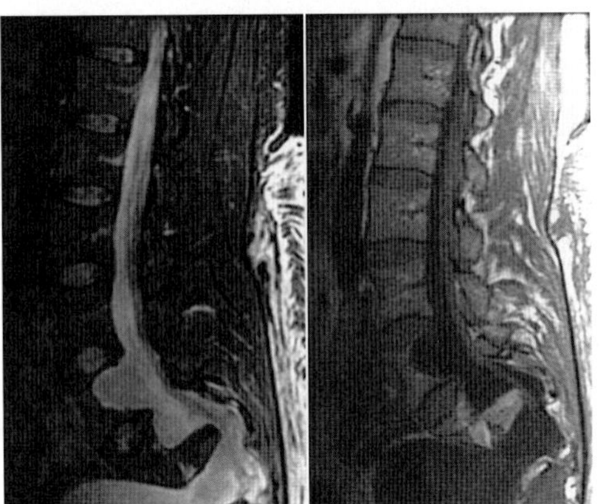

Figure 73.1

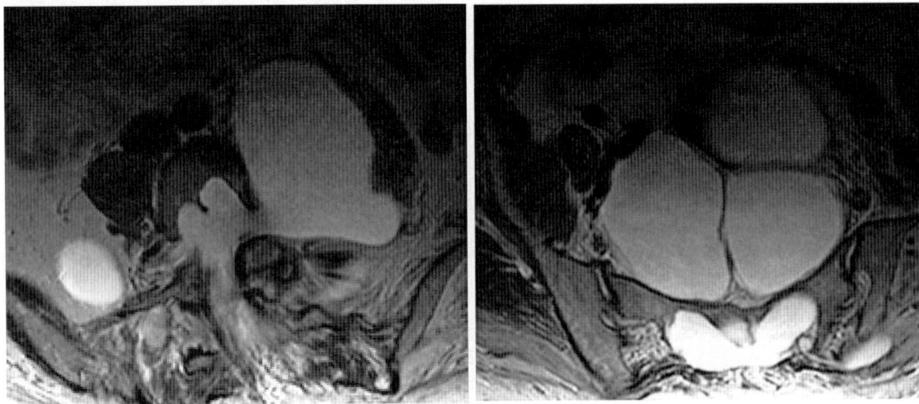

Figure 73.2

Findings

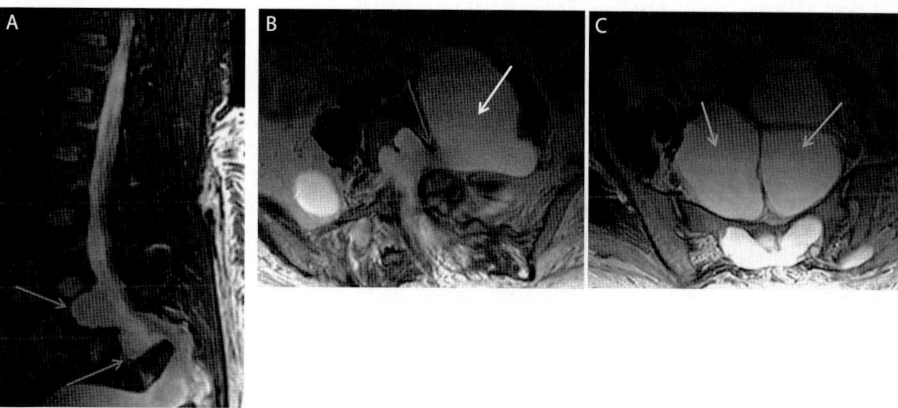

Figure 73.3

Dural ectasia (**Figure 73.3**). Widening of the thecal sac and scalloping of the posterior vertebral bodies are best appreciated on sagittal T2-weighted sequences (Figure 73.3A) or CT but may be suggested on lateral spine radiographs. There is also associated widening of the neural foramina (left arrow) and lateral meningoceles (top arrow) that are localized with axial images (Figure 73.3B). Anterior sacral meningoceles may present as intraabdominal masses (Figure 73.3C). Dural ectasia is more common in the lumbar and sacral regions.

Differential Diagnosis

Isolated minor posterior vertebral concavity can be seen in up to 50% of normal individuals. Diffuse posterior vertebral scalloping is associated with achondroplasia (though the interpedicular distance is decreased rather than increased) and mucopolysaccharidoses such as Hurler's and Morquio's syndromes. Posterior scalloping may also be seen in acromegaly due to soft tissue hypertrophy and increased bone resorption.

Discussion

Dural ectasia results from the weakness of the dura and lack of protection of the vertebral body. It is commonly associated with the following conditions and should prompt further imaging:

▶ Marfan syndrome (reported in up to 92% of patients)
▶ Ehlers–Danlos
▶ Neurofibromatosis Type 1
▶ Ankylosing spondylitis (may have associated arachnoid cysts causing cauda equina syndrome)
▶ Intraspinal tumors causing bony remodeling

Dural ectasia may have other sequelae:

▶ Spondylolisthesis
▶ Scoliosis
▶ Syringomyelia in NF-1
▶ Failure of intrathecal anesthesia secondary to greater volume of cerebrospinal fluid (CSF)

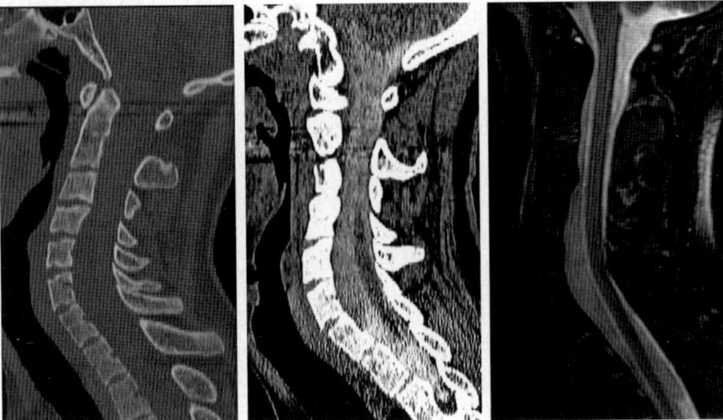

Figure 73.4

CT is a useful tool in the evaluation of vertebral body widths and the presence of pedicular thinning. MRI easily depicts enlargement of the thecal sac (**Figure 73.4**).

Cross-sectional imaging can be used in the evaluation of dural ectasia. CT demonstrates vertebral body width and pedicular thinning while CT myelography and MRI demonstrate the dural sac diameter more readily and help to assess for concomitant intraspinal tumors (Figure 73.4).

In the lumbar spine, measurements of the dural sac ratio (dural sac diameter/vertebral body diameter) can be made on midline sagittal T2-weighted MRI sequences at the level of the mid-vertebral body (Figure 73.5). Studies of patients with Marfan's syndrome have reported normal cutoffs for dural sac ratio. Utilizing these cutoffs at L3 and S1 achieved 95% sensitivity and 98% specificity for Marfan's syndrome.

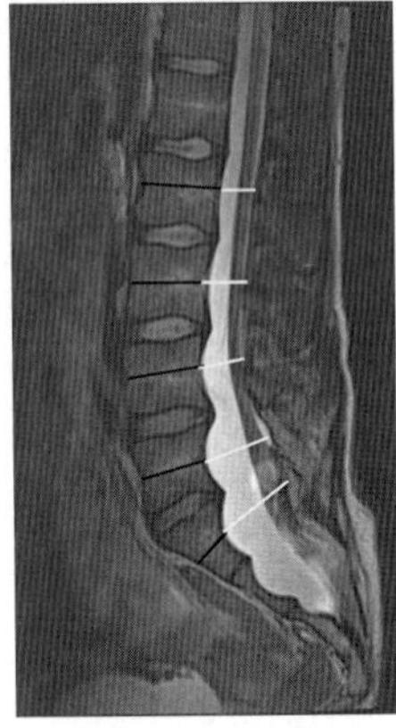

Figure 73.5

A sagittal T2 sequence demonstrates measurements of the dural sac diameter (white line) and vertebral body diameter (black line) (**Figure 73.5**). There is also a tethered cord and lipomyelomeningocele in this case.

Management

Scoliosis correction is the most common indication for surgical repair in the setting of dural ectasia. Surgical correction of scoliosis is often difficult due to thinning of the pedicles and narrowing of the vertebral bodies.

Teaching Points

▶ Dural ectasia is associated with a number of syndromes.

▶ Isolated posterior vertebral scalloping is a normal variant and should be distinguished from true dural ectasia with cross-sectional imaging.

Further Reading

1. Abul-Kasim K, Overgaard A, and Ohlin A. Dural ectasia in adolescent idiopathic scoliosis: Quantitative assessment on MRI. Eur Spine J 2010;19:754–759.
2. Oosterhof T, Groenink M, Julsmans F-J, et al. Quantitative assessment of dural ectasia as a marker for Marfan syndrome. Radiology 2001;220:514–518.
3. Wakely S. The posterior vertebral scalloping sign. Radiology 2006;239:607–609.

Chapter 74

Nima Jadidi and Sylvie Destian

History

► A 42-year-old male presents with myelopathic symptoms (**Figure 74.1**).

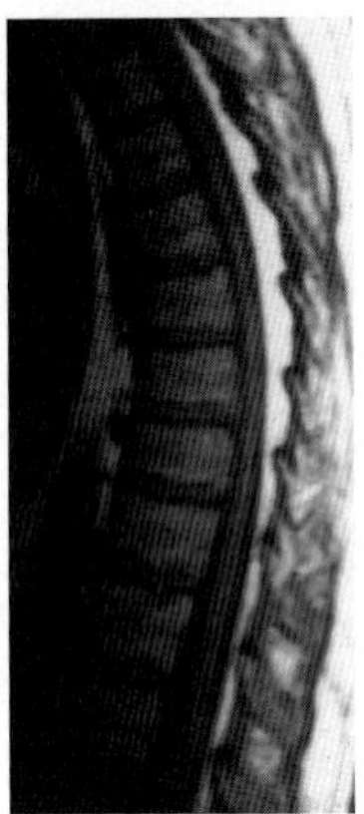

Figure 74.1

Findings

Epidural lipomatosis. A sagittal T1-weighted MRI of the thoracic spine (Figure 74.1) depicts exuberant posterior fatty tissue spanning multiple thoracic vertebral levels.

Differential Diagnosis

- ► Epidural hematoma
- ► Epidural liposarcoma

Discussion

Epidural lipomatosis is an abnormal accumulation of unencapsulated adipose tissue in the extradural space. This entity is most commonly found in middle-aged men on chronic oral steroids and in individuals with Cushing syndrome. The cause can also be idiopathic and can be found throughout the spinal column. Neurological symptoms resulting from spinal cord or severe thecal sac compression may require surgical intervention.

Radiological Evaluation

Imaging characteristics on CT and MRI will reflect that of fatty tissue. On MRI, this lesion will appear hyperintense on T1WI, intermediate intense on T2WI, and hypointense on a fat suppressed sequence. Epidural fat thicker than 6 mm across multiple vertebral levels is suggestive of this condition. Epidural lipomatosis occurs most often in the thoracic spine followed by the lumber spine (**Figures 74.2 and 74.3**). Epidural lipomatosis in the thoracic spine usually occurs posterior to the thecal sac. A unique feature of epidural lipomatosis in the lumber spine is that it can be circumferential.

An epidural abscess will enhance after contrast administration, typically around an area of central necrosis; in addition, it will not be hyperintense on T1WI. The T2WI signal will be brighter with an abscess than with epidural lipomatosis. Subacute hemorrhage is also an important etiology to keep in mind as it may have similar imaging characteristics on MRI, although fat suppression should help differentiate the two. If the patient does not have a history of trauma or clinical symptoms of an infection, hemorrhage and abscess are less likely possibilities.

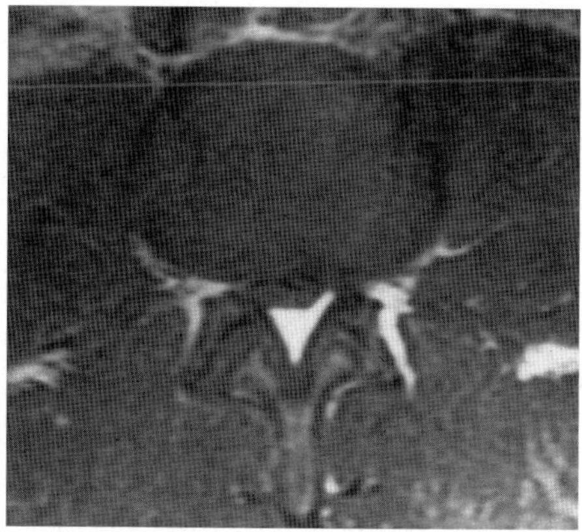

Figure 74.2

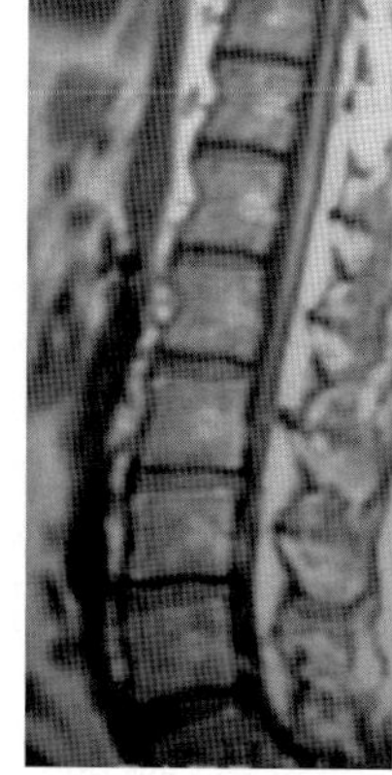

Figure 74.3

Additional patients with epidural lipomatosis (**Figures 74.2 and 74.3**). Axial T1 (Figure 74.2) and sagittal T2 (Figure 74.3) images in different patients demonstrate epidural lipomatosis.

Management

Treatment depends on the severity of the condition. Tapering of the oral steroid medication and even weight loss can potentially help. If the symptoms are severe, surgical intervention with decompressive laminectomy and excision of the epidural fat may become necessary.

Teaching Points

▶ Look for signal characteristics of fat on MRI.
▶ The clinical setting goes a long way in differentiating epidural lipomatosis from other epidural lesions. Patients are often on long-term oral steroids.

Further Reading

1. Geers C, Lecouvet FE, Behets C, et al. Polygonal deformation of the dural sac in lumbar epidural lipomatosis: Anatomic explanation by the presence of meningovertebral ligaments. AJNR Am J Neuroradiol 2003;24(7):1276–1282.
2. Venkatanarasimha N and Parrish RW. Thoracic epidural lipomatosis. Radiology 2009;252:618–622.

Brandon C. Perry and Kathleen R. Fink

History

▶ A 36 year old female presents to her primary care provider with 2 years of back pain (**Figure 75.1**).

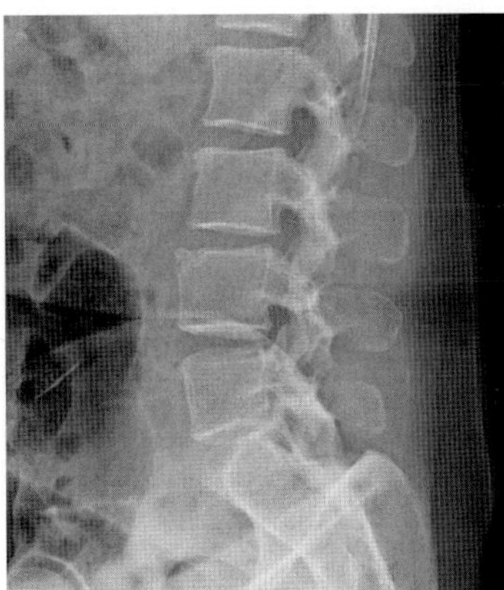

Figure 75.1

Chapter 75 Limbus Vertebra

Findings

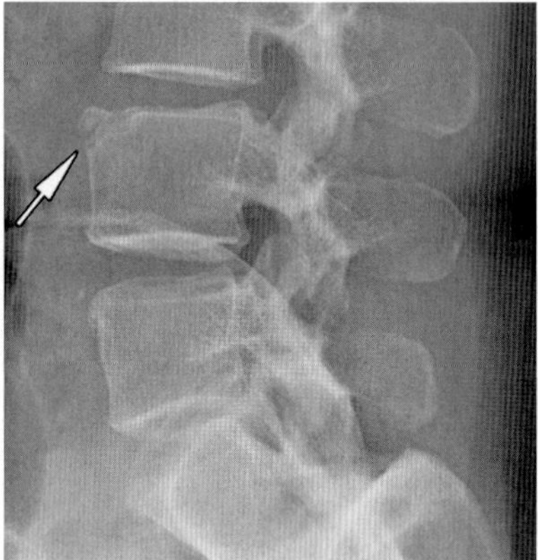

Figure 75.2

Limbus vertebra. A lateral lumbar spine radiograph (**Figure 75.2**) demonstrates a focal, well-corticated discontinuity of the anterior, superior endplate of the L4 vertebral body (arrow) with maintained vertebral body height.

Differential Diagnosis

- ▶ Acute vertebral body fracture
- ▶ Schmorls node
- ▶ Anterior osteophyte fragment

Discussion

Limbus vertebra is a common incidental finding in adults. It is thought to be due to remote injury in the skeletally immature spine, in which a portion of the nucleus pulposus herniates underneath the unfused ring apophysis. This apophysis fragment remains separated from the vertebral body, developing into a well-corticated, triangular osseous fragment. This fragment is usually located in the anteriosuperior corner of a mid-lumbar vertebral body, though limbus can occur elsewhere in the spine. Rarely, it can affect the inferior or posterior vertebral body margin.

Radiological Evaluation

Limbus vertebra is often misinterpreted as a fracture, even by experienced radiologists. The most important finding is the detection of a characteristic, well-formed osseous fragment in an anteriosuperior location (Figure 75.3). The limbus vertebra fragment roughly matches the size of the vertebral body defect and there are no other associated findings. Acute fractures will not have sclerotic, well-formed margins and there may be other associated injuries (Figure 75.4). A correlation with the clinical history is also important. CT and MRI may be used for problem solving, although this is usually unnecessary (**Figures 75.3, 75.4, 75.5, and 75.6**).

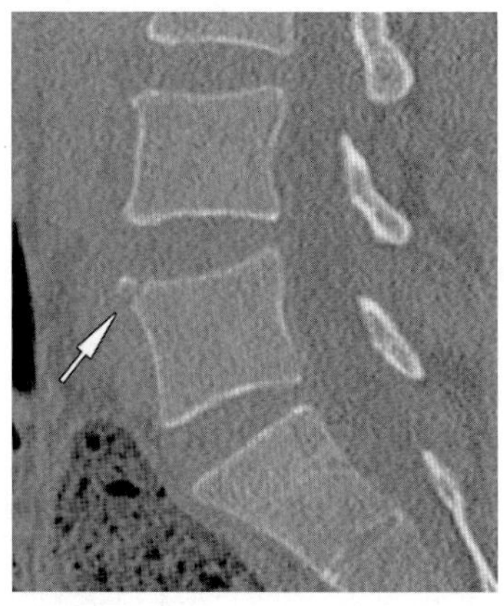 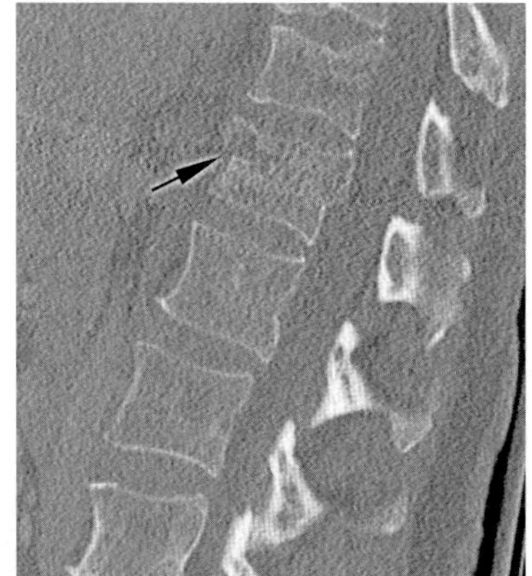

Figure 75.3

Figure 75.4

Sagittal CT images demonstrate L5 limbus vertebra (Figure 75.3, white arrow) and acute L1 anterior vertebral body fractures (Figure 75.4, black arrow). Note the well-corticated fragment in the limbus vertebra.

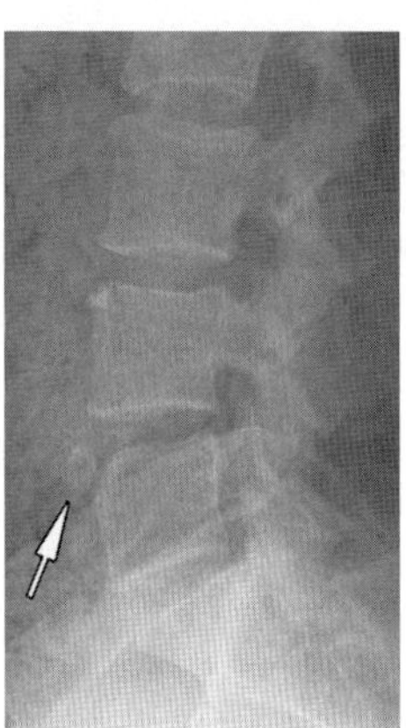 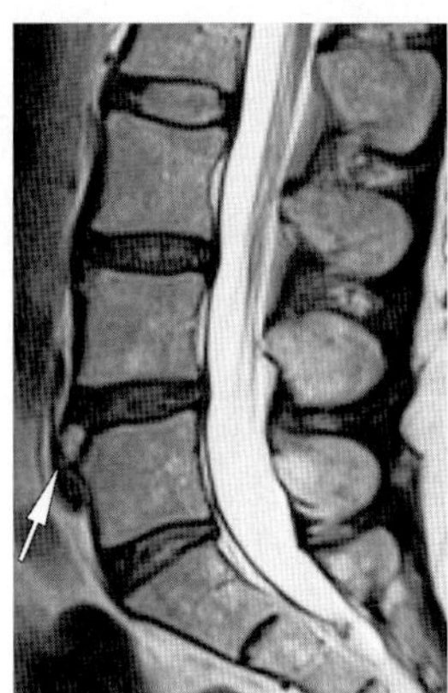

Figure 75.5

Figure 75.6

Radiograph (Figure 75.5) and sagittal T2-weighted MRI (Figure 75.6) show L5 limbus vertebra. MRI redemonstrates an osseous fragment with the characteristic location and appearance of limbus vertebra, with no associated bone edema.

Management

Anterior limbus vertebra is an incidental finding, which does not cause pain and requires no treatment. Although rare, posterior limbus vertebra may cause nerve root compression and pain.

Teaching Point

▶ Limbus vertebra is a common incidental finding that must be differentiated from an acute fracture.

Further Reading

1. Ghelman B and Freiberger RH. The limbus vertebra: An anterior disc herniation demonstrated by discography. Am J Roentgenol 1976;127:854–855.
2. McCarron RF. A case of mistaken identity, annulare mimics fracture. Orthop Rev 1987;16:173–175.
3. Yagan R. CT diagnosis of limbus vertebra. J Comput Assist Tomogr 1984;8:149–151.

Chapter 76

H. Kate Lee

History

▶ A 68-year-old female presents with increasing back pain for the past 2 months (**Figures 76.1, 76.2, 76.3, 76.4, and 76.5**).

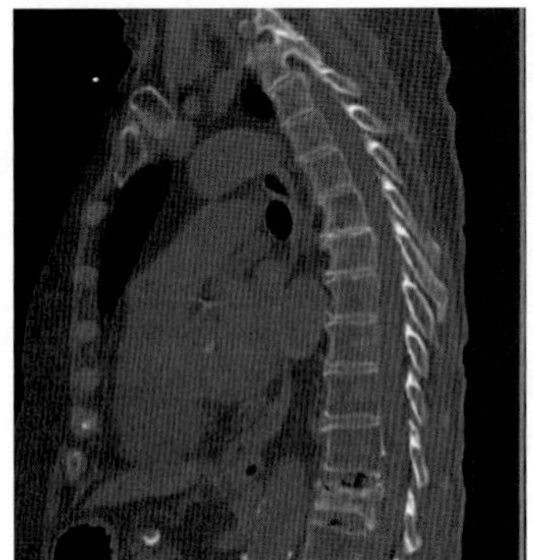

Figure 76.1

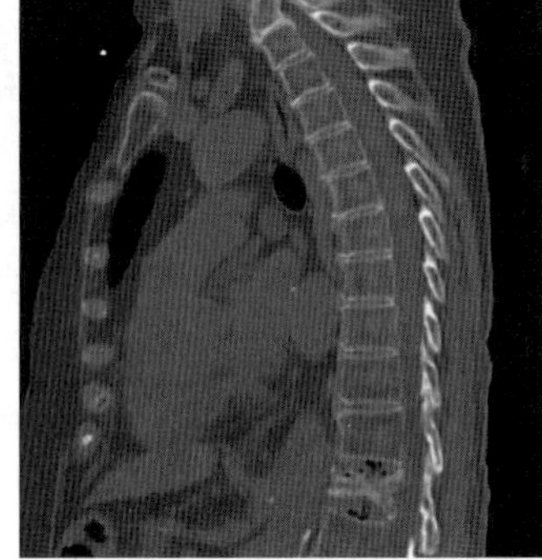

Figure 76.2

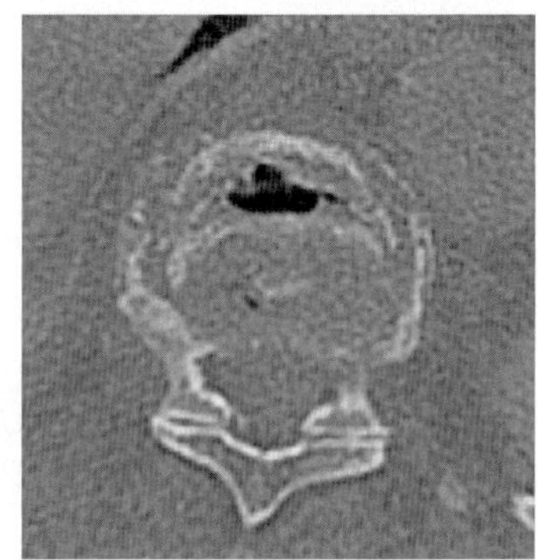

Figure 76.3

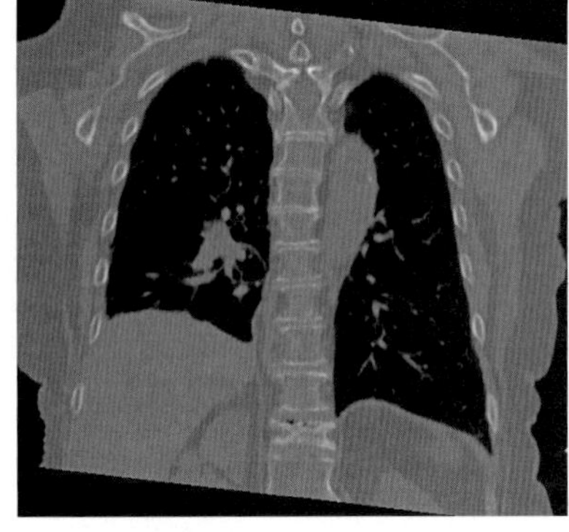

Figure 76.4

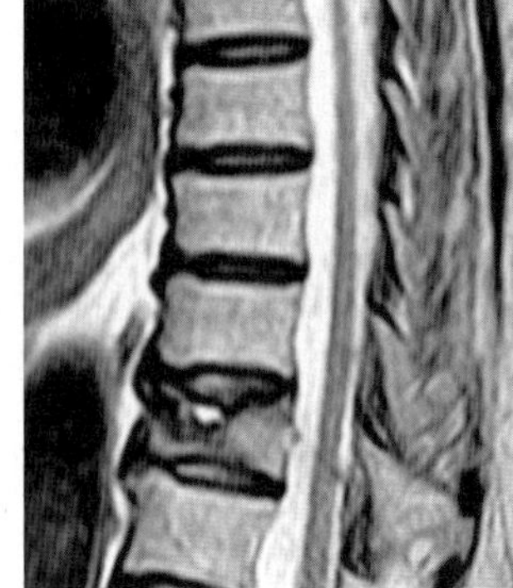

Figure 76.5

Findings

Kümmel disease (Figures 76.1, 76.2, 76.3, 76.4, and 76.5). Sagittal (Figures 76.1 and 76.2), axial (Figure 76.3), and coronal CT (Figure 76.4) reconstructions demonstrate a fractured and collapsed lower thoracic vertebral body with "intravertebral vacuum cleft sign" (air attenuation or vacuum cleft subjacent to the endplates of the collapsed vertebral body). Also note that there is a retropulsion of fracture into the spinal canal. A sagittal T2-weighted MR image (Figure 76.5) demonstrates a T2 hyperintense signal at the cleft indicating fluid ("fluid sign").

Differential Diagnosis

▶ Infectious osteonecrosis
▶ Degenerative/neoplastic vertebral body fracture
▶ Ischemic osteonecrosis
▶ Gas within an intravertebral disc herniation (can mimic an intravertebral vacuum cleft)

Discussion

Kümmel disease, also known as aseptic vertebral body osteonecrosis or Kümmel-Verneuli's disease, is an uncommon entity. It was first described by Herman Kümmel in 1891 and represents a delayed, posttraumatic vertebral body collapse due to ischemia and nonunion of the anterior vertebral body wedge fracture weeks to months following major trauma. It is most commonly seen in middle-aged and older patients.

Kümmel disease occurs in 10% of vertebral osteoporotic fractures, mainly in the thoracolumbar zone. The risk factors include trauma, osteoporosis, alcoholism, steroid use, and radiation treatment. Most patients are neurologically intact, and continued pain is a common symptom that responds well to stabilization. Spinal cord injury attributed to Kümmel disease is rare.

Radiological Evaluation

Kümmel disease is more commonly a radiographic diagnosis. Radiographs show the collapse of the affected vertebrae and an abnormal radiolucent shadow in the collapsed vertebral body. CT shows air attenuation or vacuum cleft usually in the central area or adjacent to the endplate of a collapsed vertebral body ("intravertebral vacuum cleft sign") (Figures 76.1, 76.2, 76.3, and 76.4). On MR, vacuum has a low signal intensity on all sequences with signal intensity void on gradient-echo images due to magnetic susceptibility effect. MR can additionally show a T1 hypointense and T2 hyperintense signal at the cleft indicating fluid (Figure 76. 5, "fluid sign"). The severity of the vertebral collapse has been found to be higher in those who have intravertebral gas as opposed to only intravertebral fluid. This indicates that the presence of intravertebral air is possibly a more advanced stage of the disease and intervertebral fluid occurs at an earlier stage. Histological analysis will show reactive marrow fibrosis with a high turnover rate, which indicates osteonecrosis.

Management

The treatment plan varies according to surgeon preference and the patient's comorbidities. Options range from vertebroplasty/kyphoplasty (in order to reduce pain and kyphosis) to laminectomy and stabilization in an attempt to relieve neurological symptoms.

Teaching Points

▶ Kümmel disease is also known as aseptic vertebral body osteonecrosis.

► Look for the intravertebral vacuum cleft sign on CT (air attenuation or vacuum cleft usually in the central area or subjacent to the endplate of a collapsed vertebral body) or fluid sign (fluid subjacent to the endplate) on MR.

Further Reading

1. Brower AC and Downey EF. Kümmel disease: Report of a case with serial radiographs. Radiology 1981;141(2):363–364.
2. Theodorou DJ. The intravertebral vacuum cleft sign. Radiology 2001;21:787–788.
3. Baur A, Stabler A, Arbogast S, et al. Acute osteoporotic and neoplastic vertebral compression fractures: Fluid sign at MR imaging. Radiology 2002;225:730–735.
4. Yu CW, Hsu CY, Shih TT, and Fu CJ. Vertebral osteonecrosis: MR imaging findings and related changes on adjacent levels. AJNR Am J Neuroradiol 2007;28(1):42–47.

Brandon C. Perry and Kathleen R. Fink

History

▶ A 28-year-old female presents to the emergency room following a ground level fall (**Figures 77.1 and 77.2**).

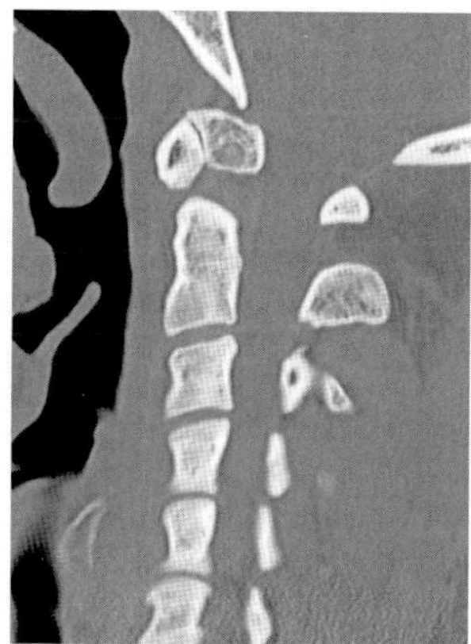

Figure 77.1

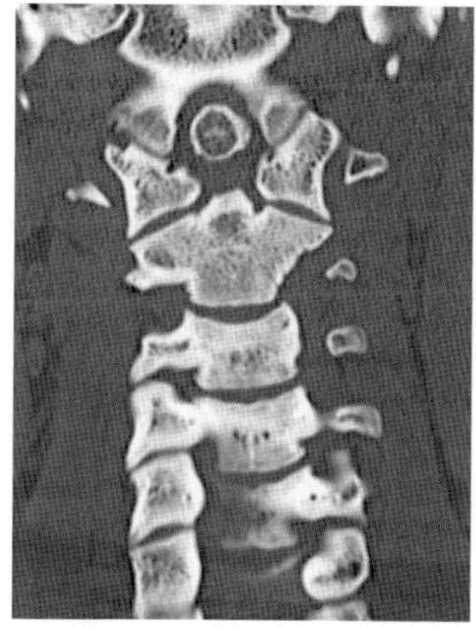

Figure 77.2

Chapter 77 Os Odontoideum

Findings

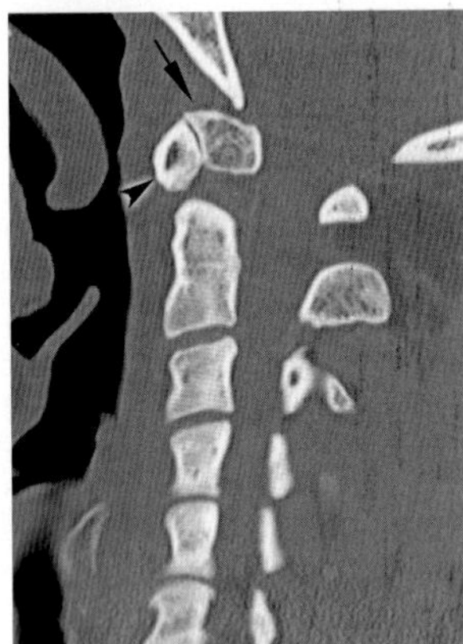

Figure 77.3

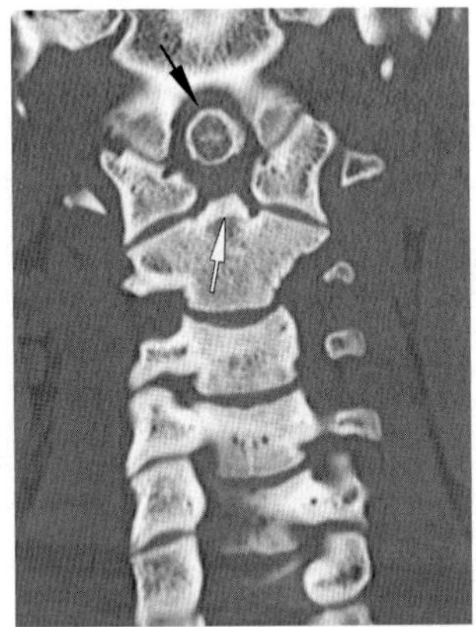

Figure 77.4

Os odontoideum. Sagittal (**Figure 77.3**) and coronal (**Figure 77.4**) cervical spine CT demonstrates a well-corticated ossicle (black arrow) superior to a small dens (white arrow, Figure 77.4) with a wide gap between the two. The arch of C1 is hyperplastic (arrowhead, Figure 77.3).

Differential Diagnosis

▶ Dens (odontoid) fracture nonunion
▶ Persistent os terminale

Discussion

An os odontoideum is a smooth, well-corticated ossicle located superiorly to a hypoplastic odontoid process. An orthotopic os odontoideum is located in the expected anatomic position posterior to the anterior arch of C1 with a gap between C2 and the os odontoideum. A dystopic os odontoideum is located elsewhere, often near the foramen magnum.

Current evidence suggests that os odontoideum results from trauma during childhood, before the age of 5–6 years, although the etiology remains controversial. A hypertrophied and rounded anterior arch of C1 is a common associated finding.

Radiological Evaluation

A distinguishing feature between os odontoideum and a Type 2 odontoid fracture is the distance between the intact dens and the ossific fragment. A fracture usually has a narrow zone of separation between the ossific fragments, and the overall size and shape of the dens are maintained (**Figure 77.5**). With os odontoideum, there is usually a larger gap between the os and the hypoplastic dens.

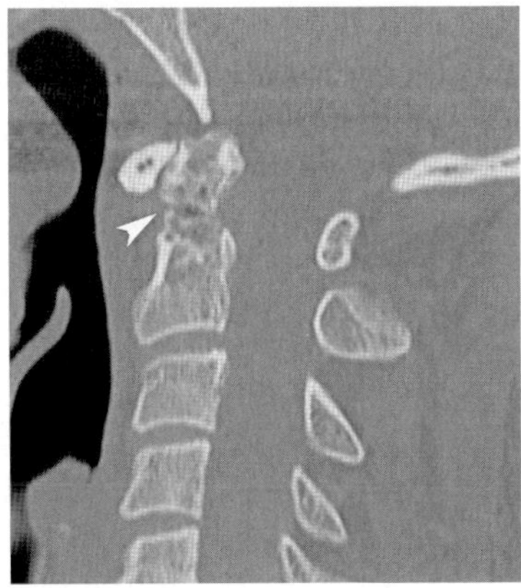

Figure 77.5

Ununited Type 2 odontoid fracture (Figure 77.5). Note the narrow gap between the ununited fracture fragments (arrowhead). The ossific fragments together form a normally sized odontoid, and the C1 arch is normal in size, not hypertrophied.

A radiological evaluation is used to confirm the diagnosis and estimate the degree of spinal instability. An initial radiological evaluation should include open-mouth, anterior–posterior, and flexion–extension lateral radiographs. These are used to confirm the diagnosis and evaluate for spinal instability (**Figures 77.6, 77.7, and 77.8**). CT and MRI are often used for problem solving or if there are neurological symptoms.

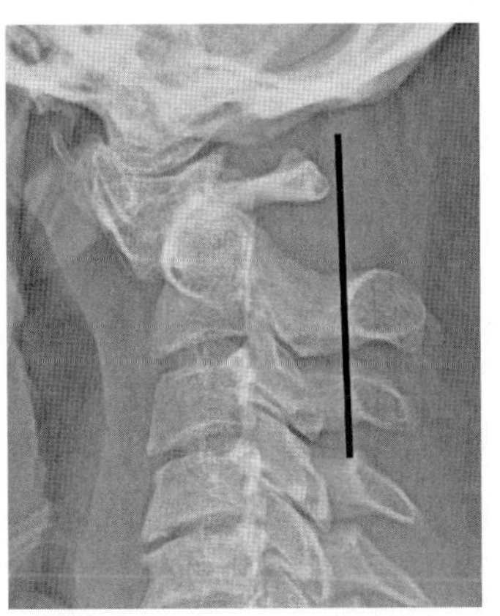

Figure 77.6

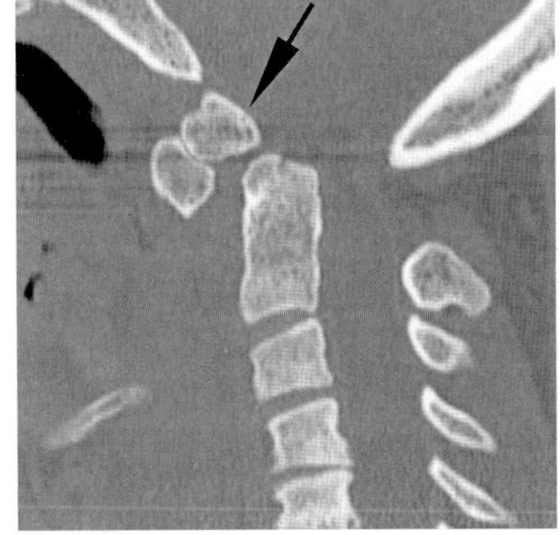

Figure 77.7

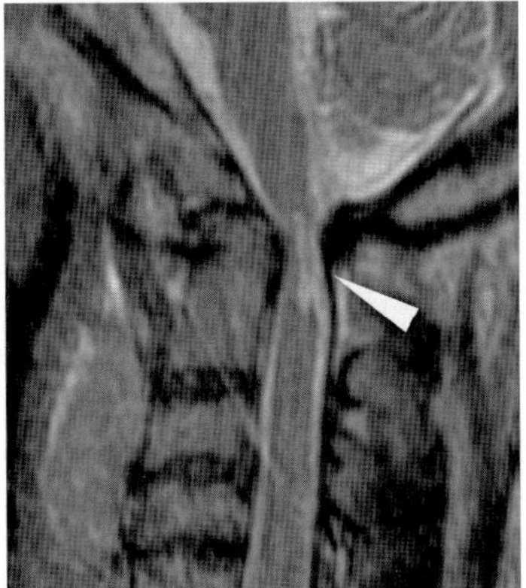

Figure 77.8

Os odontoideum resulting in spinal cord compression (**Figures 77.6, 77.7, and 77.8**). A lateral radiograph (Figure 77.6) demonstrates anterior subluxation of C1 on C2. Note the anterior translation of C1 from the spinolaminar line (black). A sagittal CT (Figure 77.7) better demonstrates the malaligned os odontoideum (black arrow). A sagittal T2-weighted MRI (Figure 77.8) shows severe cervical stenosis at the craniocervical junction with compression of the spinal cord and abnormal cord signal (arrowhead).

Management

Patients without symptoms or neurological signs are managed with clinical and radiographic surveillance. Patients with neurological symptoms or signs and C1–C2 instability may require posterior occipital-cervical fusion (**Figure 77.9**).

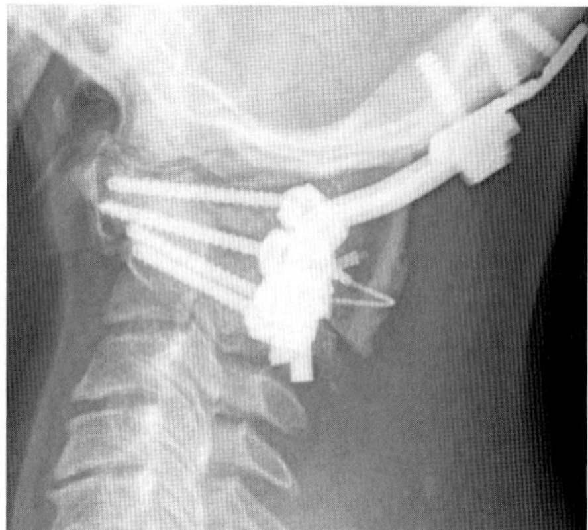

Figure 77.9

Postoperative appearance (**Figure 77.9**). Occipital to C2 posterior spinal fusion has been performed for unstable os odontoideum (the same patient as in Figures 77.6, 77.7, and 77.8).

Teaching Points

▶ Os odontoideum is believed to result from minor trauma to the odontoid synchondrosis before the age of 5–6 years, although the etiology remains controversial.
▶ It is important to distinguish os odontoideum from an ununited odontoid fracture.
▶ Os odontoideum generally requires no treatment. If there is associated spinal instability, cervical fusion may be indicated.

Further Reading

1. Carr RB, Fink KR, and Gross JA. Imaging of trauma: Part 1. Pseudotrauma of the spine—osseous variants that may simulate injury. Am J Roentgenol 2012;199(6):1200–1206.
2. Holt RG, Helms CA, Munk PL, and Gillespy T. Hypertrophy of C-1 anterior arch (useful sign to distinguish os odontoideum from acute dens fracture). Radiology 1989;173:207–209.
3. Dai L, Yuan W, Ni B, and Jia L. Os odontoideum: Etiology, diagnosis, and management. Surg Neurol 2000;53(2):106–108.

History

► A 16-year-old patient presents with back pain and kyphosis.

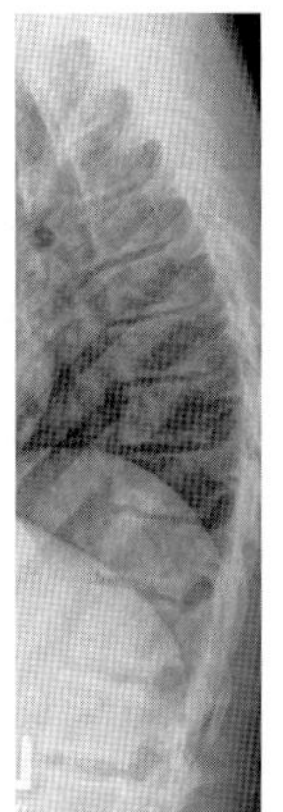

Figure 78.1

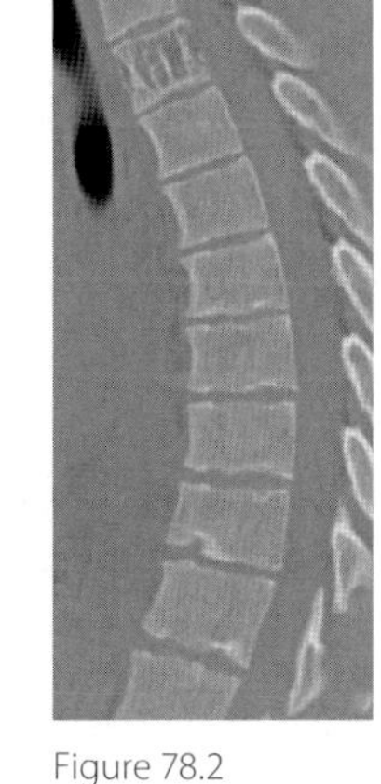

Figure 78.2

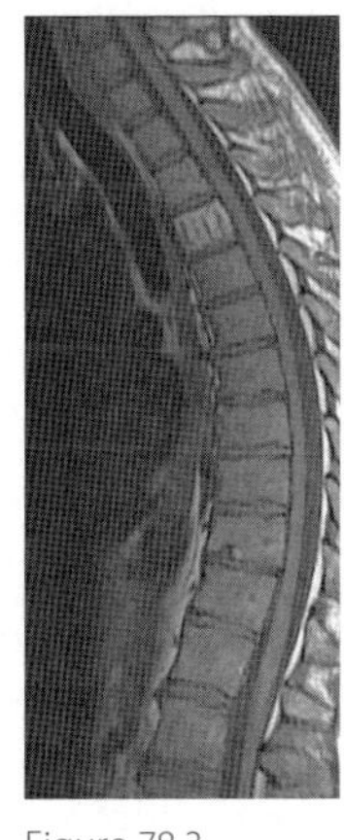

Figure 78.3

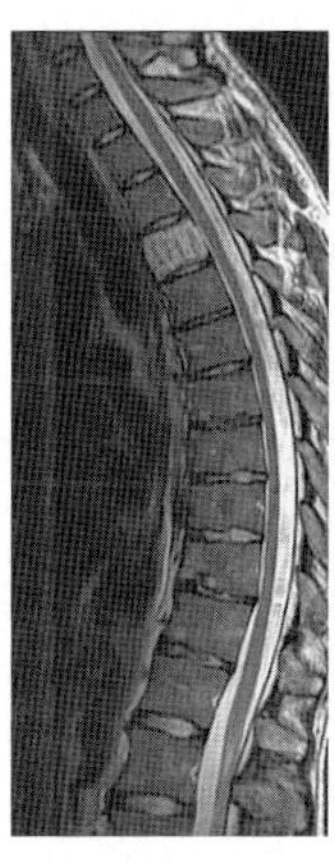

Figure 78.4

Chapter 78 **Scheuermann Disease**

Findings

Scheuermann disease (Figures 78.1, 78.2, 78.3, and 78.4). A lateral radiograph (**Figure 78.1**) shows anterior vertebral body wedging with endplate scalloping. A sagittal nonenhanced CT (NECT) image (**Figure 78.2**) shows distinct Schmorl's nodes and anterior wedging of more than three contiguous vertebral bodies with a thoracic kyphosis. There is an incidentally noted benign hemangioma in an upper thoracic vertebral body. Sagittal T1- and T2-weighted MR images (**Figures 38.3 and 38.4**) show loss of intervertebral disc signal and disc height, multilevel anterior wedging of the vertebral bodies, discrete Schmorl's nodes, and kyphosis of the thoracic spine.

Differential Diagnosis

► Postural kyphosis
► Congenital kyphosis
► Compression fractures
► Osteogenesis imperfecta

Discussion

Scheuermann disease develops in adolescents when the dorsal aspect of the spine grows more rapidly relative to the ventral aspect. This growth disparity results in premature degenerative disc disease, anterior wedging of the vertebral bodies, and a kyphotic appearance of the spine in an otherwise healthy individual. Invaginations of intervertebral discs into the adjacent vertebral body endplates, called Schmorl's nodes, are a hallmark of the degenerative disc changes. While the disease develops in adolescence, patients may remain asymptomatic until adulthood. Clinical presentation can range from kyphosis to back pain and neurological deficits, usually from associated disc herniations. This entity is clinically distinguished from postural kyphosis due to the inability of patients to voluntarily correct their posture.

Radiological Evaluation

Conventional radiography and CT are the primary imaging modalities used in the evaluation of patients with Scheuermann disease. Diagnostic criteria for Scheuermann disease include involvement of at least three contiguous vertebral body levels with Schmorl's nodes and at least 5° of wedging at each level. In 75% of cases, findings are isolated to the thoracic spine (**Figures 78.5 and 78.6**); in 20–25% of cases there is thoracolumbar involvement (**Figure 78.7**), and in <5% of patients there are isolated lumbar findings. Cervical involvement is rare. Kyphosis is a typical feature, which can be measured on radiography or CT. Greater than 40° of kyphosis is considered abnormal. The most common method of evaluating the degree of kyphosis uses the sagittal plane and measuring from one vertebra above the affected vertebrae to one vertebra below. MRI is used to evaluate for disc herniation in the setting of severe pain or neurological deficit.

The differential diagnosis of Scheuermann disease is that of kyphotic deformity in a young patient and includes postural kyphosis, congenital kyphosis, mild forms of osteogenesis imperfecta, and compression fractures. Postural kyphosis shows significantly less severe kyphosis. Mild forms of osteogenesis imperfecta are associated with osteopenia, while in Scheuermann disease bone density remains normal. Compression fractures typically demonstrate angular depressions whereas vertebral bodies in Scheuermann disease demonstrate a scalloped contour with Schmorl's nodes.

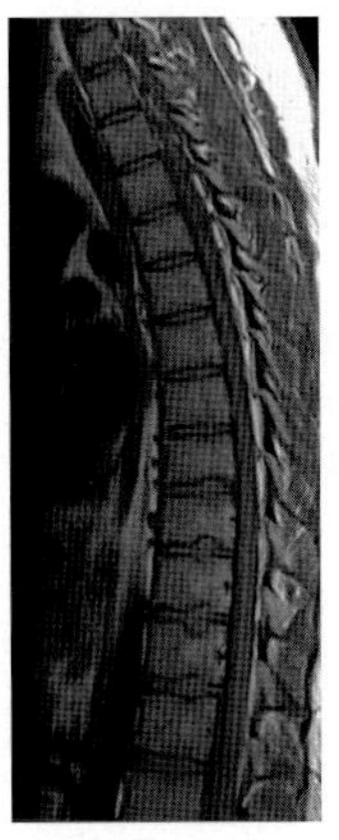 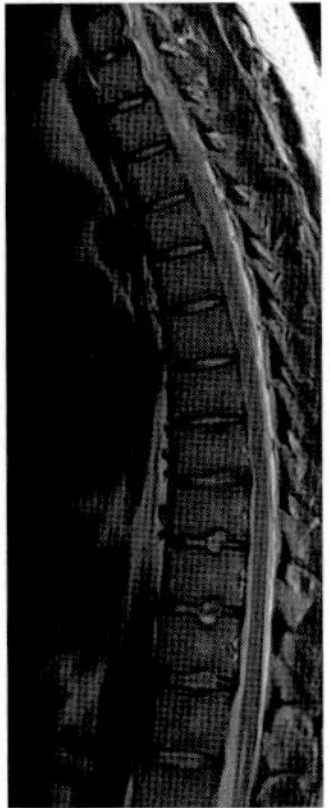

Figure 78.5   Figure 78.6

Sagittal T1 and T2 images, respectively, show disc space narrowing with endplate Schmorl's nodes spanning three levels of the thoracic spine (**Figures 78.5 and 78.6**). There is mild thoracic kyphosis. No disc herniations are seen.

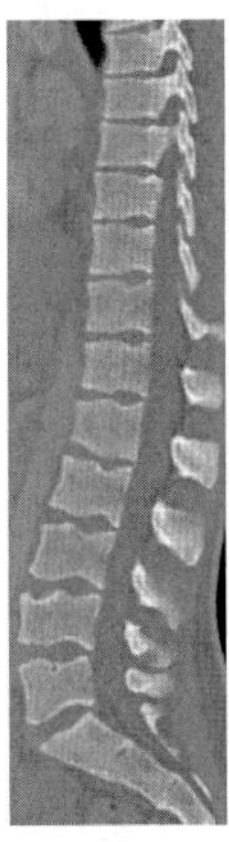

Figure 78.7

Sagittal CT shows the lumbar variant of Scheuermann disease with involvement of at least three contiguous lumbar vertebrae (**Figure 78.7**). There is diffuse loss of intervertebral disc height, mild anterior vertebral wedging, undulation of endplates, and discrete Schmorl's nodes involving the lumbar spine only.

Management

Treatment is usually conservative and includes observation and/or bracing. Surgical treatment with instrumented spinal fusion is considered when there is >75° kyphosis in a skeletally immature patient or >60° kyphosis in a skeletally mature patient, uncontrolled pain, or the presence of a neurological deficit usually secondary to disc herniation.

Teaching Points

► Scheuermann disease is a skeletal growth abnormality resulting in increased thoracic kyphosis.
► The diagnosis is demonstrated on radiographs or CT by the involvement of three contiguous vertebral body levels with Schmorl's nodes and at least 5° of anterior vertebral body wedging at each level.
► Treatment is usually conservative. However, surgical fusion or hardware instrumentation is considered in severe cases with kyphosis >75° in a skeletally immature patient or >60° kyphosis in a skeletally mature patient, or in the setting of uncontrolled pain or neurological deficits.

Further Reading

1. Khoury NJ, Hourani MH, Arabi MM, et al. Imaging of back pain in children and adolescents. Curr Probl Diagn Radiol 2006;35(6):224–244.
2. Swischuk L, John S, and Allbery S. Disk degenerative disease in childhood: Scheuermann's disease, Schmorl's nodes, and the limbus vertebra: MRI findings in 12 patients. Pediatr Radiol 1998;28:334–338.

H. Kate Lee, Ahmad Nassr, and Daniel Park

History

▶ A 73-year-old male presents with progressive myeloradiculopathy and neck stiffness. A physical examination demonstrated hand wasting and difficulty with balance and gait (**Figures 79.1, 79.2, and 79.3**).

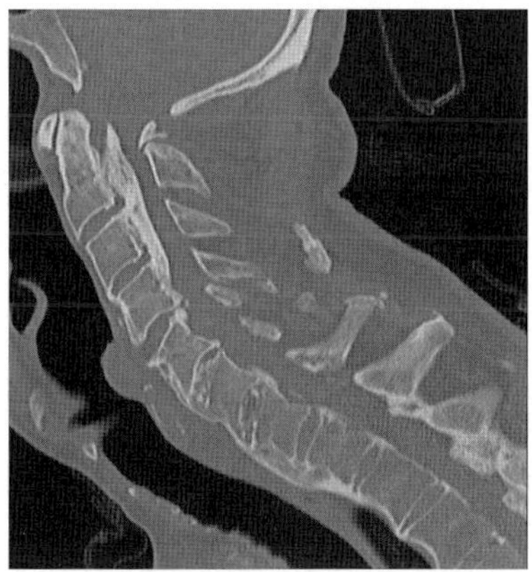

Figure 79.1

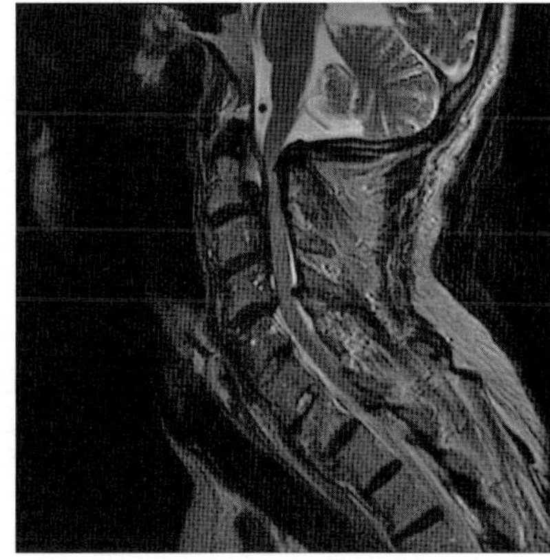

Figure 79.2

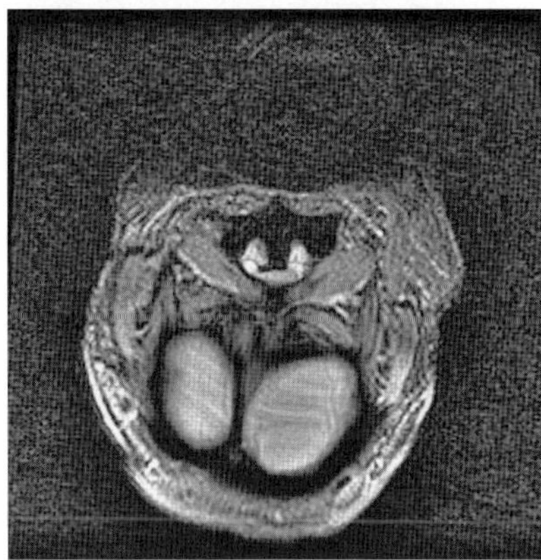

Figure 79.3

Chapter 79 Ossified Posterior Longitudinal Ligament

Findings

Ossification of the posterior longitudinal ligament (OPLL). Sagittal CT reconstruction (**Figure 79.1**) shows segmental OPLL at C2, C3, and C4 vertebral bodies. Anteriorly, there is anterior longitudinal ligament ossification from C3–C4 and C5 to T2 indicating diffuse idiopathic skeletal hyperostosis (DISH). A sagittal T2-weighted sequence MR (**Figure 79.2**) demonstrates severe spinal stenosis at the C2–C3, C3–C4, and C4–C5 levels. At the level of C2, the cervical cord is narrowed in anteroposterior diameter with a T2 hyperintense signal indicating myelomalacia. An axial T2 image at the level of C2 (**Figure 79.3**) demonstrates a thickened ligament consistent with OPLL deforming the spinal cord.

Differential Diagnosis

▶ Calcified herniated disc
▶ Calcified meningioma
▶ Calcified epidural hematoma

Discussion

OPLL occurs most commonly in the cervical spine (75%), then the thoracic spine (15%), and least commonly in the lumbar spine (10%). The exact pathogenesis is unclear. It is more common in male patients and the Asian population, especially Japanese (up to 2%). OPLL is associated with DISH, ossification of the yellow ligament, and ankylosing spondylitis. OPLL can be continuous, segmental, or both.

Radiological Evaluation

CT best demonstrates linear ossification in the spinal canal immediately posterior to the vertebral body (Figure 79.1) as it delineates the shape and size accurately. MR, especially T2-weighted sequences, detects not only ossification but also disc herniation and spinal cord changes. However, MRI has the limitation of showing unclear outline images of bone cortex (Figures 79.2 and 79.3).

Management

The natural history of OPLL has been studied extensively. The majority of patients are asymptomatic, but up to 22% of patients may present with either stiffness of the affected area of the spine, or more commonly with neurological complaints related to spinal cord compression. In patients with minimal symptoms, nonoperative treatment has been shown to be equivalent to surgical management. When myelopathy worsens, surgery intervention is strongly recommended as surgical patients maintained functional status much better than patients with nonoperative treatment.

Surgical options include anterior decompression and fusion, posterior laminectomy with or without fusion, and posterior laminoplasty (**Figures 79.4, 79.5, 79.6, and 79.7**). With the cervical spine being the most affected region in most patients, there is still controversy over the ideal approach. Anterior surgery has been suggested to have better clinical outcomes than posterior laminectomy with fusion; however, other studies demonstrate similar neurological recovery rates between posterior and anterior surgery but with higher surgical complications with anterior surgery. The degree of canal compromise dictated the approach; there were better outcomes with anterior surgery if canal compromise was >60%.

It is our opinion that if the patient has a lordotic or neutral alignment then a posterior approach is typically chosen whereas if kyphosis is present, an anterior approach may be necessary with or without concomitant posterior surgery. This may be complicated because the OPLL is often tightly adherent to the dura. The patient in this case was treated with a posterior C1–C5 decompressive laminectomy and instrumented fusion of C2–T2. Interestingly, despite surgical treatment, radiographic progression of OPLL occurred in as high as 70% of cases, but only 3% had recurrent symptoms.

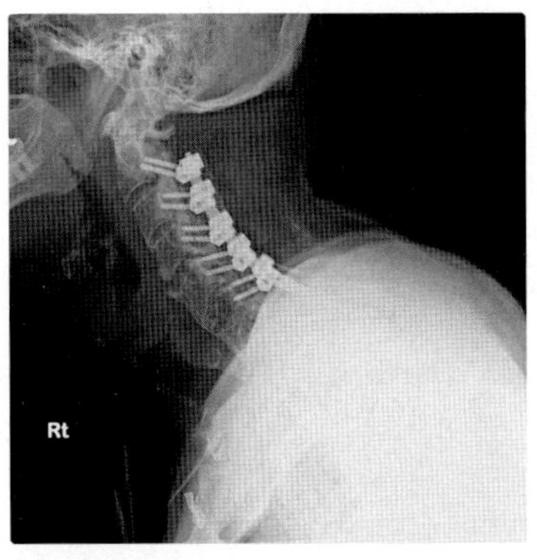

Figure 79.4

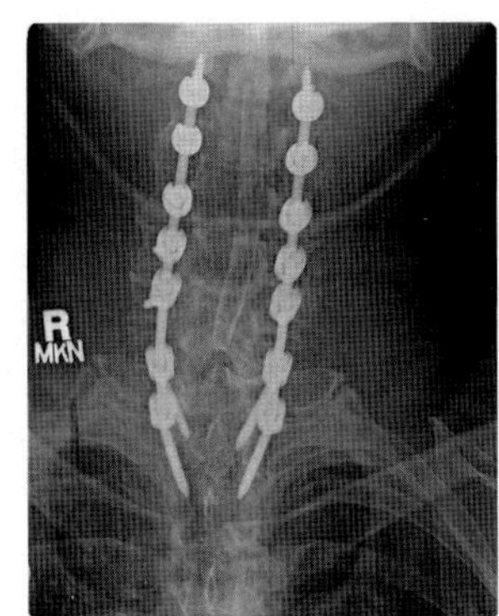

Figure 79.5

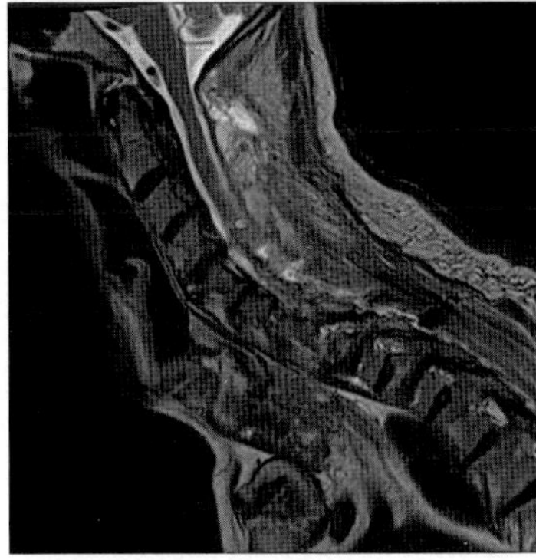

Figure 79.6

Figure 79.7

Postoperative imaging (Figures 79.4, 79.5, 79.6, and 79.7). Lateral and frontal (**Figures 79.4 and 79.5**) radiographs of the cervical spine demonstrate the expected appearance of posterior spinal fusion of the cervical spine. Sagittal T2 MR images (**Figures 79.6 and 79.7**) depict excellent decompression of the cervical canal at the level of C2.

Teaching Points

▶ OPLL is a progressive disorder.

▶ OPLL has a higher incidence among Asian patients, although any race may be affected.

▶ If there is suspicion of a thickened posterior longitudinal ligament on MR, a CT scan can be informative with regard to the surgical approach.

▶ A posterior approach is preferred to avoid the complications associated with anterior surgery. If a patient has lordotic or neutral alignment, posterior-based surgery is typically the surgical approach of choice.

▶ Surgery is highly recommended in patients with myeloradiculopathy and OPLL.

Further Reading

1. Tsuyama N. OPLL of the spine. Clin Orthop Relat Res 1984;184:71–84.
2. Saetia K, et al. OPLL: A review. Neurosurg Focus 2011;30(3):E1.
3. Choi BW, et al. OPLL: A review of literature. Asian Spine J 2011;5(4):267–276.
4. Sugita S, et al. Progression of OPLL of the thoracic spine following posterior decompression and stabilization. J Neurosurg Spine 2014;21(5):773–777.
5. Hirai T, et al. OPLL and ligamentum flavum: Imaging features. Semin Musculoskelet Radiol 2001;5(2):83–88.
6. Matsunaga S, et al. Pathogenesis of myelopathy in patients with OPLL. J Neurosurg 2002;96(2 Suppl):168–172.
7. Epstein NE. The surgical management of OPLL in 43 North Americans. Spine 1994;19(6):664–672.
8. Iwasaki M, et al. Surgical strategy for cervical myelopathy due to OPLL. Part 2: Advantages of anterior decompression and fusion over laminoplasty. Spine 2007;32:647–653 and 654–660.

Chapter 80

Cornelia Wenokor and Mark M. Mikhael

History

► A 57-year-old male after previous spinal fusion presents with several weeks of neck pain (**Figure 80.1**).

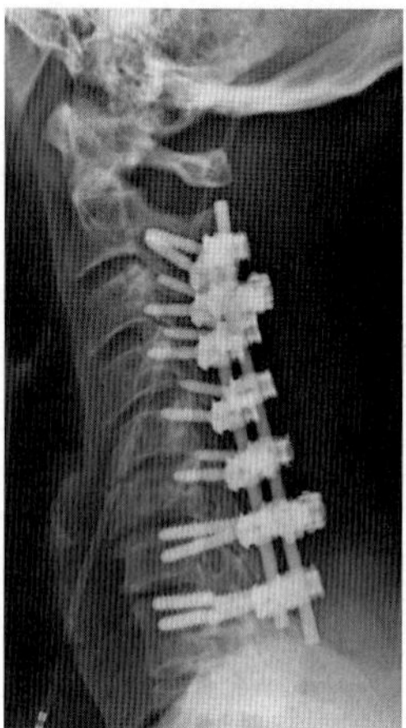

Figure 80.1

Findings

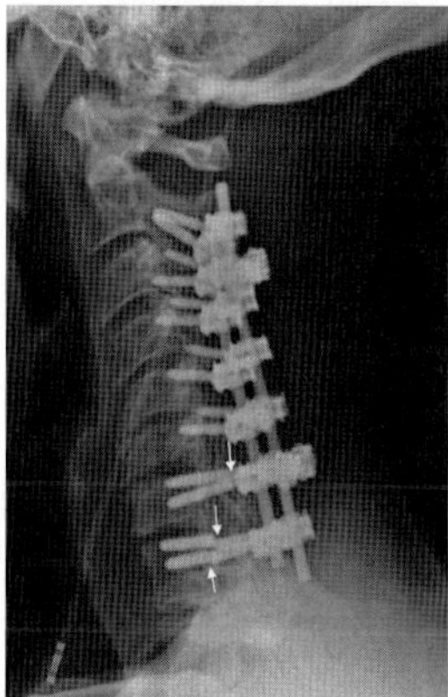

Figure 80.2

Spinal instrumentation failure (**Figure 80.2**). A lateral radiograph of the cervical spine demonstrates fractured pedicle screws at C6 and C7 (arrows).

Discussion

Spinal implants provide stability and restore alignment after operative treatment of fractures, degenerative disc disease, infection, tumor, and congenital deformities. They result in immediate stability, but if no bony fusion occurs they eventually fail due to prolonged stress and result in fatigue fractures in the metal. Fixation implants need to be assessed for adequate positioning and to ensure anatomic alignment of the fused segments on the initial radiographs. On follow-up, assessments shift toward the detection of spinal fusion or complications such as instrumentation loosening, migration, or breakage.

In the presence of chronic low-grade instability and micromotion, pseudoarthrosis may develop. Pseudoarthrosis represents fibrous rather than osseous union of the fusion mass. Without solid osseous fusion, loosening or fracture of instrumentation may occur. Early complications associated with the placement of spinal implants include hematoma formation, cerebrospinal fluid (CSF) leaks, and infection, as well as malpositioning, which can result in neurovascular injuries. Late complications include recurrent pain, new pain, and neurological symptoms due to new disc herniation, scar formation, and implant complications. Altered biomechanics after fusion increases stress on the levels above and below the fusion, and can lead to accelerated disc degeneration.

Radiological Evaluation

Imaging plays an important role in assessing for potential instrumentation failure and/or complications. The imaging appearance of implant failure varies (**Figures 80.3, 80.4, 80.5, 80.6, 80.7, 80.8, 80.9, 80.10, 80.11, and 80.12**). Comparison with prior radiographs is crucial, especially the immediate postoperative radiographs. Plain films are the initial modality but CT and/or MRI can often supplement cases in which osseous or soft tissue detail requires better delineation.

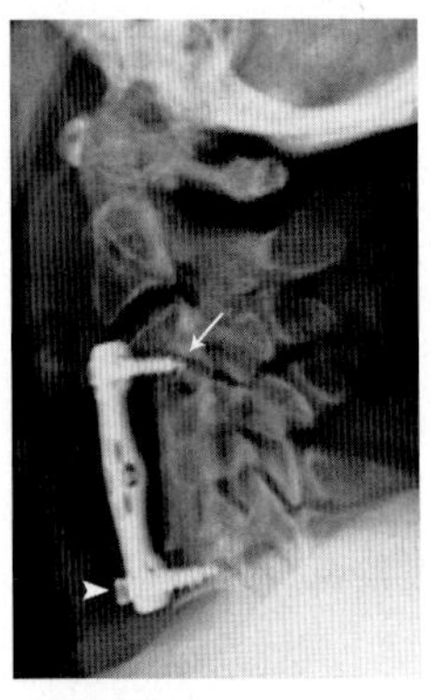

Figure 80.3

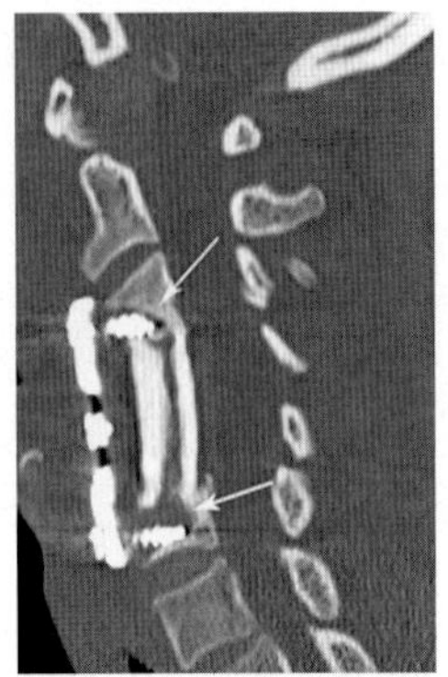

Figure 80.4

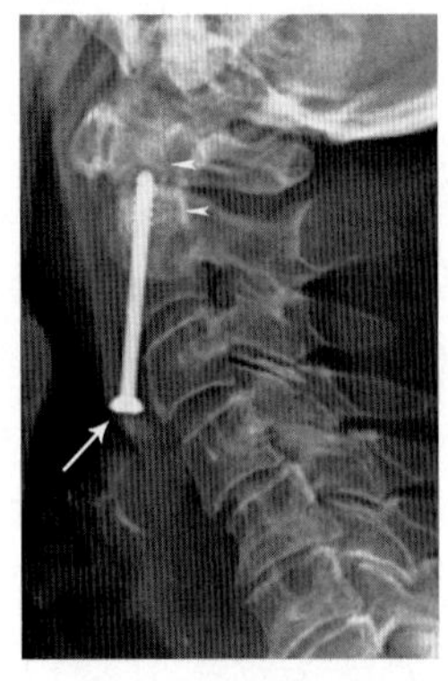

Figure 80.5

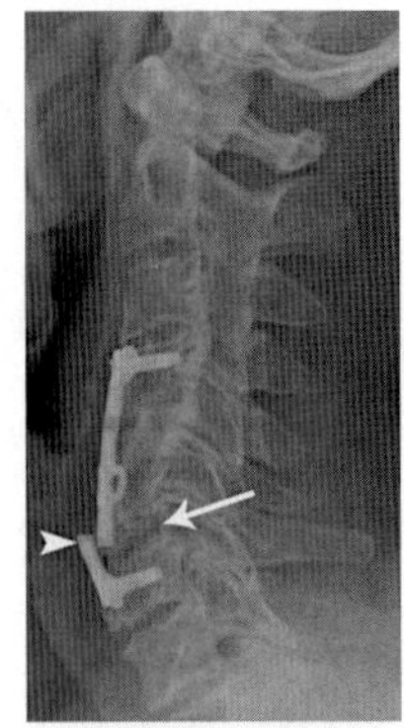

Figure 80.6

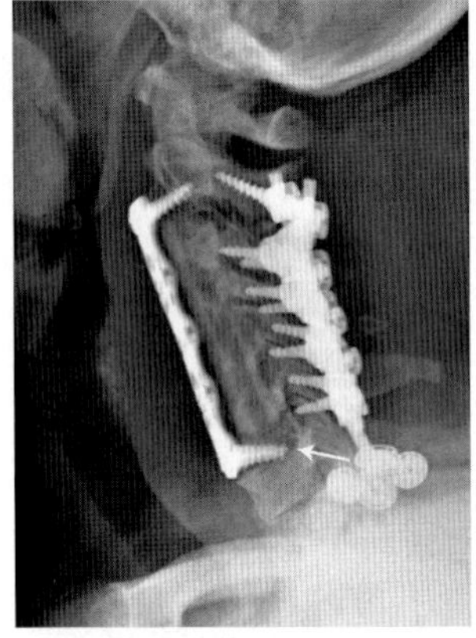

Figure 80.7

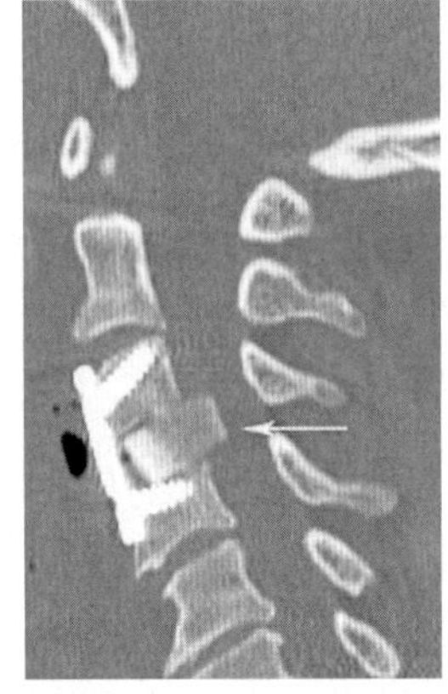

Figure 80.8

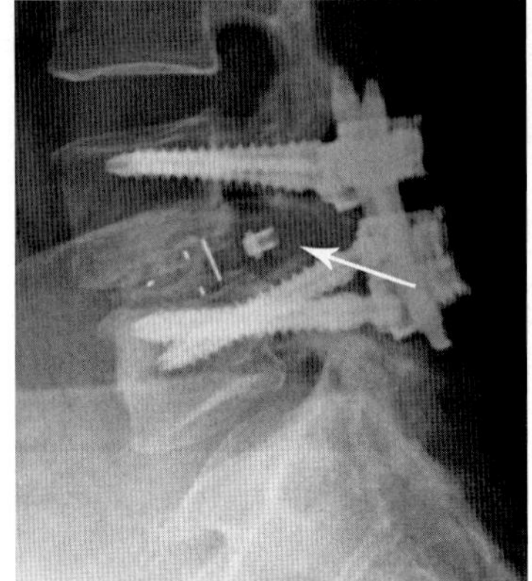

Figure 80.9

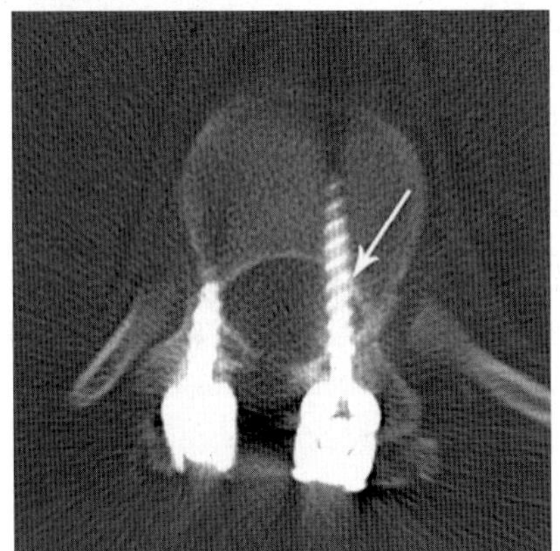

Figure 80.10

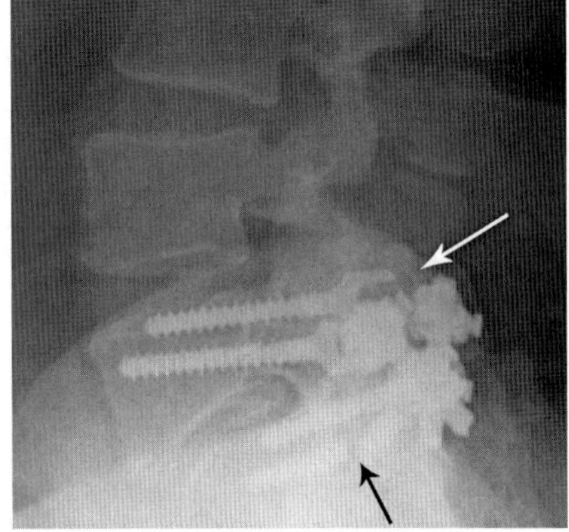

Figure 80.11

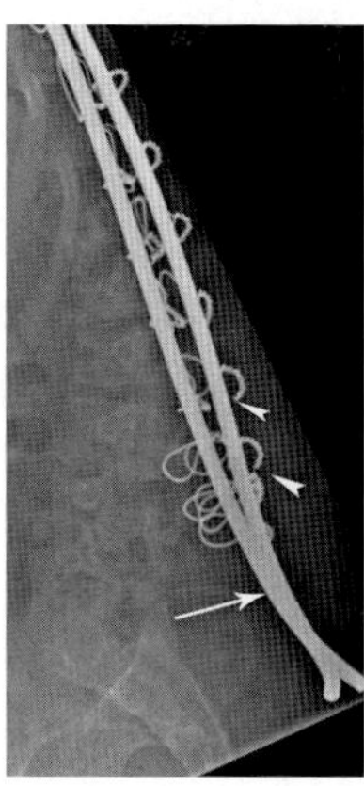

Figure 80.12

Spinal instrumentation failure (**Figures 80.3 and 80.4**). A corpectomy was performed at C4–C5 and a fibular strut graft is present, stabilized by an anterior plate at C3–C6. There is kyphotic angulation at C3–C4. The C3 screws are loose, as there is a lucent halo surrounding the screw (Figure 80.3, arrow). One of the C6 screws is loose as well and is backing out (Figure 80.3, arrowhead). This indicates lack of fusion. Figure 80.4 is a sagittal reformatted image from a CT scan also demonstrating screw loosening (arrows).

Screw fixation after Type II odontoid fracture (Figure 80.5). The screw is backing out (arrow) and now barely bridges the fracture site. The fracture is nonunited and there is slight retrolisthesis of the body of C2 with respect to the dens (arrowheads).

Spinal instrumentation failure (Figure 80.6). There is failure of strut graft incorporation (white arrow) with resultant plate fracture (arrowhead).

Spinal instrumentation failure (Figure 80.7). There is anterior and posterior cervical fusion with screw placement into the disc space at C6–C7 (arrow).

Spinal instrumentation failure resulting in cord compression (Figures 80.8 and 80.9). The interbody bone graft is protruding into the spinal canal (arrow, Figure 80.8) resulting in cord compression. The screws at C3 and C4 are close to the endplates; ideally, there should be at least a 2 mm distance from the endplate cortex. The lumbar disc TLIF spacer migrated posteriorly (arrow, Figure 80.9), with resultant canal stenosis.

Malpositioning (Figure 80.10). A malpositioned left-sided pedicle screw is placed into the spinal canal (arrow).

Spinal instrumentation failure (Figure 80.11). There are disengaged spinal rods from the L5 pedicle screws (white arrow) and pedicle screw fracture at S1 (black arrow).

Spinal instrumentation failure (Figure 80.12). There are disengaged and posteriorly displaced (arrow) Luque rods with fractured cerclage wire fixation (arrowheads).

Management

Management varies, depending on the nature of the complication. In the setting of pseudoarthrosis or lack of fusion, implants generally will be removed and revision bone grafting with instrumented stabilization will be undertaken. In cases of infections with instrumentation, thorough irrigation and debridement along with intravenous antibiotic therapy are instituted; in many circumstances, the implants can be retained unless they are grossly loose or fractured.

Teaching Points

► Radiographs are the main modality for routine follow-up examinations.
► CT is standard for postoperative assessment of hardware and MRI is essential in the work-up of infection.

Further Reading

1. Young PM, Berquist TH, Bancroft LW, and Peterson JJ. Complications of spinal instrumentation. Radiographics 2007;27(3):775–789.
2. Hayashi D, et al. Imaging features of postoperative complications after spinal surgery and instrumentation. AJR 2012;199:W123–W129.
3. Karasick D, Schweitzer ME, and Vacaro AR. Complications of cervical spine fusion: Imaging features. AJR 1997;169:869–874.

Section 9   Signs in Radiology

Eric Friedberg and Paul Harkey

History

▶ A 63-year-old male presents with chronic renal insufficiency and back pain (**Figures 81.1, and 81.2**).

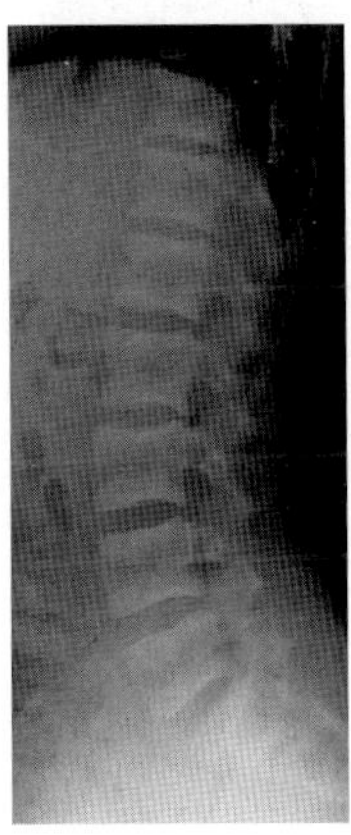

Figure 81.1

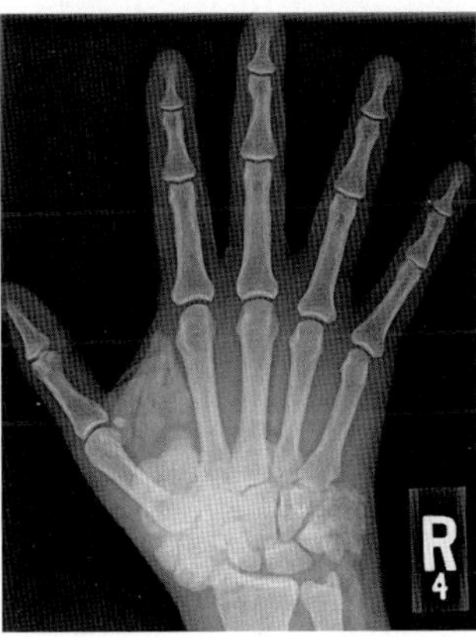

Figure 81.2

Chapter 81 Rugger Jersey Sign

Findings

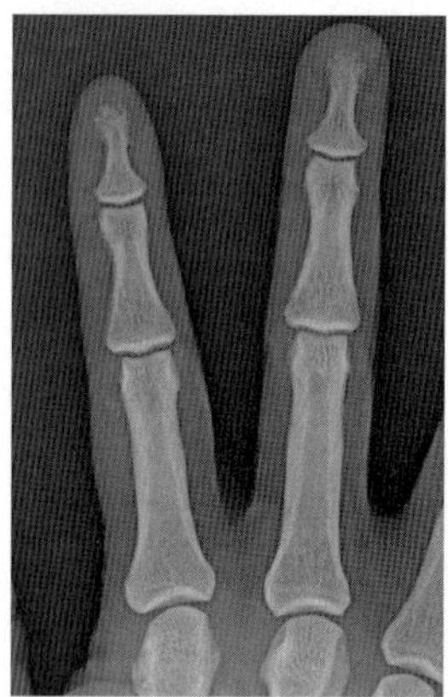

Figure 81.3

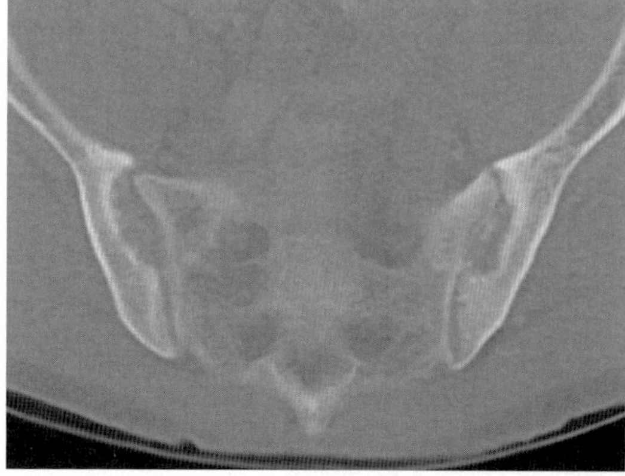

Figure 81.4

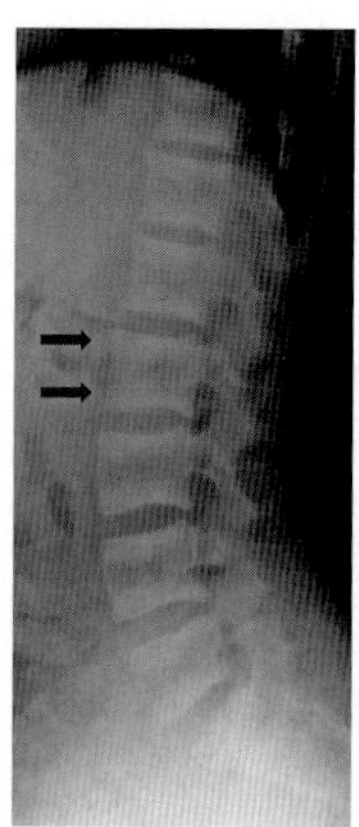

Figure 81.5

Rugger jersey spine (**Figures 81.1, 81.2, 81.3, 81.4, 81.5, 81.6, and 81.7**). A lateral lumbar spine radiograph (Figure 81.5) demonstrates alternating bands of vertebral endplate sclerosis (arrows).

A frontal right hand radiograph (Figure 81.2) demonstrates cloud-like mineral deposition in the thenar and carpal regions in keeping with tumoral calcinosis of renal failure. A coned down radiograph of the index and middle fingers (Figure 81.3) depicts classic subperiosteal resorption along the radial aspects of the middle phalanges and tuft resorption (acroosteolysis) of the index finger.

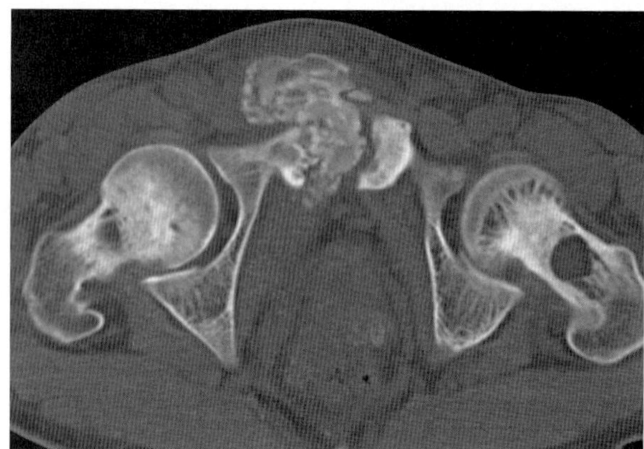

Figure 81.6

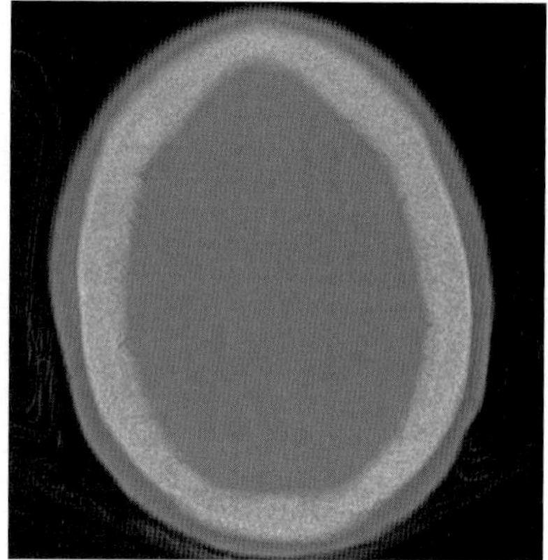

Figure 81.7

Axial CT images of the sacrum (Figure 81.4), pubic symphysis (Figure 81.6), and skull (Figure 81.7) show sacroiliac joint widening secondary to subchondral resorption, which is also seen in the pubic symphysis (Figure 81.6) where there is calcinosis of renal failure (note calcium fluid levels) with associated symphyseal resorption. The calvarium (Figure 81.7) demonstrates a granular sclerotic "salt and pepper" appearance with obscuration of inner and outer table differentiation.

Differential Diagnosis

- Osteopetrosis
- Paget disease
- Lymphoma
- Metastasis

Discussion

"Rugger jersey spine" is an osseous manifestation most often associated with secondary hyperparathyroidism in chronic renal insufficiency (CRI). The pathophysiology is complex, initiated by decreased renal function leading to an accumulation of phosphate and decreased activation of vitamin D. Increased phosphate binds serum calcium resulting in hypocalcemia. Decreased vitamin D activation leads to calcium malabsorption from the gastrointestinal tract. These processes stimulate parathyroid hormone (PTH) release resulting in bone resorption.

Radiological Evaluation

The earliest manifestation and pathognomonic characteristic of CRI involve subperiosteal bone resorption often occurring along the radial aspects of the index and middle fingers (Figures 81.2 and 81.3). Subchondral, subligamentous, and subtendinous bone resorption also occur frequently manifesting as erosions with joint space widening (Figure 81.4). Increased osteoclastic activity may result in well-defined lytic bone lesions known as Brown tumors and may be confused with more malignant processes. Granular sclerosis of the calvarium may also be seen with decreased differentiation of the inner and outer tables of the skull (Figure 81.7). Decreased vitamin D levels of CRI cause defective bone mineralization yielding osteomalacia, which may demonstrate looser zones and progression to displaced fractures. CRI causes increased soft tissue calcifications and may manifest as chondrocalcinosis (CPPD) in the knee, wrist, and pubic symphysis or may deposit in periarticular soft tissues as cloud-like densities indistinguishable from primary tumoral calcinosis (Figures 81.6, 81.8, and 81.9).

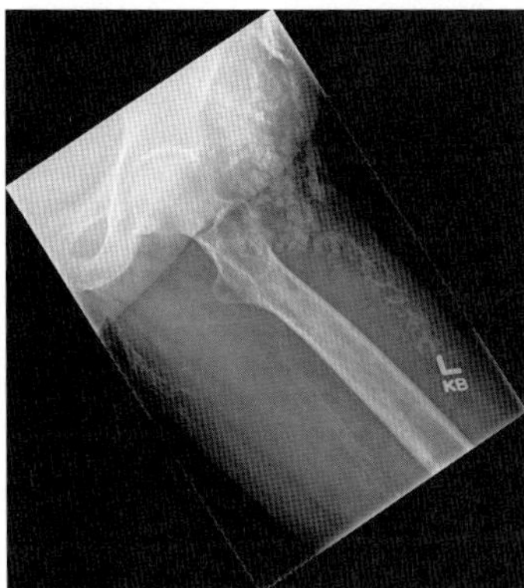

Figure 81.8

Soft tissue calcification in a patient with scleroderma (Figure 81.8). A frog leg view of the left hip demonstrates soft tissue calcification along the soft tissues, a finding seen in several underlying conditions.

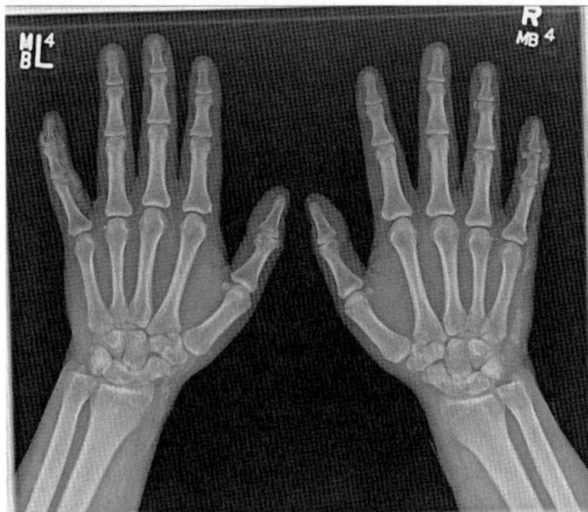

Figure 81.9

Soft tissue calcification in a patient undergoing dialysis therapy (Figure 81.9). Frontal radiographs of the bilateral hands demonstrate soft tissue calcifications mainly along the medial aspects of both hands, most robust adjacent to the bilateral fifth DIP joint spaces. This calcification was related to dialysis therapy.

Management

End-stage renal failure patients are managed with dialysis or a renal transplant.

Teaching Points

► Rugger jersey spine results from alternating bands of vertebral endplate sclerosis brought about by metabolic derangement of calcium associated with elevated PTH.
► A pathognomonic characteristic of CRI is subperiosteal bone resorption.
► CRI may also be associated with CPPD, tumoral calcinosis, and brown tumors.

Further Reading

1. Boswell SB, Patel DB, White EA, et al. Musculoskeletal manifestations of endocrine disorders. Clin Imaging 2014;38(4):384–396.
2. Jevtic V. Imaging of renal osteodystrophy. Eur J Radiol 2003;46(2):85–95.
3. Lim CY and Ong KO. Various musculoskeletal manifestations of chronic renal insufficiency. Clin Radiol 2013;68(7):e397–411.
4. Sundaram M. Renal osteodystrophy. Skeletal Radiol 1989;18(6):415–426.
5. Tigges S, Nance EP, Carpenter WA, and Erb R. Renal osteodystrophy: Imaging findings that mimic those of other diseases. AJR Am J Roentgenol 1995;165(1):143–148.
6. Wittenberg A. The rugger jersey spine sign. Radiology 2004;230(2):491–492.

Eric Friedberg and Paul Harkey

History

▶ A 34-year-old Native American dentist presents with chronic neck pain (**Figure 82.1**).

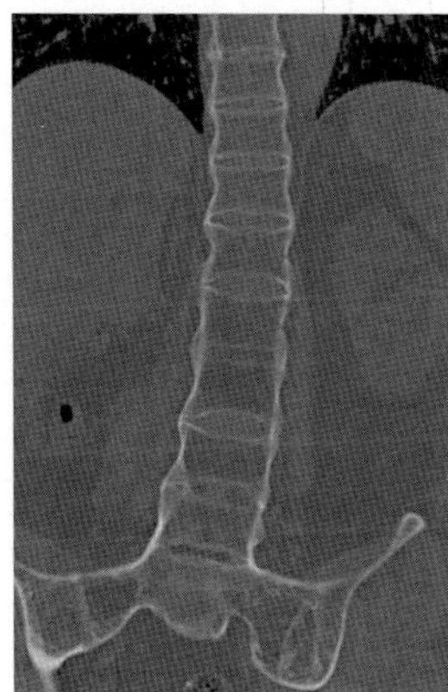

Figure 82.1

Chapter 82   Bamboo Spine

Findings

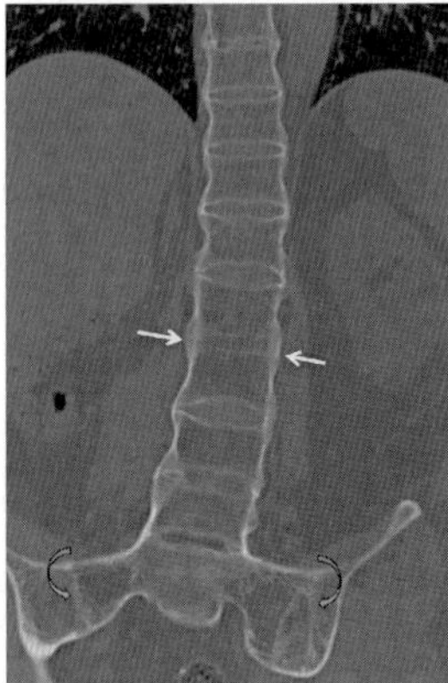

Figure 82.2

Bamboo spine: CT coronal reformat (**Figure 82.2**) demonstrates thin vertical syndesmophytes (arrows) with bridging fusion across all disc spaces ("bamboo spine") and bilateral sacroiliac joint fusion (curved arrows).

Differential Diagnosis

▶ Psoriatic arthritis
▶ Chronic reactive arthritis
▶ Inflammatory bowel disease
▶ Diffuse idiopathic skeletal hyperostosis
▶ Osteoarthritis

Discussion

Ankylosing spondylitis (AS) is an immune-mediated inflammatory process highly associated with the HLA-B27 antigen, which is four times more common in men. Commonly, AS generally presents in patients younger than 40 years of age with chronic back pain persisting greater than 3 months. AS begins with an inflammatory cascade resulting in bony ankylosis (**Figure 82.2**). Potential extraosseous manifestations include acute anterior uveitis, aortitis, heart block, and interstitial lung disease.

Radiological Evaluation

Sacroiliac Joints

One of the earliest and defining findings of AS is sacroiliitis, which can be detected at its earliest stage by MRI demonstrating periarticular edema. Classically, the sacroiliitis is symmetric and bilateral (unlike psoriatic and reactive arthritis). However, unilateral or asymmetric disease is also observed. CT and radiography are useful in identifying subchondral demineralization, erosions, and ankylosis.

Spine

Changes typically begin at the thoracolumbar or lumbosacral locations. Romanus lesions are erosions with adjacent sclerosis occurring at the corners of the vertebral bodies. The sclerosis associated with these lesions is known as "shiny corners" on radiography and CT. As the disease progresses, squaring of the vertebral bodies and syndesmophyte formation occur resulting in a bamboo spine (**Figures 82.3 and 82.4**). The interspinous and supraspinous ligaments can ossify (dagger sign) and facets can fuse (tram track sign) (**Figures 82.5 and 82.6**). Spinal fusion increases the risk for unstable disc space fractures, which maybe subtle.

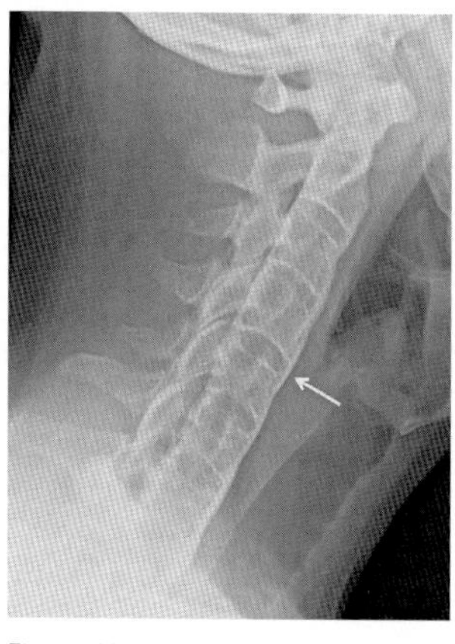
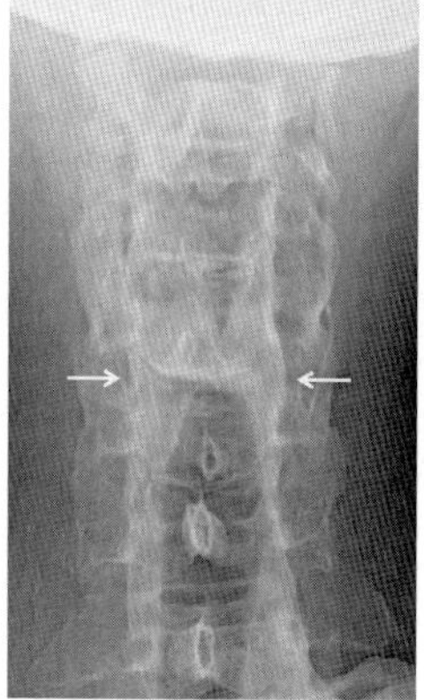

Figure 82.3

Figure 82.4

Lateral (**Figure 82.3**) and frontal (**Figure 82.4**) cervical spine radiographs demonstrating thin vertically oriented syndesmophytes (arrows) flowing along the anterior and lateral vertebral body margins representing ossification of the peripheral fibers of the annulus fibrosis and anterior longitudinal ligament.

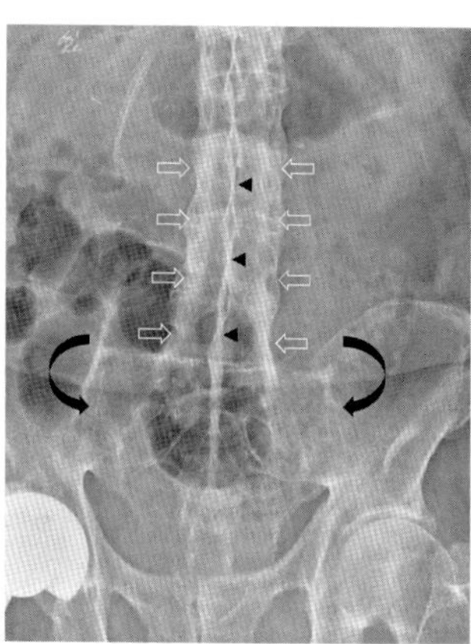
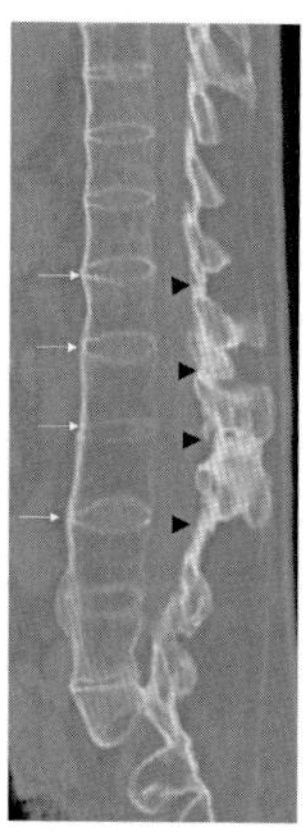

Figure 82.5

Figure 82.6

Frontal (**Figure 82.5**) lumbar spine radiograph and CT sagittal (**Figure 82.6**) reformats through posterior spinous processes depict the dagger sign with supraspinous and interspinous ligament ossification (black arrowheads). Also note bilateral fusion of the sacroiliac joints (black curved arrows), tram track sign from ankylosis of the facet joints (white open arrows), and flowing syndesmophytes anteriorly (thin white arrows).

Management

Current treatment strategies include tumor necrosis factor (TNF)-α inhibitors such as infliximab. Please refer to Chapter 33, "Ankylosing Spondylitis," for further discussion of unstable fracture management.

Teaching Points (Summary)

► Commonly HLA-B27 positive presenting in young males.
► Look for bilateral sacroiliitis with early erosions and subsequent ankylosis.
► Syndesmophytes (bamboo spine) are often seen.
► Scrutinize for unstable spinal fractures.

Further Reading

1. Jang JH, Ward MM, Rucker AN, et al. Ankylosing spondylitis: Patterns of radiographic involvement—a re-examination of accepted principles in a cohort of 769 patients. Radiology 2011;258(1):192–198.
2. Lacout A, Rousselin B, and Pelage JP. CT and MRI of spine and sacroiliac involvement in spondyloarthropathy. AJR Am J Roentgenol 2008;191(4):1016–1023.
3. Bennett DL, Ohashi K, and El-Khoury GY. Spondyloarthropathies: Ankylosing spondylitis and psoriatic arthritis. Radiol Clin North Am 2004;42(1):121–134.
4. Manaster BJ. Ankylosing spondylitis. Statdx. Amirsys, Inc. Retrieved from https://my.statdx.com/STATdxMain.jsp?rc=false#dxContent;ankylosing_spondylitis_dx

History

None.

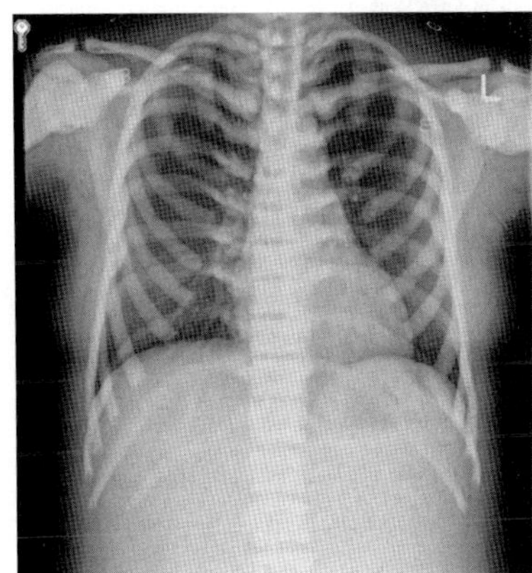

Figure 83.1

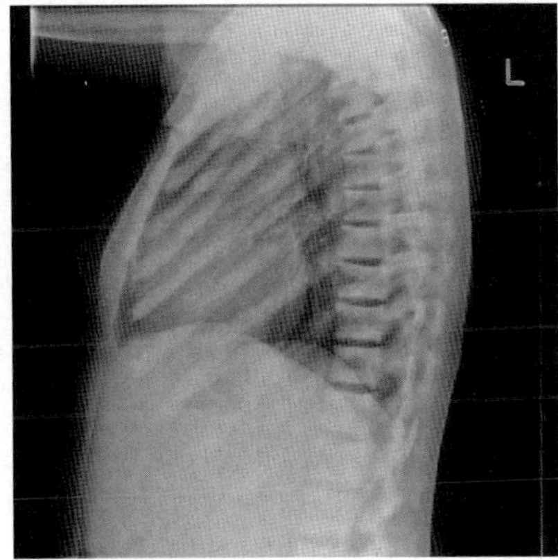

Figure 83.2

Chapter 83　"Bone in a Bone" Appearance

Findings

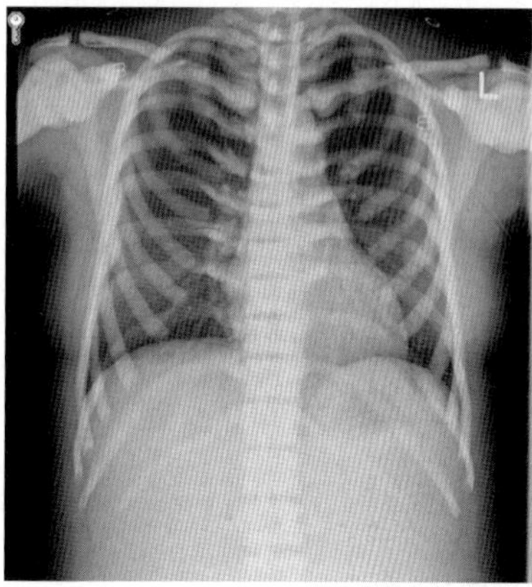

Figure 83.3

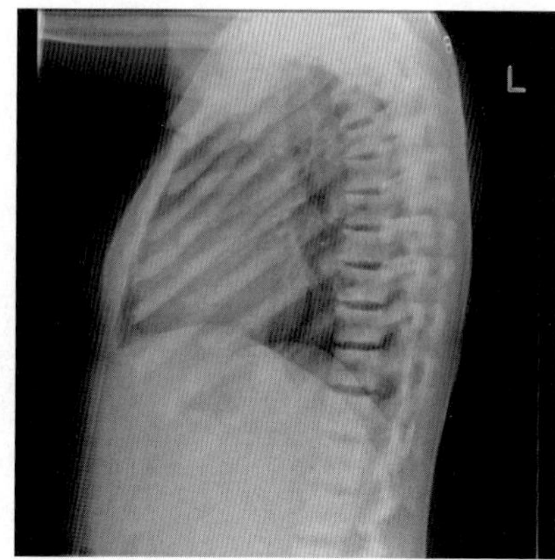

Figure 83.4

Bone in bone appearance. Anteroposterior (AP) (**Figure 83.3**) and lateral (**Figure 83.4**) radiographs of the thoracic spine demonstrate diffusely increased sclerosis, especially at the endplates. Figure 83.2 best shows the bone in a bone appearance within a few vertebral bodies.

Differential Diagnosis

► Normal physiological process in thoracic/lumbar vertebrae in infants and growth recover lines after infancy
► Caffey's disease (infantile cortical hyperostosis)
► Congenital syphilis
► Gaucher disease
► Osteopetrosis/oxalosis
► Sickle cell disease/thalassemia
► Acromegaly
► Paget disease
► Postradiation
► Thorotrast
► Heavy metal ingestion (bismuth, lead, thorium)
► Hypervitaminosis D

Discussion

Bone in a bone appearance is a descriptive term applied to bones that appear to have bone within them due to endosteal new bone formation. There are several causes (refer to the differential diagnosis).

This case illustrates bone in a bone appearance in infantile or autosomal recessive osteopetrosis (also known as Albers–Schonberg disease). It is a rare hereditary disorder due to localized chromosomal defects (11q13) resulting in defective osteoclasts that lack carbonic anhydrase. While bones appear sclerotic and thick, their abnormal structure causes weak and brittle bones, resulting in fractures with poor healing. Additionally, patients present with hepatosplenomegaly as a sign of extramedullary hematopoiesis.

There are two types of osteopetrosis: autosomal recessive (infantile or malignant) and autosomal dominant (adult or benign). Prognosis of the adult type is good with a normal life expectancy, while the infantile subtype can result in stillbirth or death in infancy with few living beyond middle age. Mortality is typically due to bone marrow failure resulting in recurrent infection, hemorrhage, or transformation to leukemia.

Radiological Evaluation

On radiographs and CT, patients with osteopetrosis have a diffusely dense skeleton with "sandwich vertebrae" with bone in a bone appearance, which shows alternating sclerosis and lucency indicating the fluctuating course of the disease (**Figures 83.3 and 83.4**). These patients can present with multiple healing fractures (**Figures 83.4, 83.6, 83.7, 83.8, and 83.9**), metaphyseal flaring with "Erlenmeyer flask deformity" (**Figure 83.7**), poorly pneumatized paranasal sinuses, hypertelorism, and poor dentition due to incomplete enamel formation. "Hair-on-end" skull and hepatosplenomegaly (**Figure 83.10**) indicate extramedullary hematopoiesis. MR will show low signal intensity in sclerotic bones on both T1- and T2-weighted MR images and intermediate signal intensity in marrow-containing areas.

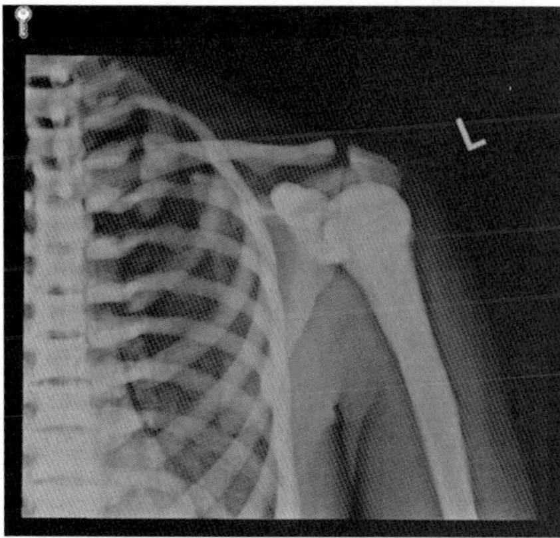

Figure 83.5

Diffuse osseous sclerosis (**Figure 83.5**). A frontal radiograph demonstrates extensive sclerosis of the bones. These patients are prone to fractures.

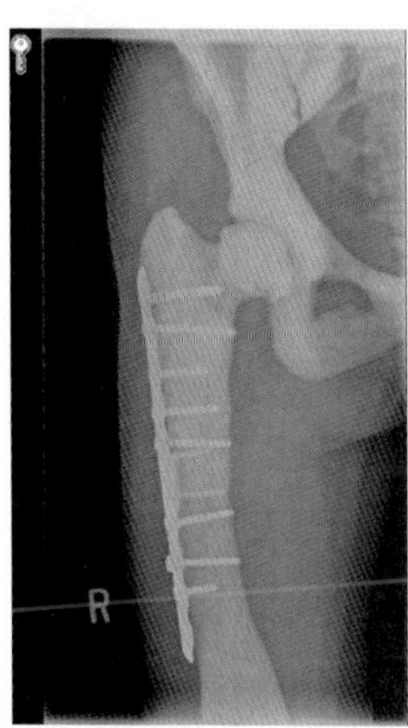
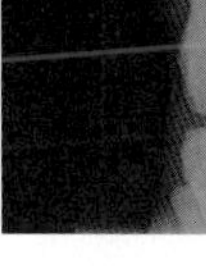
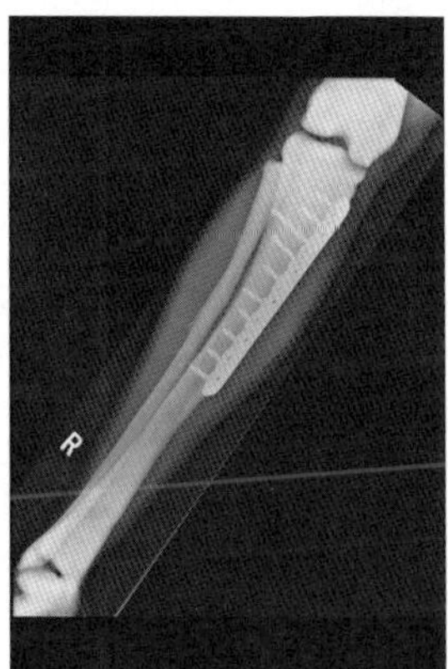

Figure 83.6   Figure 83.7   Figure 83.8

Dense bones with secondary traumatic complications (**Figures 83.6, 83.7, and 83.8**). AP views of the right femur (**Figures 83.6 and 83.7**) and an AP view of the right tibia/fibula demonstrate the diffusely increased density of the bones with postsurgical fixation of the femoral and tibial fractures.

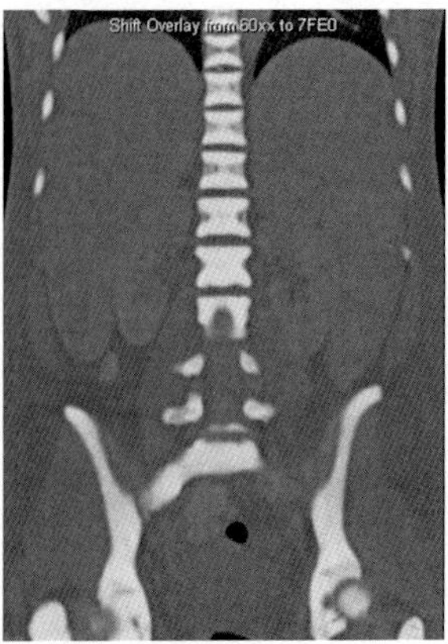

Figure 83.9

Bone in bone appearance on CT (**Figure 83.9**). A coronal CT reformat again demonstrates dense bones and a bone in bone appearance along the thoracolumbar spine.

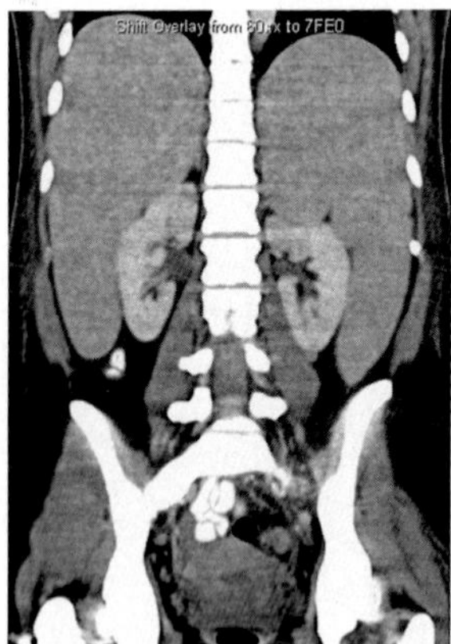

Figure 83.8

Secondary findings seen on CT (**Figure 83.10**). Coronal CT reformatted image demonstrates hepatosplenomegaly indicating extramedullary hematopoiesis.

Management

Treatment of the underlying condition is typically indicated. Surgical fixation can manage complications such as fractures. Patients with osteopetrosis may have acute leukemia and treatment involves bone marrow transplant to restore normal hematopoietic marrow function and bone production.

Teaching Points

▶ Bone in a bone appearance describes bones that have another bone within them and can be seen in a number of conditions.

▶ Management involves treatment of the underlying condition.

Further Reading

1. Wilson CJ and Vellodi A. Autosomal recessive osteopetrosis: Diagnosis, management, and outcome. Arch Dis Child 2000;83(5):449–452.
2. Gerritsen EJ, Vossen JM, van Loo IH, et al. Autosomal recessive osteopetrosis: Variability of findings at diagnosis and during the natural course. Pediatrics 1994;93(2):247–253.
3. Elster AD, Theros EG, Key LL, and Chen MY. Cranial imaging in autosomal recessive osteopetrosis. Part I. Facial bones and calvarium. Radiology 1992;183(1):129–135.

Keith A. Cauley and Christopher G. Filippi

History

▶ Fluorography was performed for an image-guided lumbar puncture (**Figure 84.1**).

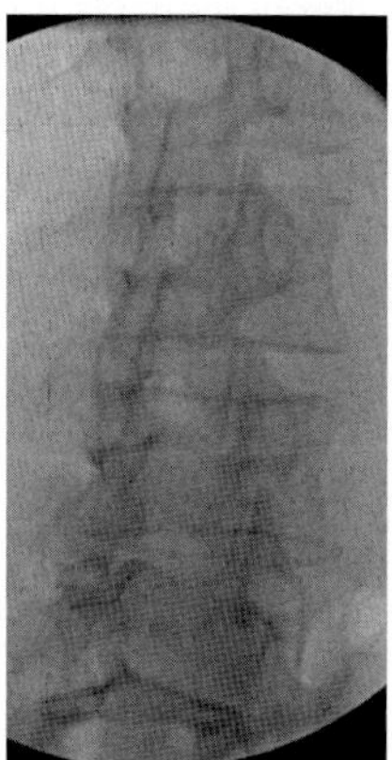

Figure 84.1

Chapter 84   Scotty Dog Sign

Findings

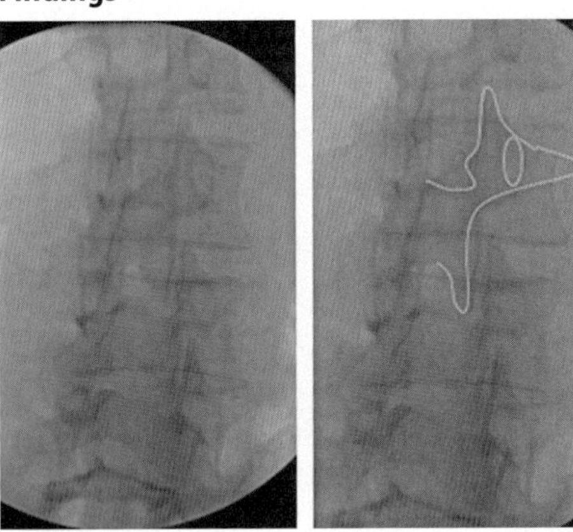

Figure 84.2

"Scotty dog sign" (**Figures 84.1 and 84.2**). Oblique fluoroscopic views of the lumbar spine outline the "scotty dog sign."

Discussion

The "scotty dog sign" refers to the normal appearance of the lumbar vertebral bodies on oblique plain film or fluoroscopic views and can be useful in the assessment of fractures of the pars interarticularis.

Radiological Evaluation

The pars interarticularis is the neck of the dog, and a fracture of the pars is well seen on oblique views when the scotty dog sign is visible. The transverse process is the nose of the dog. The eye of the dog is the end-on view of the pedicle. The inferior articulating facet is the front leg of the dog; the superior articulating facet is the ear of the dog.

Pars interarticularis defects (pars defects) will be seen as lucency through the neck of the dog, and will appear as a white or gray-white collar (**Figure 84.3**). Pars defects are seen in spondylolysis, and are a common cause of back pain.

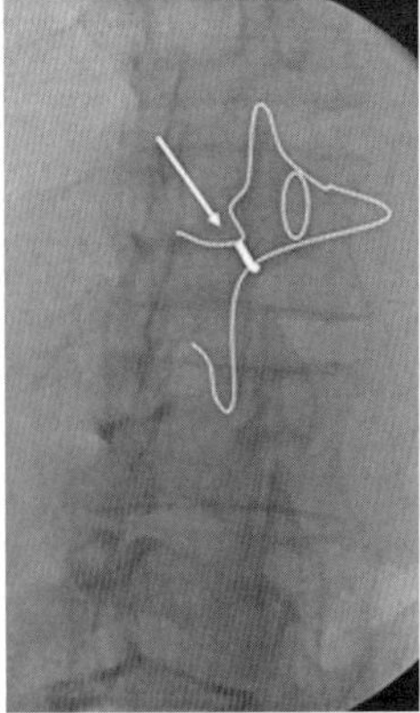

Figure 84.3

"Collar" of the "scotty dog sign" (**Figure 84.3**). Pars interarticularis defects (pars defects) are seen as lucency through the neck of the dog, and will appear as a white or gray-white collar.

Portions of the "scotty dog" are as follows:

▶ Neck—pars interarticularis
▶ Eye—pedicle
▶ Ear—superior articulating facet
▶ Front leg—inferior articulating facet
▶ Nose—transverse process

Management

Please refer to Chapter 36, "Pars Defects."

Teaching Points

▶ The "scotty dog sign" refers to the normal appearance of the lumbar vertebral bodies when seen obliquely on plain film or fluorographic studies.
▶ Chronic fracture through the pars interarticularis is seen in spondylolysis, and appears as a lucency through the neck of the dog, or a "collar" on the "scotty dog."

Further Reading

1. Millard L. The scotty dog and his collar. J Ark Med Soc 1976;72(8):339–340.

Chapter 85

Jaspreet Bajwa and Shivani Gupta

History

► See Figures 85.1 and 85.2.

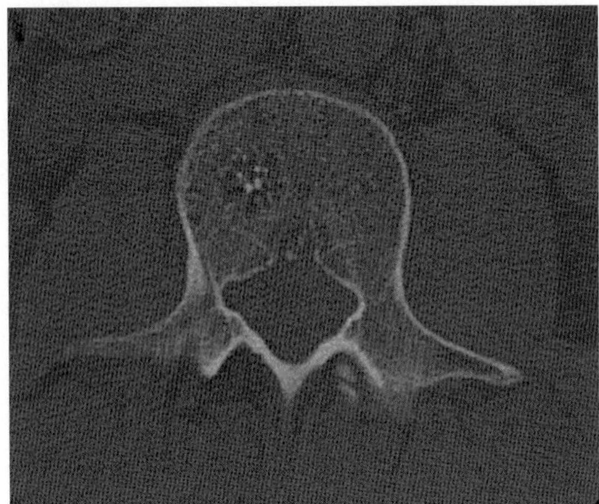

Figure 85.1

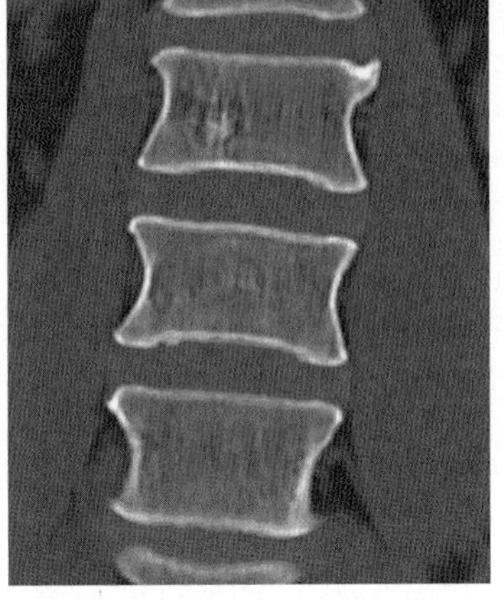

Figure 85.2

Findings

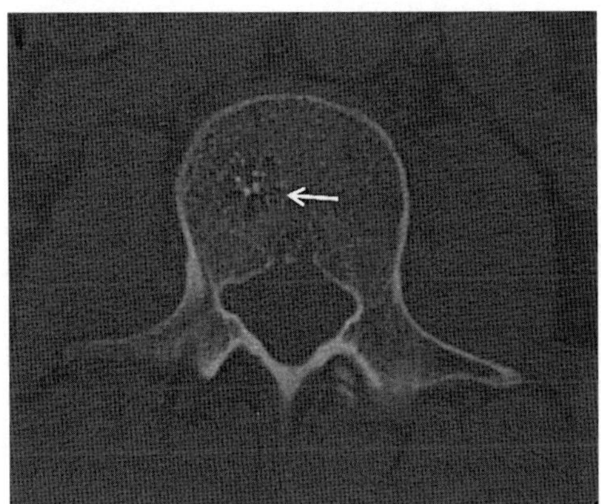

Figure 85.3

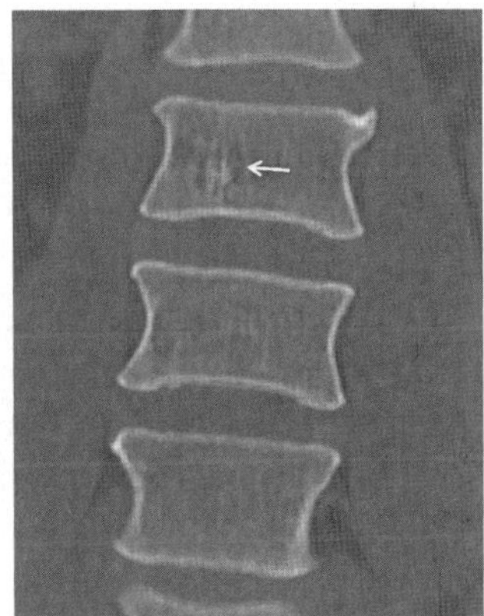

Figure 85.4

Polka-dot sign (**Figures 85.3 and 85.4**). Axial and sagittal CT images in bone windows demonstrate a focal lesion within a vertebral body. This lesion has a prominent trabecular pattern (white arrows). The cortex is not thickened and the surrounding soft tissues are normal. This is characteristic of an intraosseous hemangioma of the spine.

Discussion

The polka-dot sign refers to an imaging finding seen on CT imaging. The polka-dot appearance is seen within the medullary cavity of a vertebral body as several rounded high-attenuation foci. These foci are the result of thickened trabeculae in a vertebral body hemangioma. Thickening of the trabeculae occurs due to reinforcement of the osseous network adjacent to the vascular channels of the lesion, all of which occurs in the fatty marrow.

Hemangiomas of the spine are benign and are most common in the lower thoracic spine. They are most commonly asymptomatic and are more frequent in females. Complications are rare but include compression (pathological fractures), thrombosis, and pain (due to displacement of adjacent nerves).

Imaging Findings

On CT imaging, the polka-dot appearance within a vertebral body is virtually diagnostic of an intraosseous hemangioma. Other entities are possible, but will have more aggressive associated features such as an associated soft tissue mass, destruction of the bone cortex, or invasion of the periosteum. These lesions include sarcomas (including primary Ewing sarcoma of the spine), metastases, multiple myeloma, lymphoma, and chondrosarcomas.

MR imaging is occasionally needed in cases of atypical CT features. On both T1- and T2-weighted imaging, the lesion will demonstrate increased signal intensity. This increased signal is dependent on the degree of fat present, which can be variable.

Management

The majority of spinal hemangiomas require no treatment. If symptomatic, treatment options include vascular embolization, surgical excision, or vertebroplasty.

Teaching Points

▶ The polka dot sign is seen on CT imaging.

▶ The appearance is due to thickened trabeculae in a vertebral body hemangioma.

▶ Associated aggressive features should raise suspicion of a different underlying diagnosis.

Further Reading

1. Laredo JD, Reizine D, Bard M, and Merland JJ. Vertebral hemangiomas: Radiologic evaluation. Radiology 1986;161:183–189.
2. Bemporad JA, Sze G, Chaloupka JC, and Duncan C. Pseudohemangioma of the vertebrae: An unusual radiographic manifestation of primary Ewing's sarcoma. AJNR Am J Neuroradiol 1999;20(10):1809–1813.
3. Murphey MD, Fairbairn KJ, Parman LM, et al. Musculoskeletal angiomatous lesions: Radiologic-pathologic correlation. RadioGraphics 1995;15:893–915.
4. Karlin CA and Brower AC. Multiple primary hemangiomas of bone. AJR Am J Roentgenol 1977;129:162–164.

Bita Ameri and Shivani Gupta

History

▶ A 64-year-old woman with a history of breast cancer presents with back pain (**Figure 86.1**).

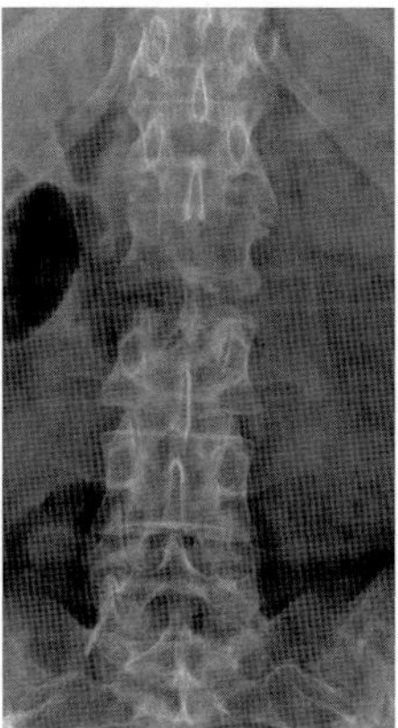

Figure 86.1

Chapter 86 Winking Owl Sign

Findings

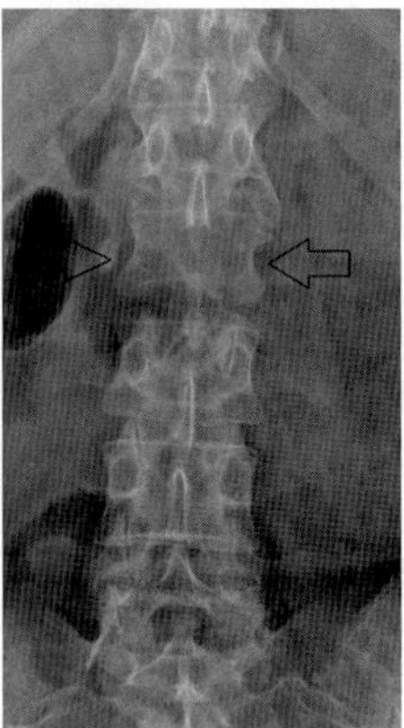

Figure 86.2

Absent pedicle sign ("winking owl sign") secondary to metastatic breast cancer. A frontal radiograph of the spine (**Figure 86.2**) shows the absence of the bilateral L2 pedicles (arrows). The "winking owl" sign at these levels is highly suspicious for osteolytic metastatic disease.

Differential Diagnosis

► Spinal metastasis
► Primary bone lesion
► Radiation effects
► Congenital anomalies (hypoplasia, complex pediculate anomaly, Klippel–Feil syndrome)
► Traumatic lesion (fracture, pars defect)
► Granulomatous lesion (tuberculosis, sarcoidosis)
► Degenerative disease
► Vascular lesion
► Neurofibromatosis
► Fibrous dysplasia

Discussion

The absence of the vertebral body pedicle on a frontal X-ray of the spine should raise high suspicion for spinal metastatic disease. The spine is the third most common site for metastatic disease, preceded by the lung and the liver. Tumors that commonly metastasize to the bone are prostate, breast, lung, thyroid, kidney, and pancreatic cancers. The majority of metastatic spinal lesions are extradural lesions, which either arise from the vertebra and extend into the epidural space, or arise purely from the epidural space and erode into bone.

Radiological Evaluation

The radiographic "winking owl sign," also known as the "absent pedicle sign," refers to the unilateral loss of a vertebral body pedicle on a frontal radiograph of the spine. This is due to destruction of the cortical margins of the absent pedicle. Abnormal sclerosis of the underlying bone, such as that seen with metastatic sclerotic disease, can also result in an absent pedicle (see **Figure 86.7** below). On a normal frontal radiograph of the spine, the two pedicles of a vertebral body represent the owl's eyes and the spinous process represents the owl's beak. In the absence of one pedicle, the face is thought to have a "winking" appearance.

Conventional radiographs are standard for the initial evaluation of a patient with back pain; however, up to 40% of metastatic lesions could be missed by radiography alone since detection necessitates a 1-cm-diameter mass or at least 30–50% bone mineral loss. An osseous metastatic lesion can be identified by CT imaging up to 6 months earlier than with conventional radiography. Thus, radiographs should be used in combination with other modalities such as CT, radionuclide bone scan, or MRI to evaluate for suspected metastasis and extent of disease (**Figures 86.3, 86.4, 86.5, 86.6, and 86.7**).

The differential diagnosis for the "winking owl sign" also includes primary bone lesions, radiation effects, congenital anomalies (hypoplasia, complex pediculate anomaly, Klippel–Feil syndrome), trauma (fracture, pars defect), granulomatous lesion (tuberculosis, sarcoidosis), degenerative disease, vascular lesion, neurofibromatosis, or fibrous dysplasia, which are essentially indistinguishable on radiography but can be better delineated using CT imaging.

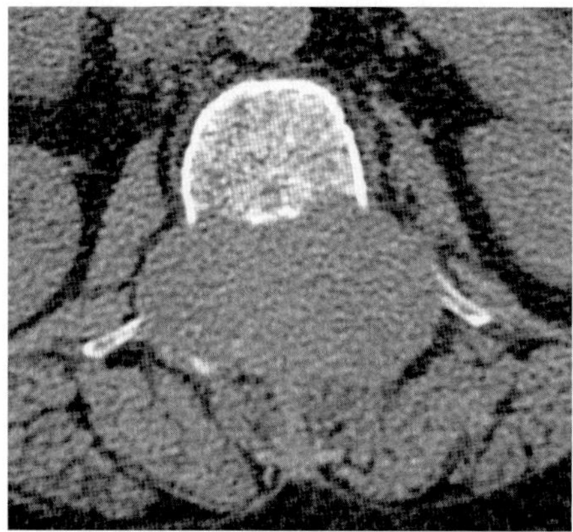

Figure 86.3

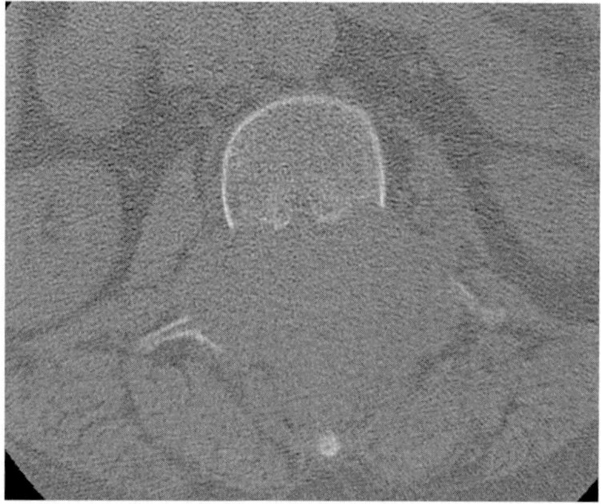

Figure 86.4

CT and MRI findings in metastatic breast cancer (**Figures 86.3, 86.4, and 86.5**). Axial CT (Figures 86.3 and 86.4) at the level of L2 confirms osteolytic metastatic disease with a soft tissue mass eroding the pedicles, transverse processes, and posterior aspect of the vertebral body with invasion into the spinal canal. A sagittal T2-weighted image (Figure 86.5) and a sagittal T1-weighted postcontrast image (**Figure 86.6**) confirm anterior displacement and compression of the cauda equina at the level of L2 by an enhancing soft tissue mass arising from the posterior elements.

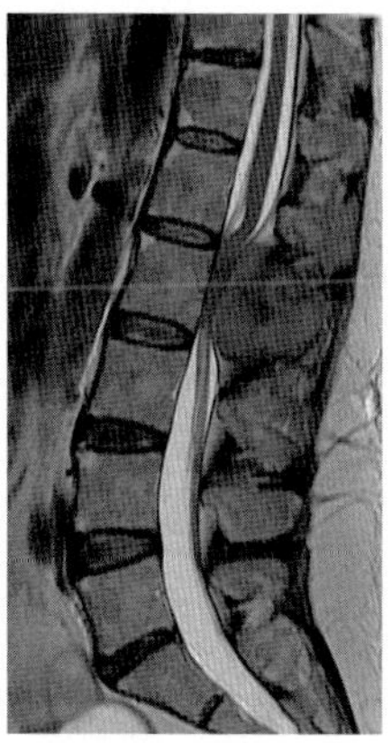
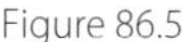

Figure 86.5

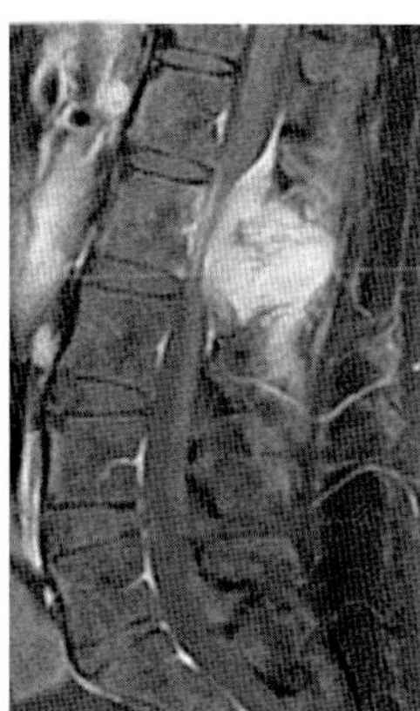

Figure 86.6

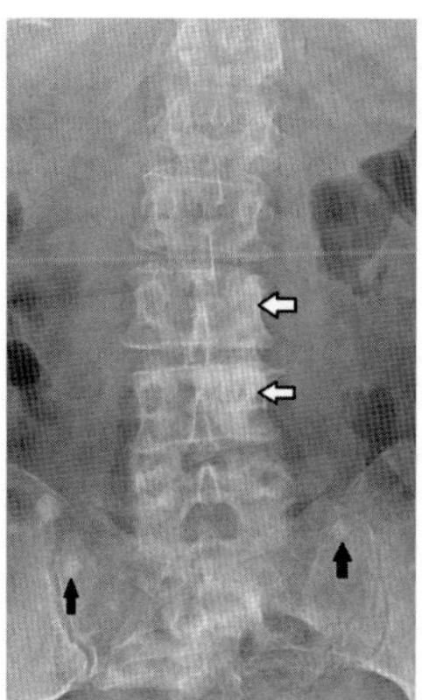

Figure 86.7

Absent pedicle sign secondary to sclerotic metastatic disease (prostate cancer). A frontal radiograph of the lumbar spine (**Figure 86.7**) demonstrates absent pedicles on the left at L3 and L4, later shown to represent sclerotic metastases (white arrows). Sclerotic foci were also seen in the sacrum (black arrows).

Management

Treatment of metastatic spinal disease is based on symptomatology and is primarily palliative. The goal of therapy is to relieve pain, prevent pathological fractures, and maintain or improve mobility. Therapeutic options include local treatment with radiotherapy and/or surgery, and systemic treatment using chemotherapy, endocrine therapy, agents to inhibit bone resorption, as well as pain management drugs. Also refer to Chapter 16 on Metastasis for further discussion on management.

Teaching Points

▶ When evaluating a frontal radiograph of the spine, it is important to look at the pedicles.
▶ The "winking owl sign" is a unilaterally absent vertebral body pedicle, which should raise high suspicion for an underlying bone lesion.

Further Reading

1. Shah LM and Salzman KL. Imaging of spinal metastatic disease. Int J Surg Oncol 2011;2011:769753.
2. Salvo N, Christakis M, Rubenstein J, et al. The role of plain radiographs in management of bone metastases. J Palliative Med 2009;12(2):195–198.
3. Patel NP, Kumar R, Kinkhabwala, M, and Wengrover S. Radiology of lumbar vertebral pedicles: Variants, anomolies, and pathological conditions Radiographics 1987;7(1):101–137.
4. Gold RI, Seeger LL, Bassett LW, and Steckel RJ. An integrated approach to the evaluation of metastatic bone disease. Radiol Clin North Am 1990;28(2):471–483.
5. Nielsen OS, Munro AJ, and Tannock IF. Bone metastases: Pathophysiology and management policy. J Clin Oncol 1991;9(3):509–524.

History

▶ A 47-year-old female presents with back pain. She has no significant past medical history (**Figure 87.1**).

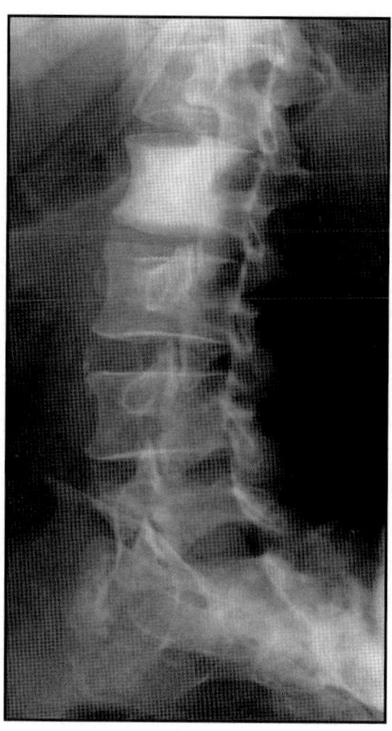

Figure 87.1

Chapter 87   Ivory Vertebra Sign

Findings

Ivory vertebral body. An oblique radiograph of the lumbar spine (**Figure 87.1**) demonstrates diffuse sclerosis of the L2 vertebral body without loss of vertebral body height.

Differential Diagnosis

▶ Malignancy (metastasis versus primary)
▶ Paget disease
▶ Chronic osteomyelitis
▶ Diffuse condensing osteoses (renal osteodystrophy, mastocytosis, osteopetrosis, fluorosis, myelofibrosis, and pycnodysostosis)
▶ SAPHO (synovitis, acne, pustulosis, hyperostosis, osteitis) syndrome
▶ Idiopathic

Discussion

An "ivory vertebra" refers to a diffusely dense vertebra by X-ray or CT that is otherwise normal (with preservation of vertebral body height and its contours). The adjacent intervertebral disc spaces are also preserved and unaffected. The patient's age is useful in stratifying a differential diagnosis. In adults, depending on the history, the underlying etiology is often metastatic (common primary malignancies including prostate or breast cancer) or lymphoma. Paget disease is also important to consider, although it typically causes expansion of a vertebral body with trabecular thickening, as well as a "picture frame vertebra" (sclerosis is most prominent at the periphery of the vertebral body with a lucent center). Chronic infection can also result in an ivory vertebral body, but often, the adjacent disc spaces are abnormal and the vertebral body endplates are irregular. Diffuse condensing osteoses can also result in this sign, such as fluorosis and osteopetrosis. Many of these conditions have associated systemic signs that help narrow the differential diagnosis.

An ivory vertebral body is an uncommon entity in children, but when present tends to be secondary to lymphoma (usually Hodgkins), neuroblastoma, medulloblastoma, osteosarcoma, and less commonly, osteoblastoma. Rarely, Ewing sarcoma can result in an ivory vertebral body.

Radiological Evaluation

Once an ivory vertebral body is detected by CT or X-ray, a nuclear bone scan is commonly performed to assess for the presence of additional osseous lesions, which would then favor a malignant etiology (**Figures 87.2 and 87.3**). Ivory vertebrae commonly demonstrate diffuse uptake of radiotracer on a bone scan or similarly are positive on PET-FDG studies due to the uptake of the radiopharmaceutical (FDG). On MRI, an ivory vertebral body tends to have a low T1WI signal and a slight increase in T2WI signal (see **Figures 87.5, 87.6, and 87.7** below). MRI is useful to help identify an associated soft tissue mass such as may be associated with malignancy or to determine intervertebral disc involvement that can occur with osteomyelitis.

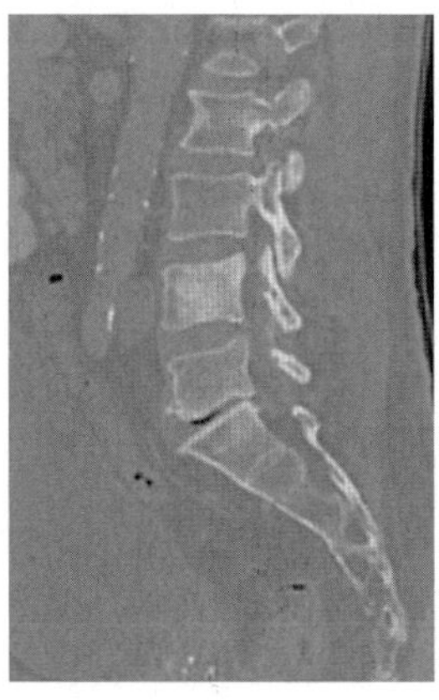
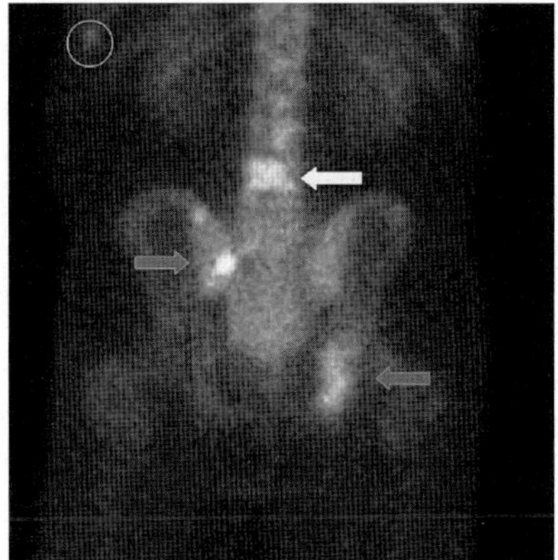

Figure 87.2   Figure 87.3

Ivory vertebral body secondary to metastatic disease (**Figures 87.2 and 87.3**). In a different patient, a sagittal CT of the lumbar spine (Figure 87.2) demonstrates diffuse sclerosis of the L4 vertebral body (ivory vertebra) without expansion or an extraosseous soft tissue component. A corresponding bone scan in the posterior projection (Figure 87.3) demonstrates an increased uptake of radiotracer in the L4 vertebral body (white arrow) as well as at the left posterior ilium and right ischial tuberosity (gray arrows), and the left anterior tenth rib (circle) in this patient with metastatic prostate cancer.

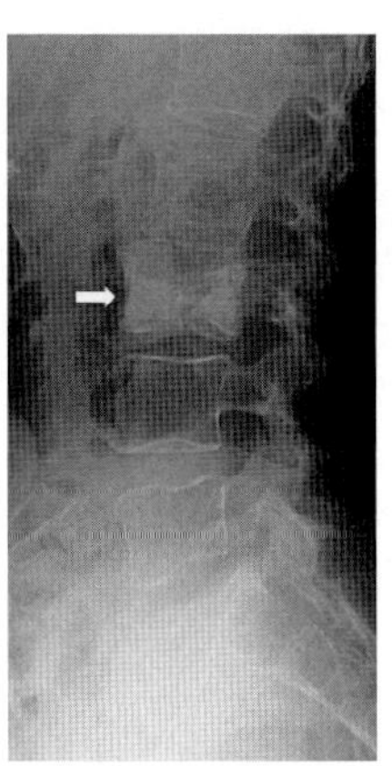

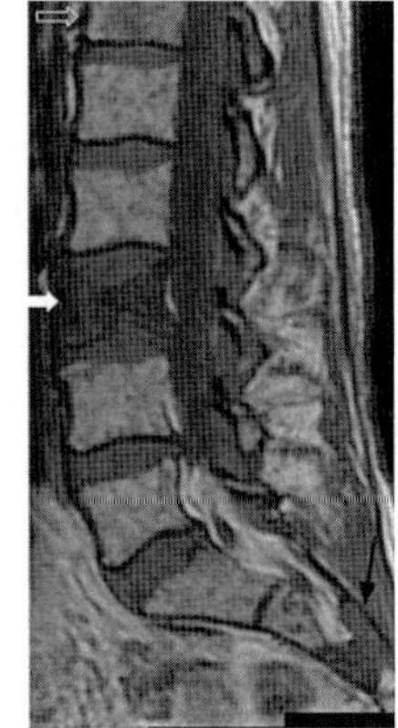

Figure 87.4   Figure 87.5

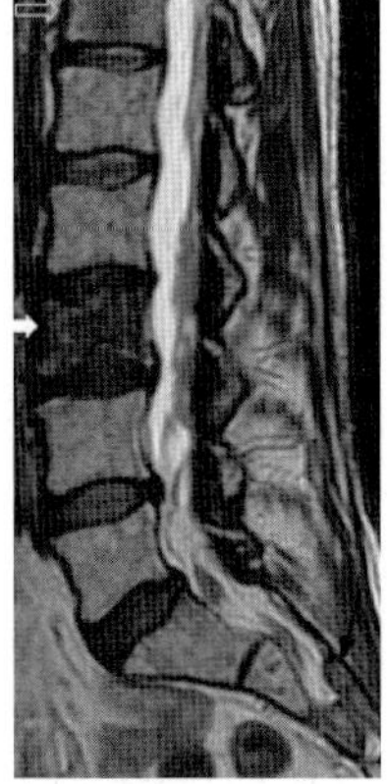
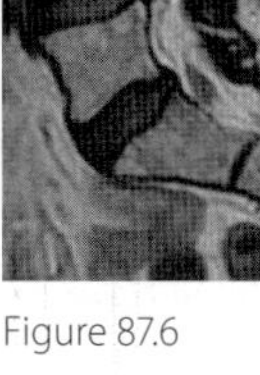
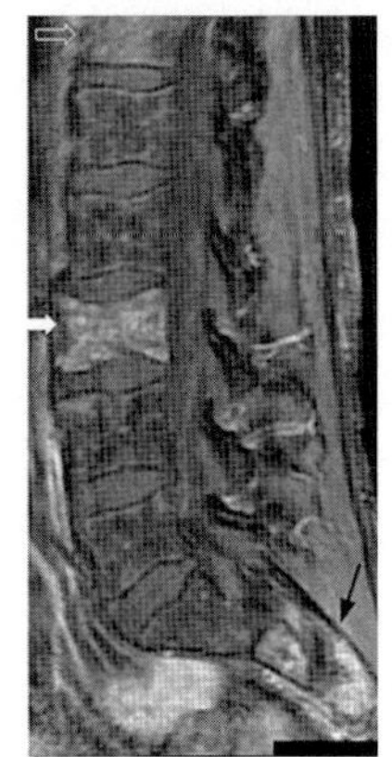

Figure 87.6   Figure 87.7

Ivory vertebral body with associated pathological fracture (**Figures 87.4, 87.5, 87.6, and 87.7**). A lateral lumbar spine radiograph (Figure 87.4) demonstrates a sclerotic L3 vertebral body with a pathological fracture. Sagittal T1, T2, and T1 postcontrast imaging with fat saturation (Figures 87.5 and 87.6) demonstrates pathological marrow infiltration involving the L3 vertebral body with an associated compression fracture. Notice the T1 and T2 hypointense metastatic lesions demonstrating enhancement lesions in the T12 vertebral body and sacrum. This patient also had metastatic cancer resulting in an ivory vertebral body.

Management

Management of an ivory vertebral body is directed by the underlying pathology. An idiopathic etiology is a diagnosis of exclusion; it is favored following a detailed history, physical examination, and diagnostic studies such as appropriate blood work, chest radiographs, nuclear bone scan, prostate-specific antigen (PSA; males)/breast imaging (females), and urinalysis for calcium and hydroxyproline. If an idiopathic diagnosis is made, then yearly follow-up with imaging is warranted until benignity is confidently established. Biopsy is a consideration when significant concern for malignancy is present.

Teaching Points

▶ An ivory vertebral body is an uncommon entity that has benign and aggressive etiologies that are best stratified by the clinical situation and imaging.
▶ An ivory vertebral body can be seen in children and a malignant etiology is most common.
▶ The three important differential considerations include metastatic disease, lymphoma, and Paget disease.

Further Reading

1. Carpineta L and Gagné M. The ivory vertebra: An approach to investigation and management based on two case studies. Spine 2002;27(9):E242–247.
2. Clifford PD and Jose J. Ivory vertebra sign. Am J Orthop 2010;39(8):400–402.
3. Graham TS. The ivory vertebra sign. Radiology 2005;235(2):614–615.
4. Silverman IE and Flynn JA. Images in clinical medicine. Ivory vertebra. N Engl J Med 1998;338(2):1000.
5. Dennis JM. The solitary dense vertebral body. Radiology 1961;77:618–621.

Philip Dougherty and Kathleen R. Fink

History

▶ A-35-year old patient presents with progressive back pain (**Figures 88.1, 88.2, and 88.3**).

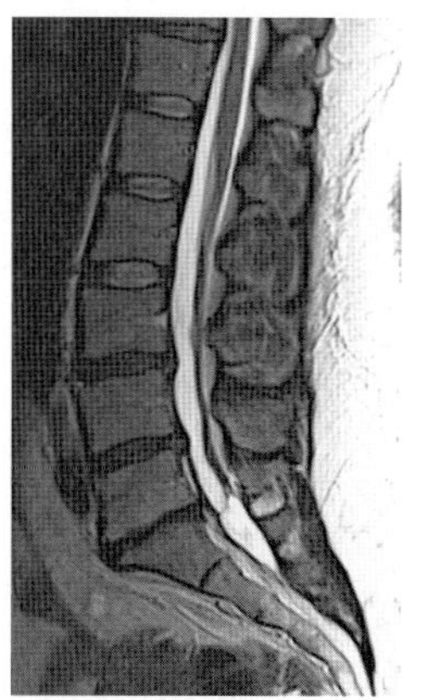

Figure 88.1

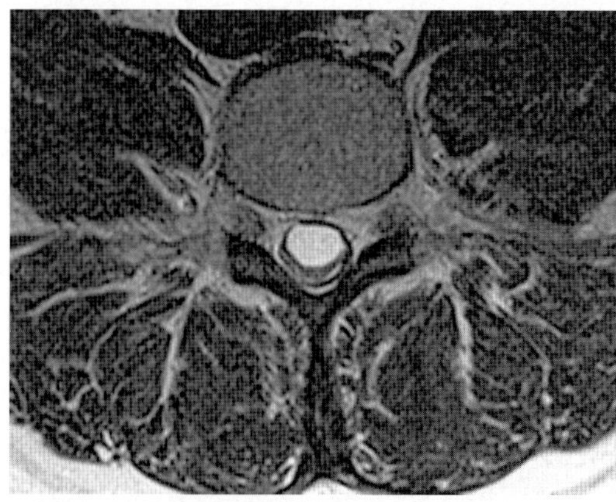

Figure 88.2

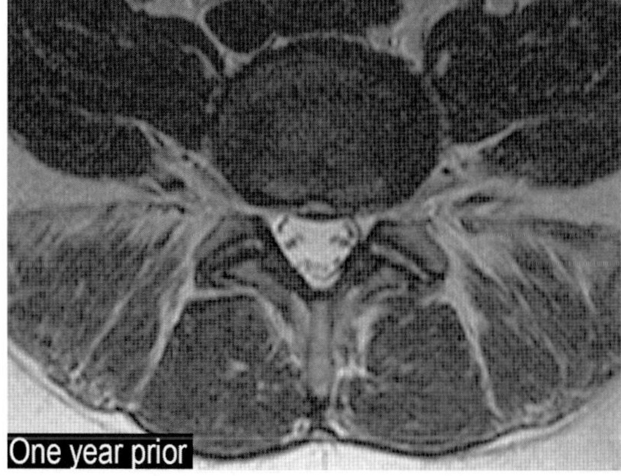

Figure 88.3

Chapter 88 **Empty Thecal Sac Sign**

Findings

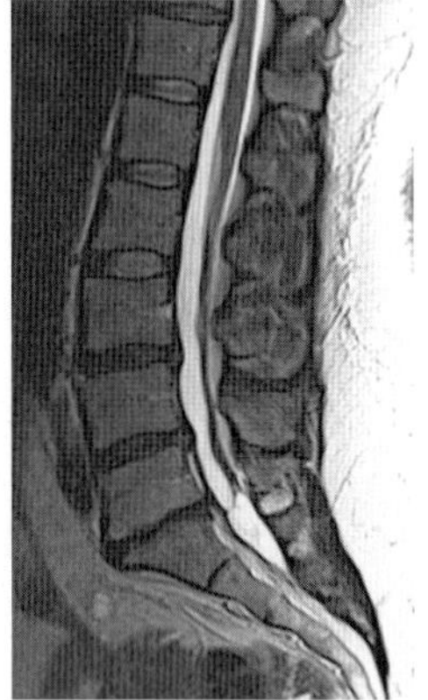

Figure 88.4

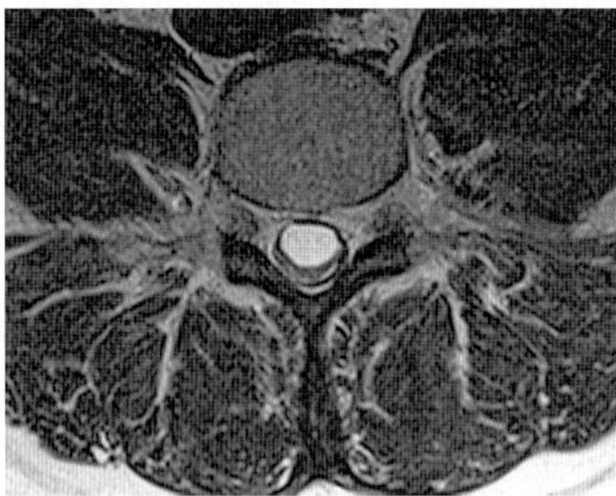

Figure 88.5

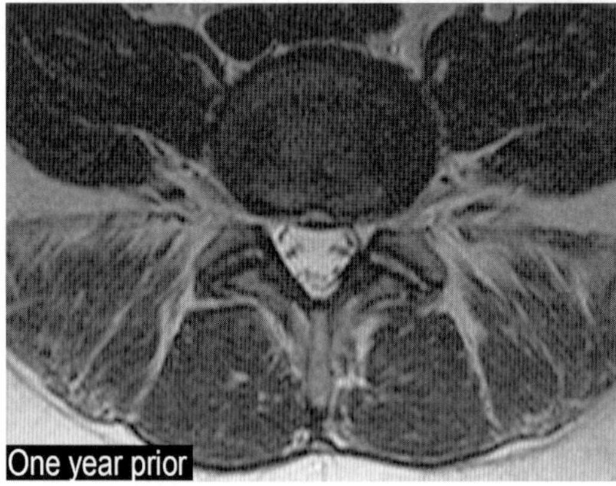

Figure 88.6

Adhesive arachnoiditis with "empty sac" sign. A sagittal T2-weighted MRI (**Figure 88.4**) shows clumping and posterior displacement of the cauda equina from L2–L3 through L5–S1 where there is tethering of the nerve roots to the ventral and dorsal thecal sac. An axial T2-weighted MRI through the inferior L4 vertebral body level (**Figure 88.5**) shows adhesion of the nerve roots to the periphery of the thecal sac resulting in the "empty sac" sign. A comparison T2-weighted MRI from a year earlier at the L4–L5 disk space level (**Figure 88.6**) is normal.

Differential Diagnosis

- ▶ Adhesive arachnoiditis
- ▶ Primary neoplasm of the cauda equina
- ▶ Spinal stenosis
- ▶ Drop metastases to cauda equina

Discussion

Arachnoiditis is an inflammatory process involving the nerve roots of the cauda equina. Inflammation rich in a fibrinous exudate covers the nerve roots causing them to stick to each other and the thecal sac. With time, collagenous scar tissue is laid down by fibroblasts, compartmentalizing the intradural space.

The causes of arachnoiditis are diverse, but typically fall into three main categories: infection (meningitis), trauma/surgical (particularly complex surgeries, intraoperative durotomies, or multiple bloody lumbar punctures), and chemical (myelograms and intrathecal steroid injections). Pantopaque, an oily intrathecal contrast agent, is also notorious for causing arachnoiditis, but is no longer in use. Cases of Pantopaque-induced arachnoiditis may still be encountered, however, due to a long latency period for the development of symptoms. Modern water-soluble intrathecal contrast has an improved safety profile, but is not completely devoid of risk.

Clinical manifestations of arachnoiditis are variable and imprecise. Typical pain is poorly localized, burning, and constant with minimal relief from analgesics. The distribution includes the inner aspects of the knees, insteps, and lumbosacroiliac areas. Patients have also reported genitourinary, gastrointestinal, and other systemic symptoms. It is important to note that not all patients with imaging findings of arachnoiditis will be symptomatic.

Radiological Evaluation

MRI is the imaging modality of choice. Both axial and sagittal T1- and T2-weighted sequences should be included. Contrast may be helpful to identify nerve root enhancement in the acute phase (Figures 88.7 and 88.8).

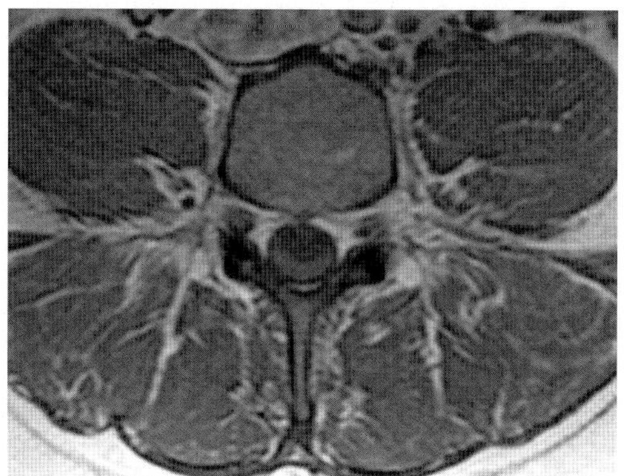

Figure 88.7

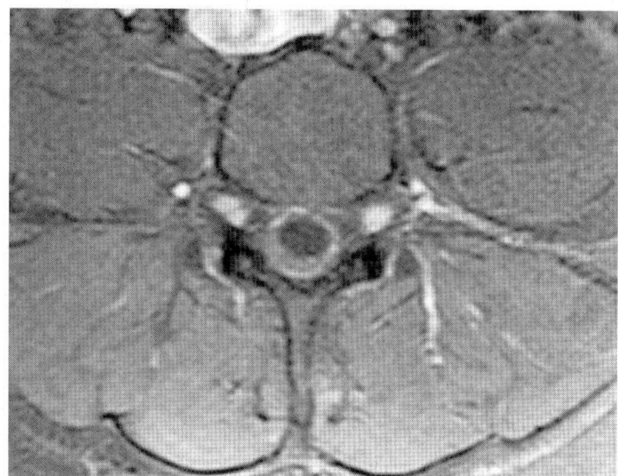

Figure 88.8

Nerve root enhancement (**Figures 88.7 and 88.8**). An axial T1-weighted MRI before (Figure 88.4) and after (Figure 88.5) intravenous contrast (postcontrast MRI is fat suppressed) shows mild enhancement of the peripherally located nerve roots, as well as normal enhancement of the dorsal root ganglia.

There are three main patterns of arachnoiditis described on imaging:

Type 1: Central clumping of roots residing centrally in the thecal sac.

Type 2: Peripheral orientation of nerve roots giving rise to the "empty sac" sign.

Type 3: A conglomerate inflammatory pseudomass filling the intrathecal sac that enhances poorly and should not be mistaken for an intradural neoplasm. This is considered the end stage of the inflammatory response.

Other imaging findings of arachnoiditis include intrathecal calcifications, nerve root enhancement, intrathecal pseudocysts, and residual oil-based intrathecal contrast (Pantopaque). If MR is contraindicated a CT myelogram is an acceptable alternative, but may be painful if the adherent nerve roots are contacted.

Management

Arachnoiditis is difficult to treat and long-term outcomes are unpredictable. Most treatments focus on palliation with a combination of medication, physical therapy, and psychotherapy. Spinal cord stimulation has shown some promising results with pain relief. Surgical intervention remains controversial.

Teaching Points

▶ MR with contrast is the modality of choice for adhesive arachnoiditis.
▶ There are three main types of adhesive arachnoiditis based on imaging findings. Type 2 gives rise to the characteristic "empty sac" sign. Type 3 should not be mistaken for an intradural mass.

Further Reading

1. Delamarter RB, Ross JS, Marsaryk TJ, et al. Diagnosis of lumbar arachnoiditis by magnetic resonance imaging. Spine 1990;15(4):304–310.
2. Quiles M, Marchisello PJ, and Tsairis P. Lumbar adhesive arachnoiditis: Etiologic and pathologic aspects. Spine 1978;3(1):45–56.

Shamir Rai, Ismail Tawakol Ali, and Savvas Nicolaou

History

▶ A 24-year-old patient flipped off of a trampoline and landed on his neck resulting in tenderness at C7 associated with new-onset C7 paresthesias (**Figures 89.1, 89.2, and 89.3**).

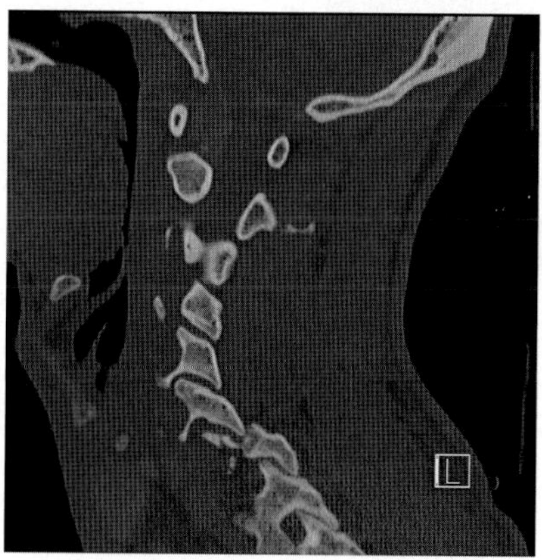

Figure 89.1

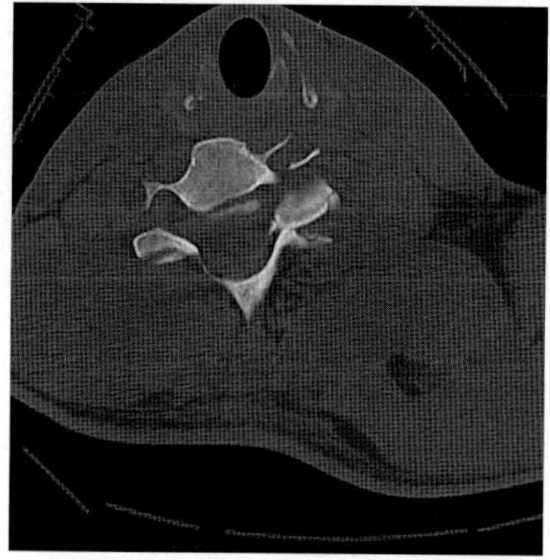

Figure 89.2

Chapter 89 Naked Facet Sign

Findings

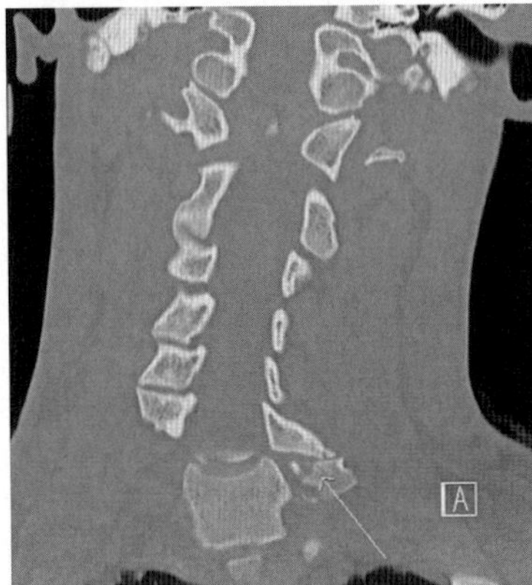

Figure 89.3

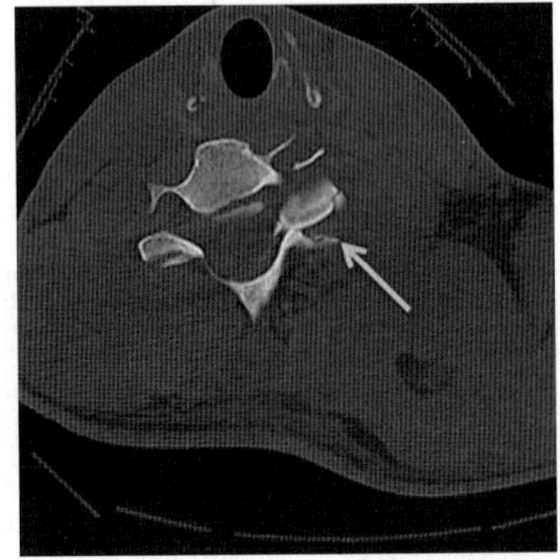

Figure 89.4

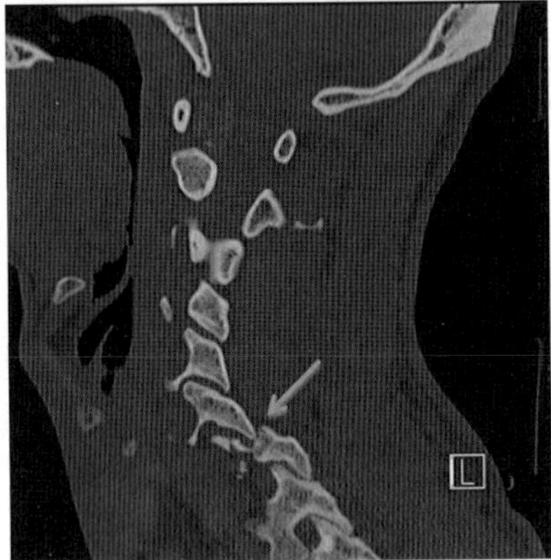

Figure 89.5

Naked facet sign. Coronal (**Figure 89.3**) and axial (**Figure 89.4**) CT images demonstrate a left unilateral facet dislocation at C6/C7, secondary to fractures involving the inferior articular process of C6 and the superior articular process of C7. On the axial image, in relation to the description of the hamburger sign, only half of the facet joint is visible on the left side. This is indicative of perching (complete facet uncovering) of the left inferior articulating process on the superior articular process of C7. A sagittal CT image (Figure 89.4) demonstrates this perching (naked facet).

Discussion

Flexion injuries of the spine are common in motor vehicle accidents. Multiple forms of injuries have been identified with flexion injuries including compression fractures of the vertebral bodies and horizontal fractures through the posterior neural arch with distraction of the bony fragments and variable extension into the vertebral body, which are dependent on the horizontal plane in which the stress vectors are resolved.

With the use of lap-type seatbelts an increased frequency of a specific pattern of flexion injury to the spine has been noted. In this pattern, there is minimal compression of the vertebral body but extensive disruption of the ligamentous framework of the posterior elements with resultant vertical distraction of the articular process. This similar process has also been described in patients who have fallen or jumped from a height, as in the case presented here. The naked facet sign refers to the CT appearance of an uncovered articulating process that results from severe disruption of ligamentous structures with or without fractures.

Normally, the facet joints are symmetrical and uniformly superimposed and are kept in fixed relation with minimal physiological movement. Various ligaments maintain this anatomical alignment: the supraspinous ligaments, infraspinous ligaments, ligamentum flavum, and facet joint capsule. The anterior and posterior longitudinal ligaments mainly maintain the vertebral body alignment and may also play an indirect role in facet stability. With severe flexion-distraction injuries there is disruption in the spinous ligaments that results in anterior subluxation of the vertebrae, with widening of facet joints and uncovering of the articulating processes. More specifically, the superior vertebra undergoes forward subluxation, with anterior displacement of the corresponding inferior articulating facet of the vertebrae below. The superior and inferior articulating processes lie "naked." The degree of facet uncovering could be partial (subluxed facets) or complete (perched facets). It is important to look for concurrent fractures, as demonstrated with this case. It has been reported that 73% of unilateral facet dislocations are associated with fractures of the involved articular processes.

Roche et al. have described the vertebral facet (apophyseal) joint space as a hamburger. The superior articular process of the vertebrae below forms the "bun" on top of the "meat patty" and the inferior articular process of the vertebrae above forms the bun beneath the patty. When the facet joint is dislocated, the top bun of the hamburger (superior articular facet) lies posteriorly and is now uncovered or "naked."

Radiological Evaluation

A plain film examination of the spine is an essential part of the primary screen for patients who present with flexion injuries. Identification of the naked facet sign is essential, as it indicates severe ligamentous injury with spinous instability. However, diagnosis of disruption of the posterior neural arch requires further evaluation with CT or MRI. Transverse CT imaging with sagittal and coronal reconstruction offers a comprehensive demonstration of osseous and soft-tissue injuries, with accurate depiction of both the anterior and posterior elements of the vertebrae, the vertebral element alignment, and the degree of spinal canal compromise.

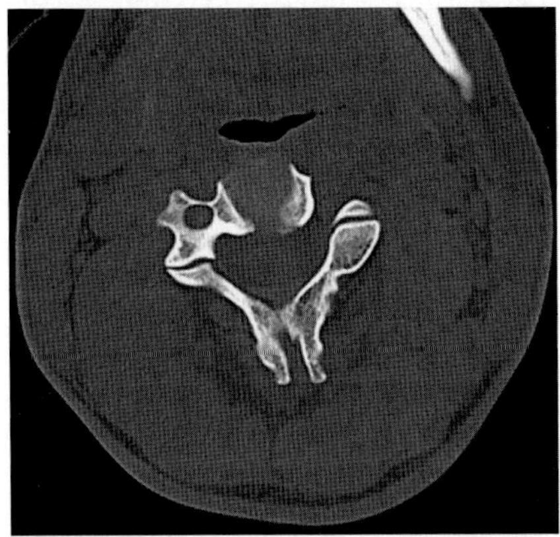

Figure 89.6

Normal articulating processes (**Figure 89.6**). The superior articular process of the vertebrae below forms the "bun" on top of the "meat patty" and the inferior articular process of the vertebrae above forms the bun beneath the patty. Note that the convex sides of the outside of the "bun" are anterior and posterior, while the flat articular portions are positioned centrally much like a hamburger bun would be positioned.

Management

Differentiation of primary bone injury from primarily ligamentous injury is crucial. Osseous injury tends to heal spontaneously if satisfactory reduction is achieved and the patient is immobilized in a hyperextension cast. Ligamentous injury tends not to heal and requires operative fixation to prevent the complication of late instability.

Teaching Points

▶ The naked facet sign refers to the CT appearance of an uncovered articulating process.

▶ The naked facet sign is an indication of a flexion-distraction injury of the spine and indicates severe ligamentous disruption and spinal instability.

▶ There is a high degree of association between articular fractures and facet dislocations.

▶ Disruption in the spinous ligaments results in anterior subluxation of the vertebrae. The superior vertebra undergoes forward subluxation.

▶ Disruption of the posterior neural arch requires further evaluation with CT or MRI if suspected from plain films or clinically.

▶ Management of severe ligamentous injury requires operative fixation.

Further Reading

1. Kaufer H and Hayes JT. Lumbar fracture-dislocation. J Bone Joint Surg [Am] 1966;48:712–730.
2. Callaghan JP, Ullrich CG, Yuan HA, and Kieffer SA. CT of facet distraction in flexion injuries of the thoracolumbar spine: The "naked" facet. AJNR Am J Neuroradiol 1980;1:97–102.
3. Green JD, Harle TS, and Harris JH Jr. Anterior subluxation of the cervical spine: Hyperflexion sprain. AJNR Am J Neuroradiol 1981;2:243–250.
4. Lingawi S. The naked facet sign. Radiology 2001;219:366–367.
5. Roche CJ, O'Keeffe DP, Lee WK, et al. Selections from the buffet of food signs in radiology. Radiographics 2002;22(6):1369–1384.
6. Shanmubanathan K, Mirvis SE, and Levine AM. Rotational injury of cervical facets: CT analysis of fracture patterns with implications for management and neurologic outcome. AJR Am J Roentgenol 1994;163:1165–1169.
7. Yetkin Z, Osborn AG, Giles DS, and Haughton VM. Uncovertebral and facet joint dislocation in cervical articular pillar fractures: CT evaluation. AJNR Am J Neuroradiol 1985;6:633–637.

Index

Myelopathy, 137–138, 264, 290–291
  HIV-associated, 145–147
  progressive sensory, 175–177
Myeloradiculopathy, 307–309
Myxopapillary ependymoma, 105–107

Naked facet sign, 348–350
Neural compression, 141–142
Neurofibromatosis (NF), 102–104, 238–241, 286–287
Neuromyelitis optica (NMO), 165, 206–208
Neurosarcoidosis of the spine, 275–278
Nitrous oxide inhalation, 176
Numbness, 88–90, 112–113, 115–116, 230–231

Occipital condyle fracture (OCF), 44–47
Oligoastrocytoma, anaplastic, 88–90
Os Odontoideum, 20, 299–302
Ossiculum terminale of Bergmann, 20
Ossification of the posterior longitudinal ligament
  (OPLL), 307–309
Osteoblastic metastases, 64*t*, 65
Osteoblastoma, 76, 78–81
Osteogenesis imperfecta (OI), 248–251
Osteomyelitis/discitis, 151–153
Osteopetrosis, 252–255, 325
Osteoporosis, 202–205
Osteosarcoma, primary, 82–85

Paget disease, 188–191
Paraganglioma, 94–97
Paresthesias. *See also* Tingling sensation
  bilateral upper extremity, 206–208
  cases, 82–85, 102–103, 177–178, 206–208,
    259–262, 347–349
  progressive painless spastic, 263–264
Pars defect, 133–136
Persistent ossiculum terminale, 20
Platyspondyly, 249, 250
Pneumothoraces, bilateral, 32
Polka-dot sign, 333–334
Posterior ligamentous complex (PLC), 12–13
Posterior longitudinal ligament, ossification
  of, 307–309
Pott's disease, 148–150
Prostate cancer, metastatic, 65, 337–338, 340, 341

Quadriplegia, 40–42

Radiculopathy, 74–76, 130. *See also*
  Myeloradiculopathy

Renal angiomyolipoma, 244, 245
Renal cell carcinoma, metastatic, 62–65
Renal insufficiency. *See* Chronic
  renal insufficiency
Renal osteodystrophy and secondary
  hyperparathyroidism (HPTH), 197–201
Rugger jersey sign, 317–320

Sacral agenesis (SA), 234–237
Sacroiliac joints, 322
Sacroilitis, 122
Sarcoidosis. *See* Neurosarcoidosis of the spine
Scheuermann disease, 303–306
Schwannoma, 59–61
Scoliosis, 226–229
Scotty dog sign, 330–331
Spinal canal narrowing, 5
Spinal cord, 3–6. *See also specific topics*
Spinal cord compression. *See* Cord
  compression
Spinal cord infarction, 259–262
Spinal dural arteriovenous fistula
  (SDAVF), 263–264
Spinal epidural abscess (SEA), 153–158
Spinal instrumentation failure, 309–316
Spondylitis. *See* Ankylosing
  spondylitis; Pott's disease
Spondyloarthropathy, 200
Spondylodiscitis, 152
Spondylolisthesis, 134, 135
Spondylolysis, 185, 330
Spondylolysis defects, 134–135
Subacute combined degeneration of the spinal cord
  (SCD), 175–179
Subependymoma, spinal, 115–117
Synovial cyst, 140–142
Syrinx, 100, 212, 213, 216–218

Tetraplegia, 28–29
Thalassemia, 266–267
Thecal sac sign, empty, 344–346
Thecal schematic, 9
Thoracic kyphosis, 303–306
Thoracic outlet syndrome (TOS), 284
Thoracic paresthesia, 102–103
Thoracolumbar (TL) kyphosis, 223
Thoracolumbar region, prominent flow
  voids in, 96
Tingling sensation, 59–60, 88–89, 230–231, 283–284.
  See also Paresthesias